Where Did i Go?

Praise for *Where Did i Go?*

"It is important work, and I commend you for putting in the effort, all while living with the effects of brain injury every day. *Where did i Go?* offers insight into the effects brain injury can have on all aspects of a person's life. It is an excellent read for both brain injury survivors and professionals who may serve this community. It is so important to consider and listen to the lived experience(s) of brain injury survivors, as is highlighted through Francene's own words."

—Marlee Smith, Navigator, Brain Injury Association of Nova Scotia.

"Francene, in awe of your spirit, your passions; love your honesty and integrity!"

—Counsellor, Carmen, Burnaby, BC.

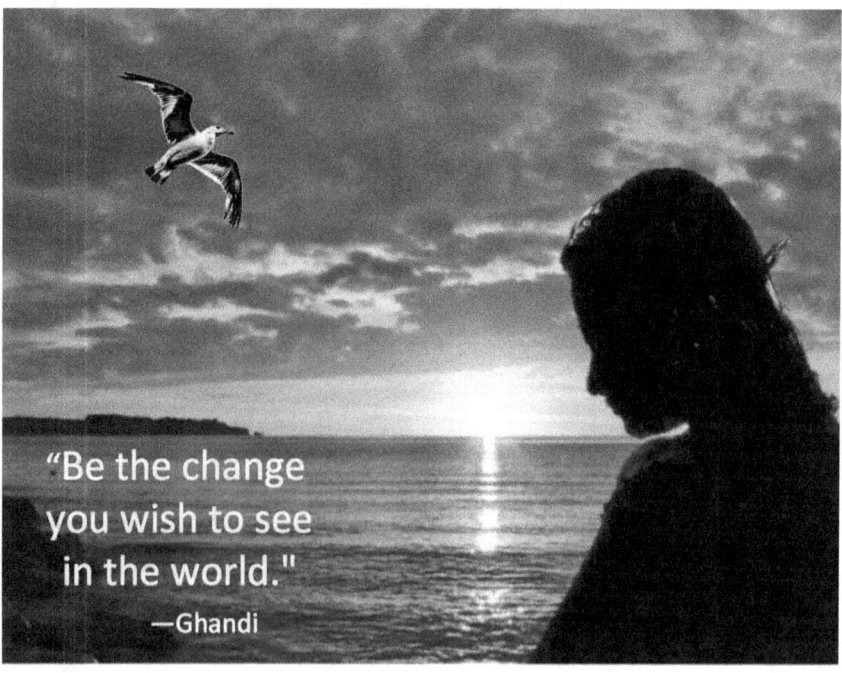

"Be the change you wish to see in the world."
—Ghandi

"Francene Gillis taught thousands of children throughout the school system in the Strait Region. She is a determined, focused, committed role model, and I found it very tough to see such a very well-spoken and educated individual struggle to pull together a complete sentence without stuttering, to stand without a weighted vest to correct her balance, and to wear specialty prism eyeglasses to correct her vision. However, we believe with all that stands in front of her, she will come through in a positive light."

— Damian MacInnis, former student

"Just finished reading *Where Did i Go?* It is an amazing blend of informative facts, insights, and practical lists to help those concussed move through the quagmire of getting the help they need and deserve. What shone through for me was Francene's sincere vulnerability in relating the rawness of her own experiences during the eight years since that life changing moment on February 1, 2016. Because of this book, I am far more aware of the hidden tragedy that exists for so many of these people not seen or heard as they suffer, often in silence. A must read for everyone including health care educators and providers."

— Anna Conner

A writer and, I believe, generally all persons must think that whatever happens to him or her is a resource. All things have been given to us for a purpose, and an artist must feel this more intensely. All that happens to us, including our humiliations, our misfortunes, our embarrassments all is given to us as raw material, as clay, so that we may shape our art."
Jorge Luis Borge

Where Did i Go?

a memoir plus

FRANCENE GILLIS

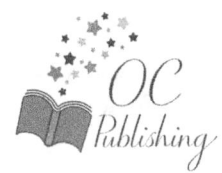

OC
Publishing

First published in 2025 by

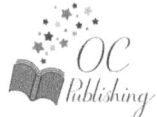

Halifax, NS, Canada
www.ocpublishing.ca

Edited by Anne Louise O'Connell
Visuals and cover design created by Francene Gillis
Cover photo by Alisha Gillis
Book design by David W. Edelstein

ISBN 978-1-989833-52-0 (Paperback edition)
ISBN 978-1-989833-53-7 (eBook edition)

Acknowledgements

Thank you to those who reshaped my life post-concussion and whiplash. A steep mountain to climb, but with learned patience and support I found my way, and the view from the summit, although different, is spectacular. To my students over the years, for keeping me young, and for being incredible movers and shakers, I thank you for the privilege. To the "plus" people added to my memoir, heartfelt appreciation, and thanks. Stories change lives.

To Dr. David Cudmore, Dr. Raymond Lok, my family, employer, therapists, and medical practitioners, your help and lessons learned will forever remain with me. I had fun creating cartoons in eye therapy as an attempt to bring humour to a dark narrative.

*"While concussion education is vitally important,
no number of resources should take the place of
medical guidance from a neurological professional
with expertise in the prevention, treatment and
management of concussion."*

— Vernon B. Williams, MD, 2017

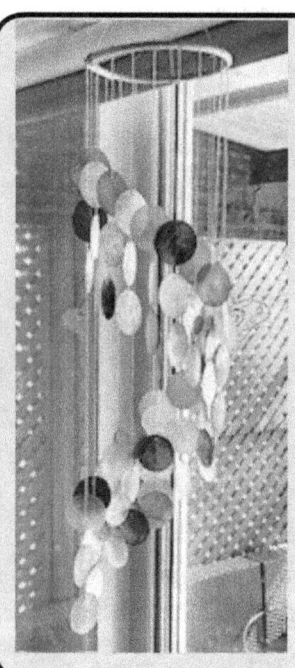

Brain Injury
How can we believe,
What we cannot see?
People wonder.
Think of the wind…
Invisible currents affecting
Depending on their strength
Clothes on a line swaying in a breeze
Leaves whispering and dancing
Hats blowing off
Weakened structures falling
Trees uprooting
We see the effects
But never the wind
Even wind chimes stir
When the invisible current flows
Like electrical impulses
In our tussled brain
Causing symptoms.

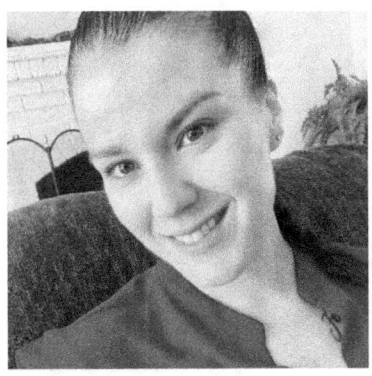

I dedicate this book to my friend and former student Rhiannon Chisholm, pictured above. What an inspiration. Warrior woman, Rhiannon faced multiple odds and critical injuries in 2022: Traumatic Brain Injury (TBI), brain bleed, and spinal cord injury yet she refused to give up moving forward, a day, hour, minute at a time. Her resilient spirit reflects all the "Plus" people in this book. Her incredible story is inside.

"Once we believe in ourselves, we can risk curiosity, wonder, spontaneous delight, or any experience that reveals the human spirit."

— EE Cummings

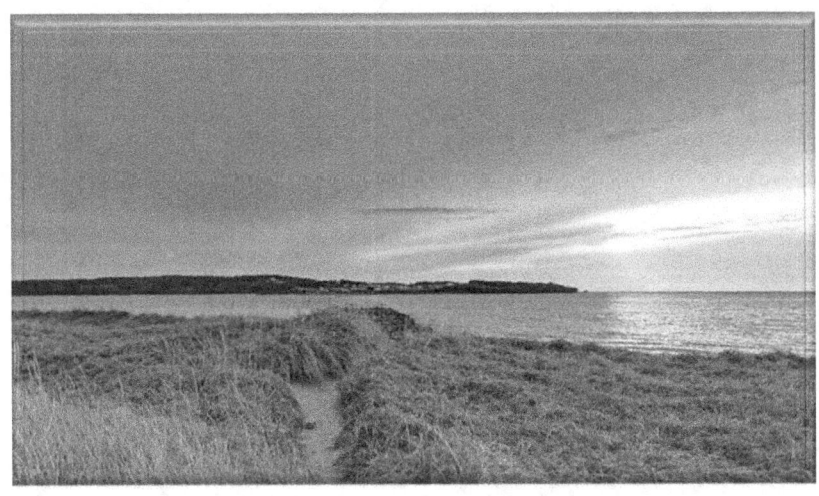

Port Hood Beach, Cape Breton, NS

Contents

Author's Note About Format

In creating this book, I chose what I needed most in my journey down the rabbit hole of panic, ignorance, fear, anger, frustration, uncertainty, and grief. I share the rough moments, and how I learned to counter them. My early mantra became, "Don't give up!"

Where Did i Go? explores my viewpoint using text and visuals to show what can happen from an unexpected brain injury. I include graphics and pictorials, easier to follow than dense text. Images summarizing main points help those of us with mild or severe brain injuries to keep our place. Visuals help with short-term memory and absorbing information.

One step at a time, I want the pages to invite interaction. The visuals within and love for my ocean speak for themselves. A big kid at heart, I try to recapture childhood creativity, thus caricatures of good-natured, medical practitioners who treated me. I smile. They are fine, caring people. Reminders of the good among the bad provide solace needed when clouds cover the sun.

Sections were born from my ignorance as one discovery piled onto another. The purpose of this book is to consider the "whole" person and how invisible injury, and trauma can affect us when we have compounding conditions. It presents strategies I discovered to help with invisible injuries, and common symptoms of post-concussion syndrome (PCS), and post-traumatic stress disorder (PTSD). I attempt to see and navigate from onset to recovery, provide perspective and insight; and answer thought-provoking queries. I share what helped me, supply uplifting quotations, and a cautionary tale of preparedness and resiliency. Credibility comes through the voice of reputable professionals. Tips and tricks to use on bad days come from excellent organizations; treatments offer starting points; and comics are my attempt at humour.

My love of nature and phenomenal Inverness County scenery, come out in photographs, a tribute to my back door and the Atlantic Ocean, my best friend even as a child going through treacherous emotional storms. The teacher in me shares lessons learned and recommends resources. Questions reflect my urgency for answers. I introduce "the claw," a pain and pressure on my forehead caused by a flooding of senses, and too many words coming too fast at me.

My Story

I share my story to help educate, improve awareness, help those with any form of head injury who might find themselves lost, as I did post-concussion, to provide a starting point and share insight on what I did not have for years. To do that I have to be completely honest and vulnerable. Please be kind. Our past can sneak in with head injury, frustrations leading to activation of the nervous system and the reliving of past trauma evoked by a word, sound, smell, image. And so, the story within includes what affected me most, both good and bad. I salute others who came before. Good on you. A slow journey to recovery, I speak chronologically, inter-mix therapies and expert advice. Because I learned so very much, I include the second part on education and awareness.

Education & Awareness

To understand concussion, we need to look at the human brain, causes, symptoms, what we can do, where we might find help, types of aid available. Questions bombard: What is wrong with me? Why does my head hurt? How do I fix this? Why am I dizzy? Why is everything coming at me? When can I get back to work?

When will I stop feeling this way? Professional organizations and specialists answer these questions floating to the surface of awareness and education.

Treatment

Where I live in rural Canada, I could not find treatment, except physio and had no idea where to go for help. I was desperate to get back to teaching. How could I get better? When? Why were my symptoms lasting so long? What treatments could help? Where could I find a specialist? It took over five years to get the answers, but I learned immediate and proper help is essential to a timely recovery.

In The Beat of a Heart

To help me understand what I could not, and to dig myself out of the rabbit holes I fell into, I relied on stories of courage. The journalist in me, to better understand myself and my struggles, interviewed others who suffered head injuries and trauma. I discovered I was on a journey of self-discovery! The seven stories within are necessary for when we need motivation, no matter our issue; it is through people who walk similar paths that we connect and do not feel so alone. May our stories bring comfort, strength, and resilience.

Finding Myself

A wrap-up and conclusion of the view from the top of the mountain.

References/Resources

These I include for further help.

Introduction

Francene Gillis (BA, B.Ed., M.Ed.)
mTBI, February 1, 2016

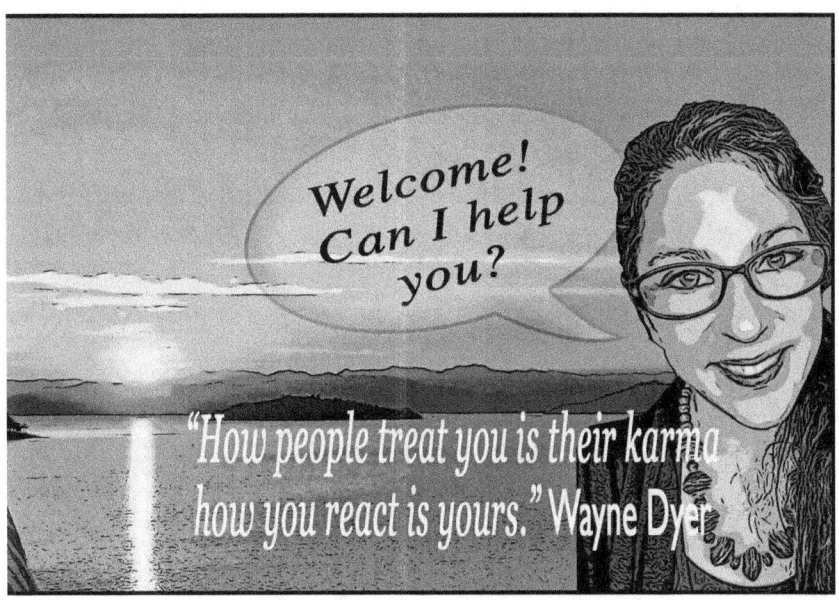

A writer from Cape Breton, Nova Scotia, I write human interest stories that centre on everyday living, family, awareness, and education. Proud mother of two daughters, two sons-in-law, and grandmother to three adorable tykes, life with my husband in beautiful Port Hood overlooking the beach brings joy, except for chronic pain, and leftover medical challenges. If I can control my environment and pace, I am okay, but some days are definitely worse than others.

A weekly columnist for *The Inverness Oran* since the early 1990s, my mantra is to show whatever challenge we face, we are not alone. Hardships experienced as a child and young woman set the stage for topics relating to self-esteem, adversity, judgment, grief, coping or not, acceptance, and moving forward through life's storms.

In 1994, I wrote *A Rose in November*, a non-fiction collection of stories about remarkable people who overcame adversity. Through my career teaching thousands of young, energetic high school students, and interviewing people for feature stories, I developed a unique lens on life's squalls and now see most everything as a learning opportunity. The beginning of a teaching semester carries suspense and uncertainty, but I never tired of student enthusiasm, queries, and challenges. Never in my wildest dreams would I have seen this crossroad in my life; the steep, sharp turn threw me off the road I was on, and nine years later resulted in this bitter-sweet book.

Life dropped me into a pile of sharp thistles. I slipped on black ice rushing into the school where I taught, fell backwards from a standing position, wrenched my neck, pulled muscles, injured my left side, and nailed my head on the pavement. Ignorant of concussion, and the other issues it can cause, I discovered an invisible beast with its own trying challenges. My struggle with acceptance imploded. No way did I want to be out of my classroom, discarded in such an undignified manner. Letting go emotionally kept me running on a ferret's wheel going nowhere. Post-traumatic stress disorder (PTSD) reared its ugly head. Frustration and inadvertent words triggered traumatic childhood memories, the brain less capable of differentiating past from present after injury, leading to the reliving of trauma. Acceptance and recovery became crucial to knowing, realizing, and living with change. It was a battle. This book came from my desperation to receive medical treatment as soon as possible, get well, and back to my classroom, students, and normalcy. It did not go as planned.

'Stay in a dark room. Wake them up every hour. Absolutely

no screen time.' These are outdated pieces of advice that are still offered about concussion. Researchers and experts know infinitely more about concussion than they did just 10 years ago. But is that information getting through to [the public] parents?" (Parachute Canada, "Concussion: It's Not All in Your Head," January 26, 2023).

Parachute is a national, charitable organization dedicated to preventing injuries and saving lives; their informative website shares uncomfortable statistics related to brain injuries and a plethora of up-to-date information. Inside you will find credible resources to help cut down on the overwhelming puzzle of concussion.

Brain Injury Canada is also an excellent website. See references. The home page divides resources into three categories from which to choose: 1) I have a brain injury; 2) I am a family member or caregiver of someone with a brain injury; and 3) I work with/support individuals and family members living with brain injury. They break these down into further topics with valuable information.

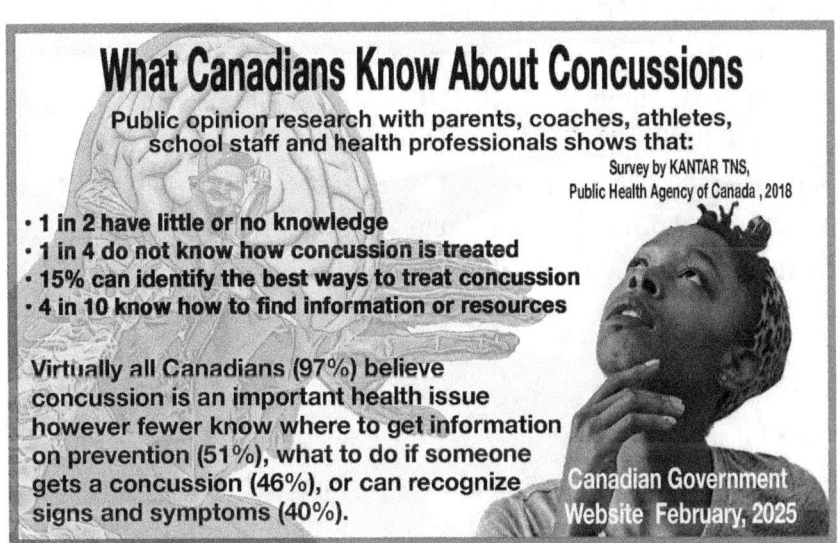

Please find courage, consolation, laughter, and healing tears within. The terrain is bumpy, less so with proper resources and tools to ensure a safe trip. I compare my journey into the world of concussion to a damaged plant. If we replenish the soil, add food, water, nutrients, place it in the sun, nurture and sing to it, as my mother did, it will have that extra boost to flourish once again. I would place the revived plant in a colourful mosaic vase, made of delicate fragments, symbolic of repurposed components of ourselves. The teacher and writer in me as well, wants to reach others struggling with an invisible injury, that which others cannot see, for we do not know what we do not know.

Sharing is paramount. My hope is that this book finds a place on coffee tables and shelves as an education and awareness tool, and as a gift for people for whom we care. Being prepared and educated is half the battle. "Concussions are the most common form of brain injury with thousands of Canadians diagnosed every year. In 2022, approximately 35,000 children and youth, aged 5 to 19, and more than 65,000 adults, 20 years and older, were diagnosed with a concussion in emergency rooms across the country." (Public Health Agency of Canada, June 13, 2024).

In the United States, the numbers are equally troubling. "There were approximately 214,110 TBI-related hospitalizations in 2020 and 69,473 TBI-related deaths in 2021. This represents more than 586 TBI-related hospitalizations and 190 TBI-related deaths per day. These estimates do not include the many TBIs that are only treated in the emergency department, primary care, urgent care, or those that go untreated." (CDC, United States government, May 16, 2024).

Government sites provide credible updates. Experts filter their information, making the BrainLine websites across Canada and the United States, vital, and evidence-based. From their "About Us" section: "BrainLine is a national multimedia project offering authoritative information and support to anyone whose life has been affected by brain injury or PTSD: people with brain injuries, their family and friends, and the professionals who work with them . . . [It] is a place where people who care about brain injury can go 24 hours a day for information, support, and ideas. BrainLine is a national service of WETA-TV, the flagship PBS station in Washington, D.C." I knew nothing of such websites when I fell, was too nauseous and dizzy to handle screens or go online.

I do not provide medical advice, or diagnosis, but a journey from not knowing about concussions and brain injury, to gaining knowledge, awareness, and understanding. This book grew from an urge to know. I wrote in snippets as brain fog, fatigue, and headaches allowed and therapists encouraged me. Desperate to know what was going on inside my head, my husband and sisters helped me find advice applicable to my injuries. Scared I was losing my mind, they researched mental wellness support, coping with mood swings, frustration, and debilitation. Adding to my upset, the computer was both my lifeline and enemy. The glare and movement on the screen had my brain nosediving, a notorious pain and pressure on the centre of my forehead as the damn claw squeezed.

This book is for people who experienced any form of mental struggle such as PCS or PTSD and ramifications thereof. It is for educators and coaches with children in their care, family members concerned about the welfare of loved ones and the risks of head injury. It guides the therapist, medical worker, parent, grandparent, and friend. Inside is the emotional tangle of living with childhood trauma, grief, and a brain injury—a condition with a mind of its own. Fear, frustration, words of battlement explode—BEFORE and AFTER injury life's new gauge creating a battle of gargantuan proportions. Before I could . . . I share, *Where Did i Go?* the lower case 'i' representing loss of my former self. It sums up ignorance of a world that robbed me of my abilities, but the question is—Do I get them back?

Often, I found myself going back to sections I had written earlier to read and adhere to my own advice, in that I recognized the value, which planted the seed to share. My symptoms morphed, and I created resources designed with various practitioners, partners, and agencies in mind, respecting their arduous research and work. Desperate, I needed to feel normal, my desire to be well and my teaching background driving me.

A combination of memoir and inspirational stories, this book deals with universals relevant to pain, the unexpected, and battles we face. It reveals anger, guilt, inferiority, and emotional triggers. It offers suggestions to make life smoother. Designed to get a few laughs, I tried to balance dark and light. A passionate advocate, silenced too long because of insecurities, I am ready to share, even as I feel vulnerable and naked. I ask that you honour the personal narratives, born out of not knowing where to turn and the thought of possibly helping others. The body heals, the proof within, but when it leaves shortfalls, knowing how to cope and respond can make the difference between a good or bad outcome.

"There are 17,000 new brain injuries annually in Nova Scotia. Most mild traumatic brain injuries (concussions) are NOT sports-related and happen doing everyday things." (Brain Injury, Nova Scotia, May 10, 2024).

In time, I realize disability does not define; it is but one fragment of a complex mosaic of who we are! I keep telling myself that even as I try to believe and gain a healthy self-esteem, but it fluctuates even with knowledge, perhaps because of insecurity, medications, or PCS leftovers. A patient's perspective, I focus on personal stories, and evidence-based strategies, and treatments designed to support and provide a starting point for those who are unaware or in the dark. Enter the world of invisible injury and trauma, and follow the emotional, mental, and physical journeys of individuals who never gave up even amidst life's worst storms when the clouds blocked the sun.

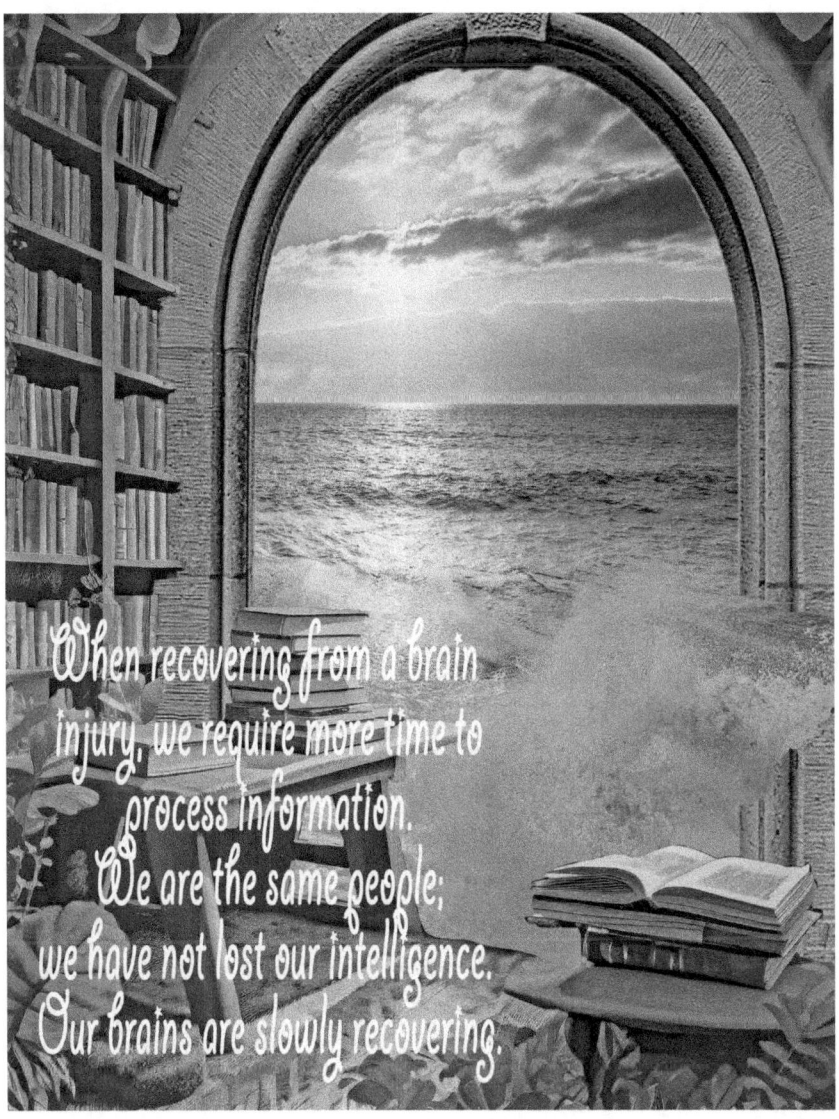

When recovering from a brain injury, we require more time to process information. We are the same people; we have not lost our intelligence. Our brains are slowly recovering.

Trauma

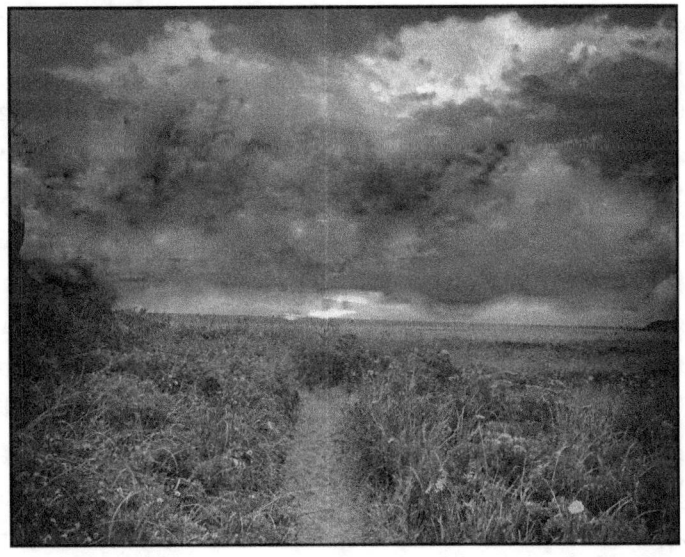

"We need little reminders from time to time that we are already dignified, deserving, worthy. Sometimes we don't feel that way because of the wounds and the scars we carry from the past or because of the uncertainty of the future. It is doubtful that we came to feel undeserving on our own. We were helped to feel unworthy. We were taught it in a thousand ways when we were little, and we learned our lessons well."

— Jon Kabat-Zinn, (American professor emeritus of medicine, creator of the Stress Reduction Clinic and the Center for Mindfulness in Medicine).

*L*et me tell you a secret. The refreshing breeze from my open, bedroom window sings to my spirit, whispering secrets and possibilities offered with getting up for the day. Thank God for nature, but my sanctuary pulls me back, a dichotomy to overcome. Will I get up or not? Isolation is a cold, dark place to be. Why am I here? Why is it so difficult to drag my widening ass out from under the cozy, comfortable covers? Why? Why? Why? Damn that three-letter inquisition; it haunts my existence ever since . . .

It is too quiet, silence screaming accusations. The boat I am on refuses to stop dipping, dropping, drowning me in rough waves, an ocean swell stirred up from a *simple knock on the head*—falling on, no, slipping on insidious, black ice, my world and identity flying into the abyss as my head bounced, pounded. What next? I remember a female hollering, "Are you okay?" Am I? Fluffy white, lost, cumulus clouds float; the snow-crusted, concrete ground is cold. I shiver. What should be my paradise is skewed by loneliness, lack of understanding, stutters, wonky eyes, dizziness, headaches. I am going to vomit. How do I get through the haze? The breeze feels sultry after the cold. It lifts my spirits. No one understands, emotions like a yo-yo. "You're not the same." Damn! What is that supposed to mean? The condescending tone suggests it is unde-sirable. Wrapped, strangled in an invisible blanket, it squeezes the breath out of me. If only I had the strength to get up. A fall. Where did i go? Lost in a foreign world of concussion and PTSD, I slip back to my childhood, which shaped me into an empath, gave me the courage and thirst to reach out but not without tremendous suffering. My philosophy shaped during my teenage years—life's experiences hold lessons. However, I am angry at myself for fall-ing, not in the mood for lectures or learning. I do not realize how much trauma affects me until my fall brings it all back.

It is a painful journey to travel within, but the most awakening trip we will ever take. Otherwise, we become distant, depressed, bitter, or angry, damaging our ability to trust, be vulnerable, true to ourselves and our aspirations. When the universe disrupted my path, it forced me to stand in stormy seas, and scurry into black holes. Bitter north winds threatened my very survival, childhood trauma surfacing, my mind travelling back.

Tragedy

An abrupt knock. I run to the stairs leading down to the front entrance, sit as a curious eight-year-old child; it is 2:00 a.m. Even at my tender age, I know something is wrong. From the top step, I eavesdrop on the exchange between two RCMP officers and my parents. A sudden chill, I hold myself in a ball, ears straining to catch the dialogue.

Sober words splatter—car crash, killed, injured, brother, dead. With the final word, my mom falls back, an excruciating yelp filling the downstairs. An officer grabs and helps her into the front room. Dad, moaning and groaning, doubles over, holds his heart. With all my being, I want to run down the stairs and wipe their tears, but it's not the right time. Curled into myself, weeping, I tiptoe back to bed shared with my younger sister.

Next morning, neighbours and extended family mull about, prepare an area in the house to wake my brother. Dreadful days follow. Sadness invades the walls and furniture. My sister and I stay with the casket throughout the night. Older adults believe you should not leave the deceased alone until after burial. Eternity candles cast a flickering glow as I study the white satin, dark wood, corpse, leaning gold-plated cross resting against the raised cover, baskets of flower arrangements. It's no place for children.

A sad house where grief lives; it affects everyone. No timeline, opportunities to talk or cry, share, or rant in safety. Too young to understand what dying means, I see what it does to my parents, enough to know the Grim Reaper's cruel, debilitating tentacles.

Sorrow leads to a snowy woods with two possible paths . . . we turn to less than savoury coping mechanisms, like drinking or drugs, in an attempt to avoid, or numb our pain. Or we learn poignant lessons in relation to empathy, generosity, and compassion. We realize our own mortality, what we do is our decision. If we treat others as if it were their last day imagine the profound shift in kindness. Do I live through rose-coloured glasses, a Pollyanna optimist? Better than living in darkness. Grief rips our soul, carries a permanency that knocks us down, leaves us searching, so lonely we doubt the sun will ever shine. If only we had those minutes back, a second chance to speak the unspoken? We need to speak from the heart in the moment, lessen the sorrowful dilemma of regret that comes with death's finality. My baby brother Frankie was the lightbulb in the family when grieving the loss of Eddie, our twenty-one-year-old brother. My parents never got over his death, and sadly, pain knows no boundaries.

As clear as yesterday, I see Frankie sitting on his two-wheeler, straw hat protecting him from the sun's rays. His legs straddle either side of the seat. He is ready to lift his leg and pedal down to Ian's Corner Store for a treat. His tanned face glows with pride as he pedals off on an errand to pick up sugar or milk, biking his second favourite activity next to swimming in the ocean and tanning on the beach.

He digs holes in the sand, shovels his heart out, buries himself with nothing but his silly grin sticking out. We laugh, dive, splash, tease, and play in the warm, salt water. Floating on our backs we are on top of the world, our cares are nonexistent. We are safe in the Atlantic's arms. We hop the burning sand to our comfortable towels and sunbathe until deeply bronzed. Dad and Mom buy him drums for his birthday; he pounds those skins playing "Wipe Out," a famous rhythmic beat. Never does his countenance beam so bright as when making noise or swimming. Oh, how we cherished our beach times. Early mornings, for chores we romp outside, pick whatever berry or wildflower is in season. He loves gathering buttercups, places them under our chins to discover who likes butter. A yellow glow tells the tale. We collect daisies, pull the petals one by one, recite so-and-so loves me, or loves me not. Mom is sad when she sees us tearing the petals. "Daisy a Day," by Jud Strunk is one of her favourite songs.

Evenings we enjoy checkers or Snakes and Ladders, but our favourite game is the stare down. Stoic, we sit opposite, glare into each other's eyes. First to blink loses. We make funny faces to see who cracks up. Precious is looking into the face of love, feeling tight, receptive hugs, hearing loving words, as a lighthearted spirit shines through the clouds. Our ritual, after hugging good night, settling in knowing we *have* tomorrow.

The afternoon of July 21 hits like a tornado. In the morning, my brother and I play catch, but I cannot take him to the beach because of my summer job. He begs and promises Mom he will not go out beyond his belly button. She gives cautious permission. About to relieve my sister working at a restaurant nearby, all hell breaks loose. His young friend, out of breath, bangs on the door, yelling, "Frankie's gone under! Frankie's gone under!" Dad, home from hospital one day after having a heart attack, rushes to the car. I jump in as we fly to the beach. A stranger searching in the salt water hollers, "I found him," pulls him out of the waves, carries my baby brother's limp body to the broken causeway where our father, certified in emergency first aid, begins CPR. An hour, among scattered boulders and sand my father pumps the tiny chest. We wait—a too slow ambulance. Wee lips are blue, body lifeless. I beg my brother to open his eyes, pray he will choke up water and breathe. I pray he move. He does not. Heartbreaking, lifelong images remain.

We wake him in our front room; my sister and I stay through the night, me coveting every second. In a white casket . . . part of me dies; I vow—in me his personality will breathe, his mischievous, kind smile and good heart live.

The torment subsides with the rolling of the seasons, although loneliness settles into the bones. I wish I had known that day would be his last. His death destroys our family. The older girls are gone. Dad's violent alcoholism rages, and Mom does her best to survive, while we two scallywags grieve and try not to get in the way. Our buffer is gone. We run and hide, do not sing at the table; if bad, "the devil will get us." "Get that buss off your face!" We are of no use. Oh, how I hate the snap of the leather belt. With time, my attention shifts from tragedies to the influence of a boy who radiated joy. I am so afraid I will forget him, but I do not; love's touch forever remains. He would not want to see me in anguish. I keep that sentiment close when sad, push ahead in his memory. The packaging might be gone, but his vibrant spirit, values, and energy, I carry forward with purpose.

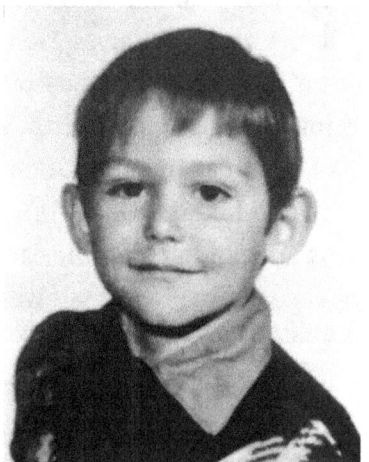

Frankie Jessome

Connected at the hip, my baby brother was my everything, my angel on Earth. His pure heart moved me to tears for decades. Rage consumed as I questioned a benevolent deity, unable to understand the loss of my soft pillow. "Why," is the most universal, problematic query. When we lose a love, we sob to the core of our very being, gut-wrenching screams, yell to the heavens trying to grasp what we cannot. Why? Why now? Unfair, if fairness relevant.

I want strength, to focus more on his life rather than his death, as the latter leads to an inability to cope.

When I am seventeen, an ex-boyfriend, driving from a Glencoe Mills dance, hits pulp on the shoulder of the road at high speed and is killed instantly. To this day I cringe when I hear of a fatal accident, tears enough to fill an ocean. I wish I could make young people slow down, the risk not worth the cost.

Junior year of university, the last weekend in January, 1978, I come home to visit Mom in the hospital, but do not realize she is as sick as she is. I leave Saturday night intending to return Sunday morning. On the way back down my boyfriend and I stop at his mom's to wish her happy birthday. The message awaits us. Mom died during the night. I am a mess. I never said goodbye, or I love you! She was fifty-seven. Throughout university grief consumes and I fight to keep my marks and scholarship. A random word, action, or comment sets me into a tailspin. I wander my beach on weekends, fall onto comforting sand, scream, shout, cry until too exhausted to breathe. Some want to fix, but nothing to fix. The why question long haunts, why some families suffer heartache and debilitating illness, while others go unscathed. Death leaves me too serious, unable to relax, aware in a heartbeat . . . I am afraid of everything; immense fear holds me back.

My heart—was a lighthearted, happy-go-lucky child proudly riding his two-wheeler without training wheels. I hear his life-giving giggles, feel his purity and unconditional love, the wonderment that comes with innocence. As I grow older, I understand the significance of his passing in a place he cherished, doing what he loved, although I wish he had lived to ninety instead of nine. A riptide seized him. We had no say. Was it an accident or meant to be? The fate versus serendipitous teapot. Will we ever know? Why do people get cancer, children die, car accidents maim, wars erupt, we sustain head injury? The brain a wondrous marvel of its own, scientists understand but a tip of the iceberg.

In glorious rainbows and sunsets, I relish my baby brother's wonderment, the message he left in the importance of little things. His probing, coffee bean peepers, twinkled as if holding celestial stars, catalysts for change, opportunities to find a reason beyond ourselves.

As a teen, I met renowned Cape Breton author Alistair MacLeod at a writing workshop on Port Hood Island. He shared a memorable adage: "What is most personal is most universal." I never forgot. No truer words have I heard. A mentor over the years, he offered to write the introduction to my next book, but teaching consumed my life. When I was ready, sadly, he had passed. I hold his advice close to my heart, his genius on my keyboard.

In 1985, I almost died giving birth to my youngest daughter. No need for details, but what I experienced, the pain and horror after she was born increased my PTSD and for months and years I had nightmares pulling me apart. In the moments of that overnight I kept saying, "No one dies giving birth in this day and age; no one dies from childbirth." But, I learned later I was wrong. The nurses really did not think I would make it through, having to call a known blood donor in town because I immediately needed transfusions and they did not have enough blood. Awake through the entire ordeal, my blood pressure tanked, and a second doctor was called in to put me back together. Through excruciating pain, I screamed and prayed; they could hear me one floor below. The doctors couldn't give me pain meds because of my critical condition. My husband said it became a bloody battlefield before the nurses asked him to leave.

Daybreak was a gift that I will never forget. It took a few days before Dawn became our baby girl's second name. As long as she was healthy, I was happy, and what a scrapper she turned out to be. I love her and our family to death and beyond! Gifted with another chance, in those early years I took it for granted but in my older age I have realized how tenuous life is, and that it is what

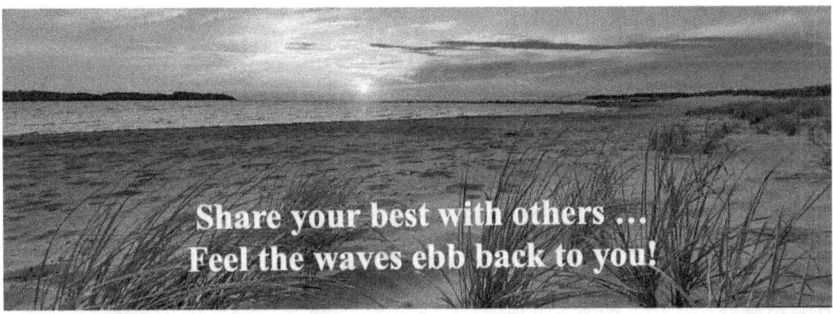

Share your best with others ...
Feel the waves ebb back to you!

we make of it as well as how we choose to walk or run through the hurdles. When the body suffers tremendous turmoil, shock, and pain, the brain protects and cushions it from another fall. I think that is why they say the journey within is difficult. Within are hidden rooms and dark corners we put aside for another day. But I discovered that it is when we can face ourselves that we can improve and grow. I realized with my mild traumatic brain injury (mTBI), that what may seem small to onlookers can be big to us. It is not up to others to judge the degree, but to realize that no matter the interpretation, we need validation without analysis. Pain is pain and validating and loving someone through it is the best approach, maybe with some TLC. Everyone needs to talk and share their hurts so they can grow, learn, and move on instead of getting stuck. And if shocks lead to health issues, we do better if we get the needed, appropriate treatment. It is a sign of strength not weakness to open up or reach out. When you are patient, driven by desperation, you learn so much! And then you educate. I did not realize how traumatic my childhood, delivery of my youngest, or head injury were until months after my fall. Trauma resurfaced when I least expected it. That winter, I refused to go outside. The fear of falling paralyzed. Nightmares kept me awake, always having to do with mix-ups at school, tumbling down a black, bleak tunnel of chaos and confusion. I was irritable, frustrated, incredibly upset, unable to do simple tasks without symptoms. My husband said I was not the same; that scared me to death, had me

hiding in the clothes closet sobbing for hours. On a dime, tragedies and pain resurfaced; my brain could not sift present from
past and so I relived what had been set aside as if it were presently
happening. Basic, daily living was a task, communicating a mine-
field, and debilitating fatigue crushed every attempt to improve. It
was impossible to accept what happened. Anger and resentment
burned. My life was different, patience essential. I had none. Was
furious. Had enough already.

As reputable organizations rally for the concussed, the public
remains uninformed and misinformed. I stretch and stretch the
elastic band to the point of snapping before finding the aid I need.

> "Females are . . . an unseen part of the concussion story
> even though they suffer more than males, have more
> severe symptoms and are slower to recover." (Roehr, Bob,
> "Concussions Affect Women More Adversely Than Men,"
> March 9, 2016).

Identity

"Be Curious, Not Judgemental."

— Walt Whitman

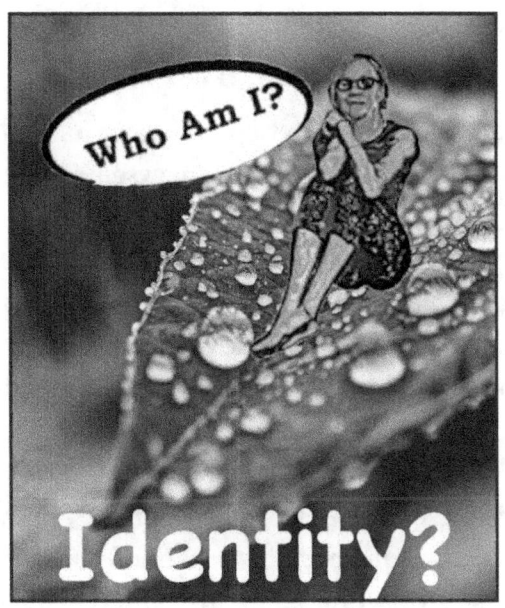

*O*ver the first few months, I write jumbled reflections to help wrap my head around a shattered existence. A concussion ripped my passion out from under me, placing me in an alternate reality where things are not as they seem, not as they once were. I spend my time wondering what specialists and therapists might help put cracked Humpty Dumpty together again. Too much to deal with. Desperate to get back to the career I love—I miss my students, busy environment, multi-tasking. Instead, I live in solitude, worthlessness gnawing my spirit, pulling me farther down a pitch-black, rabbit hole.

The Accident

February 1, 2016, the air is crisp and raw; hardened, icy snow covers the ground. Excited to begin a new semester, I walk toward the school, weighed down with a bag full of corrected exams, balancing a mug of hot coffee. I look forward to energetic teenagers. I am meeting the grade 12 Advanced English students to see their final projects. My feet slip and slide out from under me. Black ice! No way of stopping myself, I fall—straight back and down. I brace! Head hits and bounces. Blackness.

Blinding lights pollute. I shield my eyes. Where am I? Dazed, confused, a distressed voice reverberates off the ground. A Cyclops, annoying and stubborn, bangs his vexatious hammer, pounds my forehead. Please stop. I am going to vomit. Give me a corner, a quiet nook, a deep bunny hole—place to escape and hide, anything to stop the light from flashing, racket from murdering my resolve. Am I in a gruelling tug-of-war? Dense fog wraps an unfocused periphery, my head about to explode. Cannot block the spinning, my memory cracked eggshells. The ground is cold, snow and ice my bedsheets. Am I on a boat? Too much effort to think. Through a funnel a faraway female voice. I open my eyes, squint from the glare, close them. Do I reply? Only clouds. Footsteps. A colleague stands over me, grabs her cell, calls the school, which makes no sense; it is steps away. The vice-principal and another teacher hurry out. Sheepish, I peer up from a sprawled position on the ground, embarrassed. Am I okay? My reply, nonsense. What the hell? I do not sound right. I panic, try not to show it as terror grips.

Puzzled glances, they do not understand my verbiage. Syllables fly fast. Please, I can climb the stairs to my classroom. Why feelings of idiocy? My students must wonder what is going on. Two men, on either side, take my elbows, pull me to my feet. Everything whirls as they haul the barge up. Light-headed, I need a moment to adjust, wobble. Where did my glasses fly, my school bag, coffee? The female teacher gathers my belongings from the driveway. I am off-kilter, in a dinghy on rough seas.

The school is toasty warm; I had not noticed the coldness. Had I? A first responder examines for injuries, has me follow a moving pen. Is he holding one or two? I am outside myself looking in. Why am I blinking so much? Light is intense, a band squeezes, wrapped around my forehead. Cannot focus or track. My judiciousness and discernment fail me, left as fallen imprints in the snow.

I am too long in the principal's office. But I did nothing wrong! Curious teachers flow in and out. Can they hear me stuttering, repeating nonsense? Faces blur with sounds, which blur with lights, which blur with motion. Everything stop! My head throbs. Please slow everything down. The principal asks what happened. I try to explain, but once again, my utterance confuses. Cannot remember past the point of falling and my head bouncing. When I glanced down for a millisecond, black ice laughed and loomed. After that is fuzzy. Did I lose consciousness? The smack did knock me out. Others check in—want me to go to emergency. No need. My students are waiting. The peculiar aura will pass. I have much to prepare for the semester even though I hammered my noggin. Taught once before with three broken ribs. They monitor and talk to me, but the lights, noise, and nausea wear me down. The principal urges me to go to the hospital. Teachers share revealing looks. I must look as bad as I feel. I concede. They call my husband. I need a bed, silence, darkness.

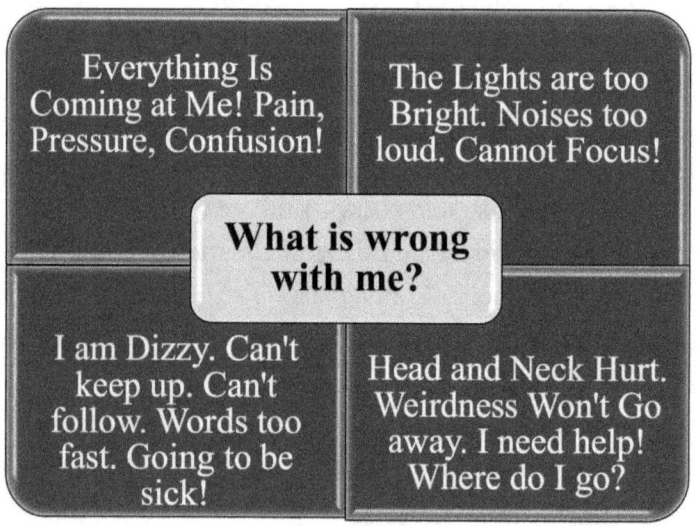

Everything Is Coming at Me! Pain, Pressure, Confusion!

The Lights are too Bright. Noises too loud. Cannot Focus!

What is wrong with me?

I am Dizzy. Can't keep up. Can't follow. Words too fast. Going to be sick!

Head and Neck Hurt. Weirdness Won't Go away. I need help! Where do I go?

Get me out of here! I am on a vessel swaying off balance in a choppy sea. My responses garbled. Am I crying? I cover my tears. My body is not cooperating. Is that me spea-king? Sounds flow fast and furious, excited, and high-pitched. Whose convoluted voice? Why so much effort? Stop the pressure and whirring in my brain. Do not ask questions. The boat climbs sizeable waves, dips, rises, rocks, refuses to settle. A wall of fatigue knocks me back. Tears drop. I wipe them before anyone notices. Do they catch the fear on my face? I brace myself. I remember my foot sliding, then my head bounced.

The hospital drive is long. I close my eyes, lean on the seat, searching for darkness so my stomach will calm. My husband and a teacher who followed us down, help me to a chair to deal with admittance. I must rest in darkness for the headache, pain, and nausea to fade. A nurse asks questions, but I cannot focus. Going to be sick. She takes me to a room with a bed, turns down the light. Small reprieve. The doctor on call examines, mentions concussion, whiplash. My spouse answers queries: my speech is a profound stut-ter with me stum-b-ling o-ver al-most e-ver-y word. Exam, X-rays. No broken bones. No *serious* injuries. They keep me until evening, little direction except to take Tylenol. If worse, return. Relief is instantaneous; I will be back working by week's end. Teaching is my passion. I want students to learn, experience fun, discover, go outside their comfort zones. They allow me to set high expectations, meet and embrace their potential. For that, I assume I must be the one to teach them. With rest and painkillers, I will recover.

The next morning, I wake to a screaming body and brain. A cartoon character splattered on a wall; a fly smacked by a fly swatter. I wrenched every part of my body. If I move, even my toenails wail. My neck, under my rib cage, arms, hands, back; I strained muscles when I tensed, tried to protect myself from falling, then hit, not just my head, it seems. How far to the pavement? I am five-foot-five. Later, I realize my puffy coat collar broke my fall, preventing a brain bleed or fracture.

My husband spends the day filtering calls from family and concerned friends, telling and retelling what happened, how I am doing, while I rest by a barf bag and bottle of Tylenol. It is a rough few days. My younger sister, who lives in the same community, comes to visit and help. The rest of my family living elsewhere, check in. We downplay my symptoms so not to alarm, figure after a week I will be fine. They send well wishes. We underestimate the impact of concussion. Although my body feels terrible and my head is in a loop, we expect a quick recovery.

One day, two days, three days, four . . . bundled in my bed or on the floor. In a dark room, I fight to come to terms with what happened. I cannot get comfortable. The pain under my rib cage keeps me awake at night, searing if I twist or turn. An achy band of pressure squeezes around my forehead. I am nauseous, cannot eat. Do not put food near me, smell of cooking makes me barf. My days get worse. Everything COMES AT ME! Noise, voices, music, light. How do I calm my brain? All over the place, thousands of ideas flash in a fast-forward movie. So many thoughts criss-cross; I cannot sleep. Pain weaves across my forehead, up my back and neck, squeezing tighter when I try to think, try not to think. I do not want to move. I restrict movements, confine activities, anything to ease soreness. For a long arduous week, I fight strange symptoms, get irritable and frustrated. Cannot concentrate, focus. I cannot focus on anything moving, listen to more than one voice at a time, sort messages without confusion. I cannot walk without bumping into things, losing my balance, dropping food.

The Hospital

I visit my family doctor . . . he admits me into the hospital. I do not put up a fuss. Just make the bizarre symptoms go away. They give me intravenous, clear liquids, a soft diet to help with nausea. I darken the room, hold the pillow over my ears to muffle the intensity of noises coming from the hallway. My husband brings down an eye mask. Stop the world from spinning, lightning speed yanking me into a vortex.

Agitated and overwrought, I wake early morning, emotional, stuttering ninety miles a minute. An older, wiser nurse calms me. Others probe my gibberish responses. How come? I limit talking to answering. Utterly embarrassed about my speech and my balance, I go no farther than the bathroom. They consult a neurologist. Shipwrecked on a massive, lonely rock in the tumultuous ocean I try to stop the craziness. I am supposed to be in my classroom not a hospital. No one stops to visit, padding a low sense of worth.

Electronic devices make my head spin. The principal hires a

substitute. I go into a tailspin, down, down, down, cannot stop crying. The fall knocks me out of commission, but I am determined to return to my classroom when released. The notion is ludicrous.

Symptoms keep me from getting out of bed, let alone returning to a busy school environment. Fear escalates. I am alone, seeking a way back, but how? The ocean continues to push me side to side; I cannot get my bearings. My family doctor discharges me after ten days, puts me off work for two weeks, which to me is too long, provides a referral to a neurologist, and a speech pathologist. People get concussions, recover within seven to ten days. None of this makes sense. As soon as I am up to more, I will search for help, fight back, regain my faculties and employment. Once upon a time, I was a communicator and teacher, a professional columnist, and writer—at least, once upon a time. A perfectionist . . . still am.

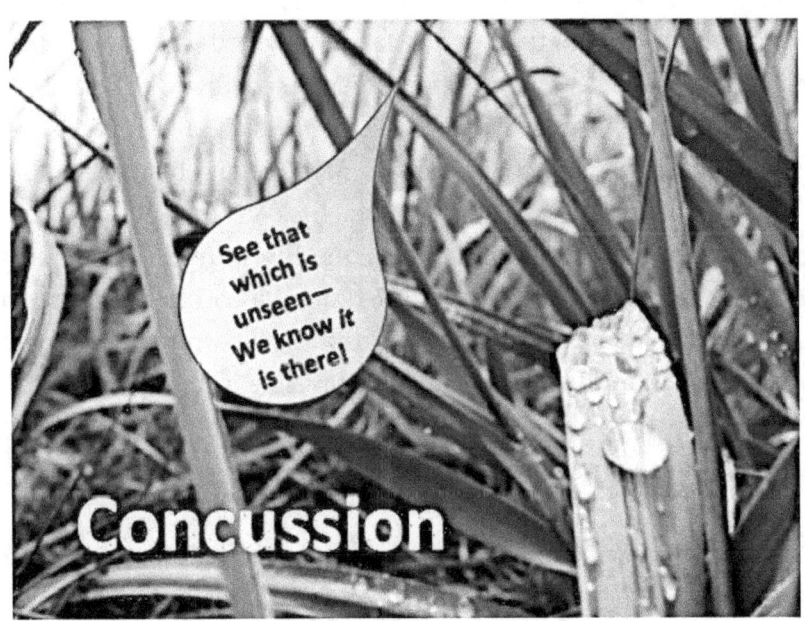

Home

My husband, and girls from afar sympathize, express concern. They investigate head injuries. The strange, foreign world of a concussion overwhelms, leaves us feeling lost. I just hit my head. "Turn your wounds into wisdom," says Oprah Winfrey.

In an instant—life can change . . . we must protect what we have, be vigilant. I left my identity on the cold, hard ground of February, beside black ice, a blue sky. Can I re-establish an identity that no longer exists? Tears well. Must I accept it to recover? I cannot face losing part of myself. Please! I need me! The way I used to be. I try, feel useless, lost without my job as a teacher and educator, can do little before the notorious claw grips my forehead. It takes little to totter near my threshold, symptoms escalate. "Hello, darkness, my old friend," say Simon & Garfunkel. "Go placidly amid the noise and haste, and remember what peace there may be in silence," says Max Ehrmann. His insights and lessons help. I want to scream.

Am I moody? A hateful word. I am exhausted, frustrated, mentally fatigued. Please name it for what it is—without judgment. If we feel judged, we shut down. Make us feel safe and loved, so we will have the best chance of recovery. My head did not hurt before. It served me well, allowed me to teach several grade levels and many topics. I loved reading, analyzing literature with students, and being around the energy they exude. We had a great rapport. They gave me life, a reason for being that flowed from deep within. One slip on black ice, and it all dried up "like a raisin in the sun," a line from the poem "Harlem," by Langston Hughes. A sudden moment altered my path, left me stranded near a mountain without proper gear.

Back home with little guidance, I am seasick, desperate to find an exit from the riptide. I want to be better; I want it NOW! Take me off this damn boat! Prior to my accident, anyone who knew me would tell you I was/am a workhorse. Those existence verbs send

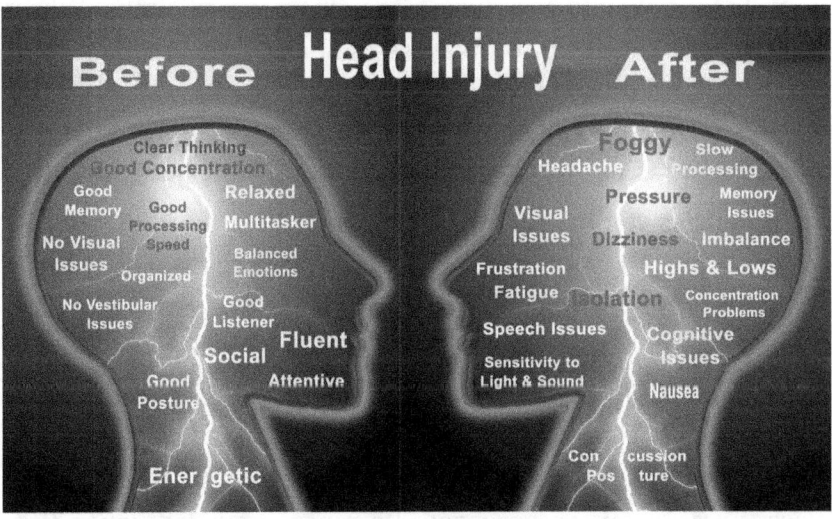

me into a hurricane. I hate before and after. Constant comparison leads to a dark spiral. "If you compare yourself to others, you may become vain and bitter; for always there will be greater and lesser persons than yourself," says Max Ehrmann in "Desiderata." Difficult to not go to that place where I juggled several balls, taught dozens, dealt with issues, finished one draft, began another, wrote a weekly column, picked at provincial, educational pursuits. I need to keep busy, my coping mechanism to distract my body from the claw exacerbated by chronic, fibromyalgia pain, diagnosed when I was twenty. I also suffered from endometriosis and interstitial cystitis, as well as irritable bowel. Still, I ran a business for three years, went back to teaching full-time for twenty-three, while raising a family, and being involved in community organizations and provincial projects. Now, I close windows and blinds, block the sun, shut my eyes, plug my ears, curl in an unsettled ball on a sofa or bed, a washed-up jellyfish stranded on burning sand.

A silent jail cell, no physical bars, I battle unfiltered senses. How depressing to not go out in the sunshine and lap it up! Earlier summers had me stretched out on my deck tanning. Not an option with PCS. Too bright, despite sunglasses and a ball cap; I cry angry tears. Is that okay to say? I cry often when overwhelmed. Where do I get help to return to my classroom and life? This is not my future. Rewind the reels; back it up. I want to go home . . . Take me *home*. My fall creates debilitating new symptoms and exacerbates pre-existing medical conditions. I feel guilty knowing how severe brain injuries can be. Although enough to stop me in my tracks, mine is minor. Desperate to get back into my classroom, I overdo appointments, ignorant of the healing time. By refusing to slow down, it becomes too much for me. I am ill-informed.

Recovery from my injury is turtle-slow. I chomp at the bit to get moving, invent cold coffee/tea, get distracted, bruise from bumping into furniture, forget, have to search for items, which places pressure on my forehead. I am not organized; when I try to be, I forget where I put my now-dead phone, shoes, earplugs. Self-criticism wails unrelenting. My fault I am disorganized, my fault my phone is missing, my fault, my fault . . . my fault I fell. And there it is! My fault. The list is endless. If you reiterate you chip more fragments off. I search, cannot remember, fall in tears. As the months move forward, my husband encourages me to ask for help instead of getting frustrated.

First hit—being off work, the second nails me to the wall—I cannot drive without fatigue and nausea, cannot look out the windshield when moving. If I want to get out on my own for a change of scenery, I cannot. Looking at moving objects is impossible, things come too fast, my depth perception shot. Difficult to see things on the periphery. I vomit. Gone is my primary activity to relax. I loved getting behind the wheel, stepping on the gas pedal, turning the SUV in whatever direction, feeling a sense of freedom, controlling when and where my vehicle went. Heartbroken tears flow, reliance now on my husband to chauffeur me.

Driving, a part of my identity allowed me to meet people, shop, visit, enjoy nature's offerings. A hard blow, it stays with me too long. I lost my independence that frightful morning. My freedom was wiped away, increasing isolation—losing an artery to the real, outside word, placed in a surreal, grey cloud of loneliness, one that I cannot express to anyone for fear of what they might think. Grey turns black. My girls are concerned, as are my sisters. They realize I will not recover as fast as we thought. They can tell from the "way I am," I have a mountain to climb before I can get back to my classroom. As the weeks and months pass, they absorb how stealthy a head injury can be.

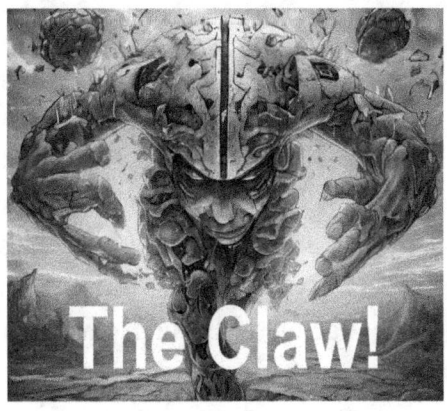

The "knock" on my head worse than expected, brings unknowns. My words come, slowly, like an inchworm struggling along at great expense. I used to be articulate. Stuttering kills me and I do not understand. Symptoms escalate whenever I try to do anything. That headache pressure in the centre of my forehead becomes known as my notorious clutching claw, always appearing with increased effort. Unsettling NOISE has me begging mercifully for silence. As a teacher, I was confident and respected, had a deep desire to help students and younger teachers; I put on workshops, shared resources, worked as a consultant. I am utterly tired, cannot shower without extreme fatigue and grief. I slip to my bathroom floor until I muster fortitude. The cold tiles on my face ground me. I am safe, comfortable, alone in the dark. It is bound to get easier . . .

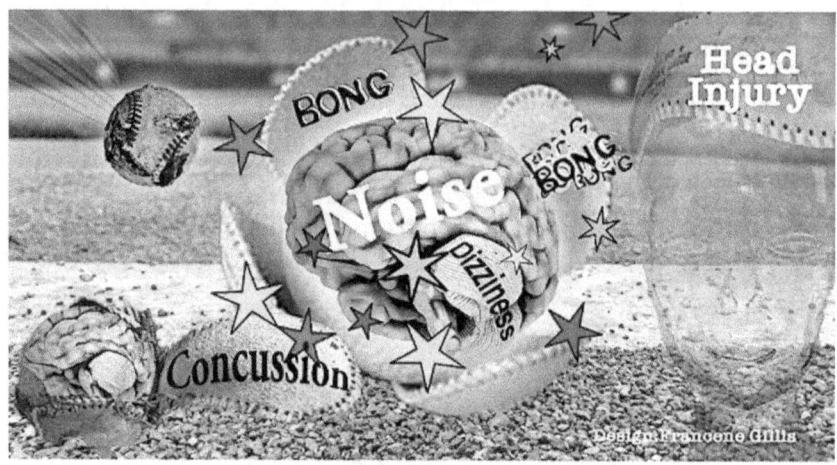

Consider a baseball, stitches holding together the figure eight seams. Tear the stitches. Place the cowhide flat on your head. The subtle, soft texture of leather replicates a silky scalp; stitching holds matter in, conversely keeps signals out. If the stitching lets go, everything gets in, placing the brain in chronic overload. It tries to filter, keep up with an enormous demand, simultaneous signals, multiple messages, senses, audio and visual stimuli. When damaged, it cannot. The stitching underneath represents interrupted nerve pathways to the brain's centre, affecting functionality rather than structure. Messages enter an unstitched brain as NOISE at high speeds amid the ruckus of thousands of fans screaming. If the parts of the ball are separate, is it still a ball?

The damage from head injuries can be cumulative. When my oldest daughter was in upper elementary, she sustained a concussion when she and her class were going down a steep hill in winter. She slipped on ice, cracked her skull, but did not realize she had a concussion. Later, she could not understand why she felt sick. When her teacher asked if she was okay, she complained of a sore belly and headache. The class continued to the rink to play broom ball. They put her on the ice to play! Bizarre, and extremely dangerous were she to fall and hit her head a second time, while still experiencing a concussion. Everything was coming at her. A severe headache, nausea, classic signs of concussion, not picked up by her teacher or any of the others gathered in that arena. She could remember nothing from early morning. Confused and sick, she called us. We took her to the hospital. The doctor diagnosed a concussion. In the 1990s, they did little for a minor head injury. She never regained her lost memory, forever writes lists. Schools and staff should be more aware. We were clueless about follow-up, except to have her rest in a dark room. Even years later, as a teacher myself, I was unaware of the extent of concussions. Few are until we experience it or educate ourselves. Migraines remained off and on for years. She felt different, could not articulate in words how. I wish I knew then what I know now. A concussion's tentacles spread farther and wider than most realize.

Searching for items drives me crazy, adds extra steps to what should be easy. I cannot find things put away minutes before for safekeeping. Tired eyes, I close them to rebuff an overstimulated, maniacal world. Thinking requires excessive effort; ideas rush in on a roller coaster. Filtering through flooding senses is a massive undertaking. Please take the constant whirring, whizzing, whistling away. The buzzing fills my thoughts. Tinnitus. What is that? A constant ringing in my left ear. Give me silence. It refuses to let up, shuts me down. Seems when I turn left, I trigger the suction down the Alice-in-Wonderland hole. A tunnel pulls me down at such a dangerous speed, I cannot handle it. I am going to hurl. Need to be cognizant, avoid left turns. A physiotherapist explains I have left-positional induced vertigo.

Symptoms bombard. I need my classroom. Please God, how long will this insanity last? In unfamiliar territory, I do not know what to expect. Why am I not better? Lights and noises grate. I cannot follow conversations. My brain cannot process what people are saying, as fast as they say it. Memory is gone unless cued. I ask the same question five times, forget I asked, am ashamed,

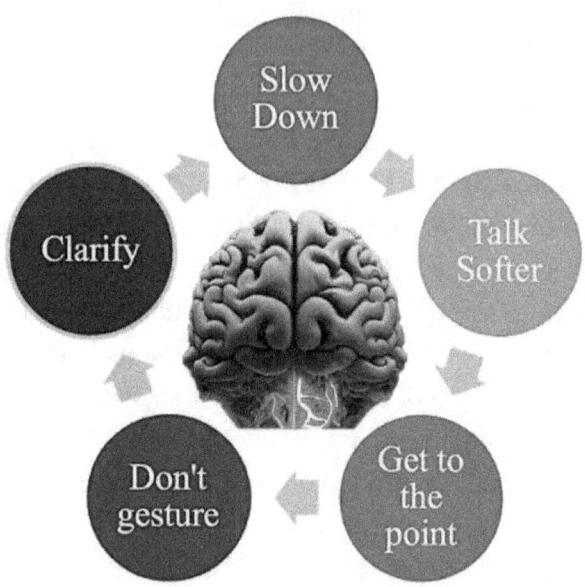

flustered, mad at myself for being so stupid. Taking medicine is a gong show. I request a blister pack with the pills packaged for morning and night, still I manage to mix them up. Did I take them? Did I put the tea bag in my cup? Hot water tastes okay. They tell me I am hard on myself, cannot speak a proper sentence without murdering my words. Few understand. I don't understand. Why do I feel such shame?

Talking tires. Stuttering tries. Wrong word, same first letter. My husband chuckles, a habit when unsure of what to say or do. He tries to lighten the mood. I tell him it is fine to be an expert, just not at everything. He laughs; we tease. Sometimes it works and sometimes it doesn't. Fatigue hurts. My Type A engine wants to push and pull, refuses to quit. My students ask for my return. They miss me. Effort and exertion increase symptoms. Is this normal after a head injury? Who has the answer? I am desperate. The why question burns a hole in my clothes. My sphere shrinks.

Trying to do multiple tasks leads to symptoms. Distraction kills my ability to listen. I cannot view loud clothes with patterns and converse at the same time. My brain fixates on oddities like humming noises no one else can detect; I seek glorious silence—no talking, background noises, questioning, chit-chatting. Pressure like a vice grip gnaws my forehead, tightens, squeezes. Kill the bright lights. Block the sun with clouds. Neutralize what provides nourishment, motivation, and growth. I wear sunglasses over my prescriptions, block the glaring sun, go outside on cinereal days, am a sad country song begging to be written. The boat tips side to side, sickening waves. I am spent. Writing, eating, showering, breathing tires. Baby steps. But I AM NOT A BABY! A veil of exhaustion and loneliness exacerbates an excruciating, slow recovery. What I once did shaped my identity, now . . .

Do not remind me what you said. If I ask, I cannot remember. Be gentle. I try to deal with changes but stagger through one drawback after the other. I do not recognize myself. Grief of losing my job in such an insidious manner takes its toll. Who am i? My students kept me going, but I am no longer a teacher. I miss them like crazy, their laughter, sunshine, exuberance, willingness to do their best. I grieve, pound my pillow, scream, yell because I cannot get up early, dress, drive to school, and teach. Tears stream for what was. When with them I did something worthwhile, knew who I was but at home, unable to do chores or tasks, even basic care without severe fatigue, I crumble, miss the cheery affirmations of my pupils. An irritable grain of sand I scratch under a wet bathing suit or grind in a beachside peanut butter sandwich.

Reminding me of what I cannot do is abrasive, triggers an overreaction as I am hypersensitive, my self-esteem rock bottom. Let me rest. Let me feel, get my fear, frustration, anxiety out. Validate my emotions. If I need to cry, scream in a private place, let me. Give me time to be more rational, release my feelings and apprehension, or I will suffer in silence, cut off from all I love. A voice screeches—I am useless without skills or abilities. Self-consciousness rears, ridicules, blames, triggers ugly outbursts.

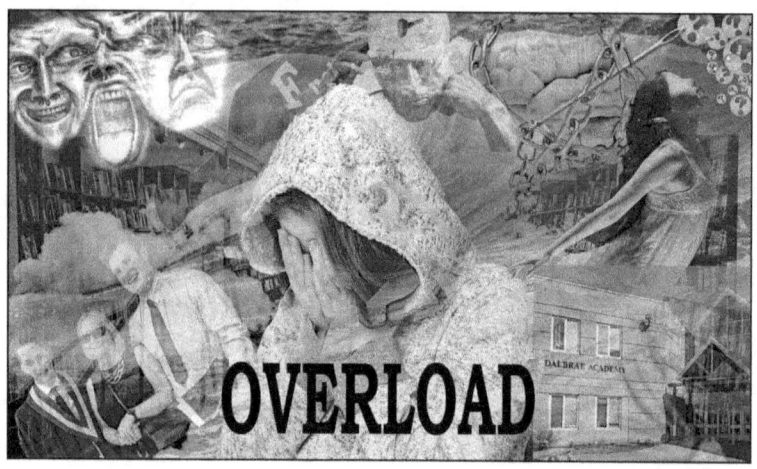

Confession

Growing up, I was self-conscious of my face, my long nose, fang teeth, fine hair, poor complexion. As a teenager, I fought battles with blemishes, a scarlet flush when I spoke to people. I was not comfortable in my body. Stuttering focuses attention to the face, brings up those excruciating feelings. I flush beet red. Will I ever be free?

Worthlessness screams. I cannot go among crowds, morph into a wallflower, multiple senses triggering symptoms. Each rebellious day, I hang onto my core, fight to bring her back, reclaim my classroom, return to the profession I love. No longer feeling complete, I struggle to regain that which was based on what I can do, rather than who I am, thus an epic explosion. A monumental piece of me is missing. I cannot get her back. Can I? I wish I could do more, be less of a concern for family. They watch, scared.

My identity—where did i go? I do not recognize myself. It hurts to think. Why focus on shame and fault, like a broken rag doll missing her limbs? Please, someone, sew them on, prove people care. I am furious at the notion of a substitute in my classroom.

I want to be greeting my students, discovering who they are, doing informal assessments, teaching them the fundamentals of our classroom. Instead, I wear dirty pyjamas, rock on a damn boat in rough seas, unable to tame the fierce ocean around me as waves push the vessel left, right, up, down, repeatedly. Mundane days crowd one into the other with no change. Left, on my own, wrapped in an itchy, obscure blanket, not knowing which way to turn, how do I get stronger? Most days, a dense fog hovers. I cannot get through.

How to describe brain fog? Pressure, fighting to get through a malleable wall. Your arm goes through, reaching into an obscure grey cloud that surrounds everything and nothing. Thoughts crowd in on each other. I reach and stretch . . . for what? Thoughts crowd in; remembering hurts. Distraction, forgetfulness, confusion, fatigue. Where am I going? Where was I going? Eye mist fills my days. Too many signals. My Raggedy Ann flops on the floor, head down. Too much COMING AT her!

I get stuck playing strange messages in my brain. Do others see me as stupid or incompetent? I cannot process what they say as fast as they say it, flounder in deep water, pretend I understand the words, nod my head while not having a clue. Multiple signals create a gelatinous glob for a brain. Naive people assume a bump on the head is nothing to worry about, unaware of the interconnected possibilities when the brain jostles inside the skull—the potential for debilitating ramifications and complications.

Specialists assess my noggin to see if, like Humpty Dumpty, they can put me together again. Please, no cracks. Are my symptoms in my head? No pun intended. Is that what unversed doctors believe? The elephant appears when medicine cannot provide answers to invisible illnesses. I enter stormy seas without a compass, the stars, my navigation, the passage foreign, pray I do not sink.

"One of the problems patients with functional and dissociative neurological symptoms experience is a feeling they are not being believed . . . research in these areas is poor. The answer, you are not imagining or making up your symptoms and you were not 'going crazy'. You have functional/dissociative symptoms. Getting your head around this takes time. Your symptoms are real, even if doctors and others make you feel as if they are not!" (Stone, Dr. Jon, MB, ChB, FRCP, PhD, neurologist, 2009)

It is reassuring that Dr. Stone considers functional aspects of the brain, which seems to be missing in mainstream neurology. New on the horizon, functional neurologists concerned with functioning of the brain rather than structure. A comfort to those with invisible injuries.

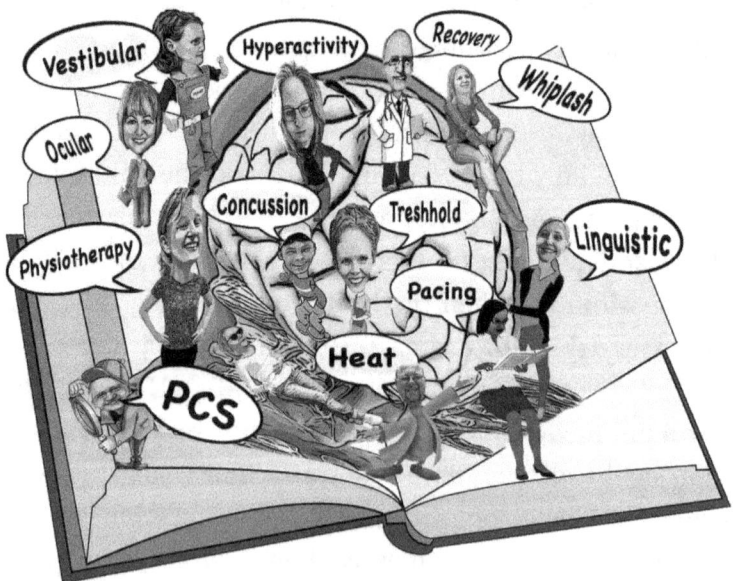

Comparing leads to sadness and depression. I used to be full of life, driven and capable. Used to be . . . a dangerous phrase. I must be mindful of how I react to situations and people. Since my head injury, I overreact because of sensory overload and an inability to filter. My voice gets loud without realizing it. I am worse if tired, which is always. Trivial things to others grow exponentially, culminating in frustration, cognitive function slowing down, and processing speed, a tortoise-slow, centurion driver.

I stagger when distracted, try to talk and walk. Concentration twists and wrings my forehead into a mayonnaise jar. Light and sound pollute, cannot even listen to instrumental music. For my lingering, painful neck, I alternate between ice and heat, depending on swelling. Extra-strength Tylenol and muscle relaxants help as do anti-inflammatory drugs. Fatigue cripples, compounds pre-existing chronic health conditions. I cannot do eighty percent of what I could do before. Preparing meals drains any energy in my gas tank. If I try to cook, I am too sore and tired to eat. My husband takes over.

Ugly voices haunt when I am depleted: I am no good to anybody, cannot teach, cannot nurture friendships, cannot help anyone, cannot, cannot, cannot. So lost and alone. Is this a result of my fall—dark thoughts? Reoccurring nightmares concerning school, my past? No one comes to visit. Why not? Did my accident erase me? Never would I have believed such dire repercussions from a fall. I crumble into tears, curl on my bed, bawl my eyes out, because I cannot do what I once could. Someone else instructs my students, makes the meals, cleans the house, walks along my shoreline. What must I do to heal? I cannot continue this way. I long to see my eager students engaged in academic pursuits, challenging each other. How do I rediscover myself and find my way back?

Identity is precarious in a world where we covet roses. Striving to find one's identity after an injury or sickness requires picking up the petals getting through the thorns. I have learned not to make assumptions, to be careful of judgment, to open the crack in the door so the view does not limit. In the willingness to revisit the ordinary, the extraordinary is born.

In 2014, during my Master of Education program, a professor recommended that I do less. I had discovered an absolute love for learning. Without sharing, what is the point? I challenged myself with everything I did until my fall stopped me cold. Extended career opportunities flew out the window, screeched to a halt. I had planned to go for my PhD; those goals fell into quicksand. Crushed plans, proposals, writings flashed red on a digital ten-foot screen, dreams flushed down the toilet because of one life-changing, idiotic step on black ice. Who knew such danger lurked on the walkway into my school?

PAUSE! While We Steal Years of Your Existence!

My inferiority complex explodes. Why? Is it my fault I fell? Should I feel shame because my symptoms lasted longer than typical? What is typical? I feel bad, as if it were my fault, failure an arch-enemy. If I expect the best from others, I better step up. But no one was at fault. It was an accident. Did/do/did/do—nasty troublesome verb dilemma. Normally, I set towering expectations and work to achieve them. Feeling deflated, I search for answers, try to understand what happened. My house cries for attention; closets look like cyclones hit. Specialists, where are they? I know so little; no one to advise me. Terrified with each passing month, what if I do not recover? I cannot handle that ball-and-chain thought. Not an option.

In trying to be *positive*, a word I do not like for its connotation, I memorize mantras, smother critical dragon voices that creep in when tired. One hundred percent I gave, a far cry from when my head did not hurt, world did not spin, light did not blind, noise did not reverberate, effort tax me. I tried to skip before I could walk, sing before I could talk, write before I could print, speak my name without stuttering.

Willpower alone cannot swing me across jungle trees and

bridges like Tarzan. Hear my war cry. Patience is a virtue I have yet
to master. Who would believe? I try to accept what is in front of me.
Humour helps, as does pacing and remembering to breathe. An
easy strategy for cooling our jets, we negate its power to settle the
hyperactive nervous system. I need to learn how. My skyscraper
expectations hurtle me into an abyss. My hands clench as I type
this. Knots twist my stomach. I am not ready to face, accept what
happened. Angry at the ice, myself . . . my body is nuclear reactive.
Why am I snail-slow in recovering? Finding helpful information
is tedious, hard, exhausting. Why are the concussed individuals
left to rely on their own resources? Does this lead to an increase
in individuals being mistreated for headaches, fatigue, mental fog,
and depression, as they come to terms with the fact that they can
no longer work or pursue their chosen career?

My concussion disguises the real me, leads to less-than-stellar
performances as I try to deal with daily pain, roadblocks, and
flare-ups. A fire-breathing dragon, scales of fear and frustration,
surrounds me. The brain must relearn to categorize and juggle five
senses. To cut down on visual and audio stimuli, I close my eyes.
Can I ask Mother Nature for camouflage to protect me from multi-
sensory predators? Red flags are everywhere when first diagnosed:
I get it. We must prioritize therapy to address loneliness, feelings
of inadequacy as suicide rates escalate. We need to listen to family
and friends, for we may not realize our own mental state. Four
awful months, I do not know where to turn, cannot find what I
need. The boat dips in fog, my journey to recovery hindered, no
guidance, a lack of knowledge and awareness of concussions.

Sickness or injury forces us to rethink everything. Reflection
helps us figure out what our new self might look like, re-establish
goals. By having a lodestar—someone or something that serves as
a guiding model—we can gain purpose within limitations.

Inspiring words, I plaster everywhere! Make connections. I
meditate on the gifts in my life, how a sunny attitude and mindset

can help. That is when I see glimpses of me buried underneath the shell, a ray of hope reappearing in the darkness. I evaluate my strengths and interests, redefine myself to accept the reality of good and bad days. The sooner we embrace our world, the sooner we can focus on reinvention. My determination falters. Youth entangles my identity. I grieve, scream, cry. No good to anyone. I miss my energetic students. They provide life and purpose, now destroyed. A flash, a mere second, a not-so-mere slip and . . . POOF! Gone! Before I fell, I was an energized professional, excited to start a new semester. Seconds later, I am on a blind journey, looking for the light.

After months of swaying on tumultuous waves, I send out a family distress call. *"Someone, help!"* I write through spilling tears. *"Cannot take it anymore. Don't know what to do. Am exhausted. My head squeezes in pain if I try to do anything. Need relief! Am going crazy. How do I recover? Need to get back to work, been too long, takes all my energy to get out of bed, write this, shower, dress. I cry every day, need someone to help. Please?"*

Immediately, my sisters make me their mission. The road is bumpy, filled with potholes and blind spots. Are there specialists nearby? I cannot drive. My husband offers. My older sister, agrees to look after the bloody paperwork, navigate financial issues, red tape fight of being off work "longer than I should?" My younger sister keeps me level-headed, gems of wisdom in her pocket she delivers every other day. I need her empathetic words. My oldest sisters offer comfort, kind words. My husband supports me but feels lost as he sees my struggles, does not know how to help. As caregiver it is tough. He does the best he can, difficult when fatigue or lack of energy activates my central nervous system. My daughters offer advice and encouragement. So thankful I have them in my corner.

One, two, three, four . . . I will deteriorate into a black ball, unless I remind myself to focus on the people and things I love.

Coping with physical pain, trauma, loss, and frustration takes a certain mindset. When we falter, we need support and reassurance. Many ask, "Can I help you?" A better question, "What can I do for you?" A question with no frayed edges attached. We fray easily. Affirmation helps as does good TLC, tender loving care. I applaud caregivers, their patience, understanding, encouragement.

One, two, three . . . Words will not come to me. On the tip of my tongue. Cannot remember a STUPID word! An English Language Arts teacher living in a lonely, cardboard box; that is my life. Who was i? Who am i? Where did i go? I must keep going until I find my identity and my healing path. Can I? Years after my injury I begin to write what I need—a collection of valuable information and resources that would have been helpful to have had when I fell, my identity stolen in mere seconds. Can I get it back?

Nature's Kisses

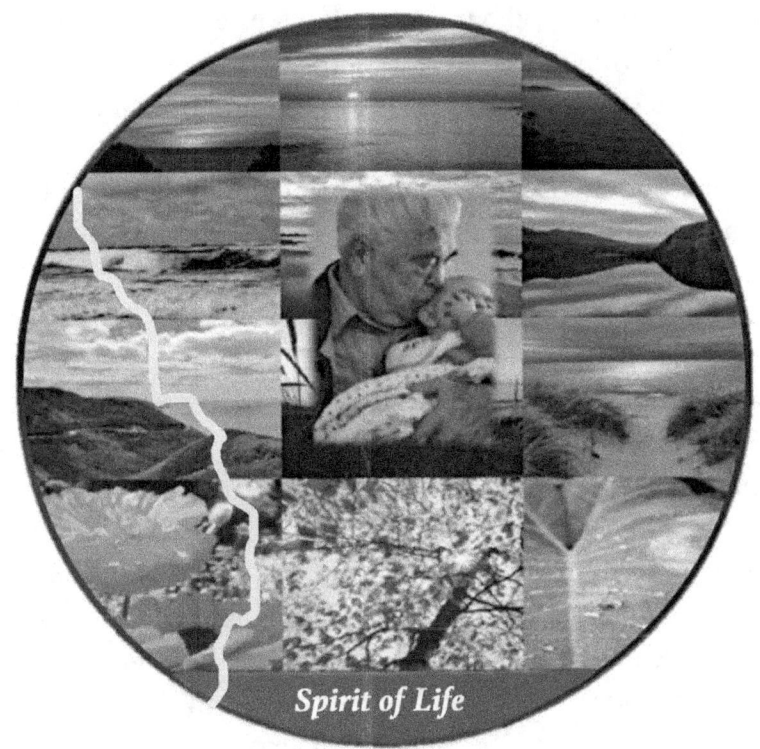

Spirit of Life

*"There is a crack in everything.
That is how the light gets in."*

— Leonard Cohen, 2011

*T*he illumination seeping through the crack calls us. Concussion and chronic illness can be dark; sharing our struggles and learning lightens the load. We are not alone. The trees whisper and murmur morning secrets through my bedroom window, stirring the desire to join them; I hear them breathe as the breeze flutters the sheer curtain separating me for a brief time from my symptoms. In my master's program two years before my injury, a professor introduced our class to the four elements of air, fire, water, and earth, sacred elements of the Indigenous People known as the Spirit of Life. That and their Medicine Wheel, which depicts wisdom, love, respect, bravery, honesty, humility, and truth, provides instruction. Our professor smudged with us—an ancient offering of burning tobacco, cedar, sage, or sweetgrass for a variety of cleansing purposes, such as to clear the mind and open the heart. I hang onto that ritual through my journey.

My love for writing and nature are lifesavers. Both bring solace. From my bed, I see my temperamental best friend, dawn to dusk. The ocean reminds me of myself, same unexpected mood swings triggered by outside forces. A metaphor for my trials and tribulations, frustration as waves crash, comfort when she rests mirror-perfect and tranquil. And who has seen the wind driving her temperaments? Nature is the backdrop of my writing. Themes in literature involve overcoming difficulties that develop determination, fortitude, commitment, and strength, which when painted through the canvas of the outdoors, take on symbolism. We can quiet inner stirrings, by sitting on a tired, worn wharf with our feet dangling, water caressing and cooling our toes. Inhale the scent of salt air and burning driftwood. A walk along the shoreline focusing on footprints in the sand, or a hike through the crackling woods, nourishes what is deep within, exercises, massages, and nourishes the soul. I do not need to walk far to experience nature's kisses. We must find that which soothes, whether people or place, and remain nestled until revived.

A favourite analogy for overcoming adversity is the patient, fluttering butterfly. The monarch exemplifies Mother Nature's wisdom through its transformation. We too undergo metamorphosis when injured. Not all things stay the same. Foolhardy to think life is static. Embracing the truth brings us closer to our desired destination; easier said than done. Should we try to emerge early? Removing a butterfly from its cocoon, kills it. Why hurry when our body screams not ready? Like dutiful soldiers, we march onward, even if frustrated to find wisdom, welcome nature's kisses to carry us along.

When frantic, I stop and stand in solitude, gaze at chestnut-brown and spotted beige cows chewing grass in an open field. Their frisky tails swish back and forth, pushing away annoying deer flies. Not a care, they saunter, minding their own business, no worries about anything else except the farmer, milking, and feeding.

Mesmerized by sunsets and gangly trees, I sit and stare at branches, limbs, and twigs, follow the curves, nuances, pathways, nobs with fresh growth. I imagine the growth at various stages, marvel at the strength and nourishment in the roots, the branches' ability to move and combat violent storms. They bend and sway, forgivingly flexible. Leaves bud, unfold, provide a green canopy, shelter from the rain. Trees reach higher into the sky. Chances are they will not snap, even with ferocious gales, smaller limbs pliable, trunk strong and sturdy. I wish I were a tree. Once upon a time I could rhyme off famous poems and poets discussing trees, now my mind goes blank.

Late morning, my husband driving me home from a doctor's appointment, dark greys blanket the upper sky in all four directions. Sunlight peeks out from behind the clouds like a gleeful grin, fanning golden-white rays. Such a small manifestation of the universe, yet my heart skips a beat. Tremendous beauty rests on the canvas of the horizon; each day a distinct snapshot. A gift! Nature offers dynamic skyscapes, landscapes, cityscapes hand-painted with masterful artistry and virtuosity. Every view is a 3D master-piece. Even with head injuries, we can view what nature gives. In time, the sun will not bother me. I love artwork and outdoor fresh-ness, cloudy days best.

Amidst injury and sickness, we lose sight of the present. Symptoms drain energy. While longing for greener pastures, we miss the pansy struggling to peek between the stones in the drive-way. Even though it should not exist, more determined it plows through, desperate to display its colours of white and yellow swirl-ing through delicate, purple petals. The simple things speak the deepest, sitting on the sandy beach, toes curled under warm sand, at the edge of the vast ocean, breathing the salty air, walking hand in hand along the shoreline admiring the majestic setting sun, while drinking in the vibrant colours that leave you breathless in their intensity and creative design. I define serenity as wispy, red clouds reflecting and hugging a glowing scarlet orb, casting pro-fundity as she sinks to sleep behind Port Hood Island, tranquil in her *ocean* bed for the night.

To help with a sense of inadequacy, I buy houseplants; caring, watering, and nurturing them provides value. With nutrients they grow strong compared to those left unattended, sowed in rocky soil, shade or too much sun. They become weak, brittle, die. All living things need sustenance, and hibernating in the safety of my house, slows my recovery, exposure necessary for progress. I am scared to let others see my issues. I under or overwater my plants. Hard to get the right balance. Some die. Microcosms in macro-cosms, lifetimes captured in minutes, hours, days, weeks. The world spins, inviting us to change perspective, see more than the view outside our window.

I never tire of the splendour along garden paths sprinkled with loving care and wonder. Flowers play peekaboo in golden mead-ows; purple and pink lupins sway wild in ditches. Greenery along dirt roads, estuaries hidden through an opening in dense woods. I stop to sniff the balsam lingering on boughs. Nature heals the soul, or at least speaks to it. The Atlantic Ocean reminds me of adversity, waves pushing forward, pulling us back, and sometimes under.

The sun, even on dreary days, is a topic of conversation. We know its power to cheer. Rain too, I enjoy. Raindrops rhythmically play drums on the roof, providing contentment in the musical melody as warm and dry we rest inside and remember childhood rain songs. I appreciate what I have; so many others have less. Guilt overcomes me for sulking. A Catch-22, the pendulum swings.

Ends and beginnings intertwine. A riddle by Confucius teases until enlightenment. We sit before a sage oracle searching for answers, search for the eureka moment. I am not giving up. Awareness is critical. An onerous mistake to walk among thistles and poison ivy in bare feet. When walking in tall grass or on a woodland hiking trail, we must be careful of ticks. Adapting to new realities and gaining knowledge presents an opportunity to educate. If folks do not understand, an excellent chance to enlighten. In nature, we find parallels to life lessons.

A common theme. In literature things not being as they seem and assumptions when we meet people a spinoff. Without prior knowledge we do not know what a person is going through, and everyone wears an overcoat that covers pain, injury, or trauma. Are we a weed or a flower? Does it matter? Depends on perspective, true of most situations. I talk in riddles, but tremendous brain exercise in examination as opposed to staring at a blank wall and seeing nothing. Divergent reasoning comes from considering multiple perspectives; we see the entire garden in its splendour, embrace the sweet fragrances, touch beauty and softness, and rationalize our way through recovery.

Acceptance is a journey, grieving one way of life for another. From Greek mythology, I need Odysseus to shepherd me through the dangerous current in the Strait of Messina, to protect me from Scylla and Charybdis, immortal creatures who live in the narrow waters. They will devour me, and I cannot control them as I do not understand. Scylla, a female creature, lumbers out of her cave to devour whatever comes within reach. Charybdis lurks under a fig tree on the opposite shore, personification of a whirlpool. I am sucked under by attacks and flare-ups throughout the day.

Both Greek monsters symbolize what, according to the *Encyclopedia Britannica*, is a poetic expression of the dangers confronting us. To be between "Scylla and Charybdis" is to find ourselves between two unpleasant alternatives. Either struggle against escalating symptoms in an overwhelming, work environment, or take rest in a confining, mysterious cage. Without proper treatments, we suffer prolonged difficulties. Nobody fully understands the functioning of the brain although scientists are close. I hope employers, in general, will learn more about head injuries to help employees with concussions ease back. For me, the path to return is frightening and unclear. Being a classroom teacher demands reasoning on the spot, the ability to multi-task and articulate, which I cannot do without strain, headaches, and forehead pressure. I would not last an hour with multiple sounds and visual messages coming at me. Scylla has me in her clutches and I am stuck until someone helps me out of the nightmare.

With support, the sun can shine again, despite clouds and unexpected delays. I must accept that, or the sea monsters will eat me. Some days the tumultuous ocean calms, reflects the sky, tranquil, but unpredictable. Life is full, even with hardships, loss, and startling turns. I must focus . . . "Keep your courage," wise words from a school classmate, Ronnie MacEachen, who shared his lovely grandmother's sage advice.

Depleted when I wake, I get mad as hell at myself. The mountain verse makes me feel better. Thank goodness for uplifting quotations. Knowledge comes with experiences, that which creates a smile or laugh, from leisurely walks, moments alone, a self-embrace, or from talking to others with comparable stories.

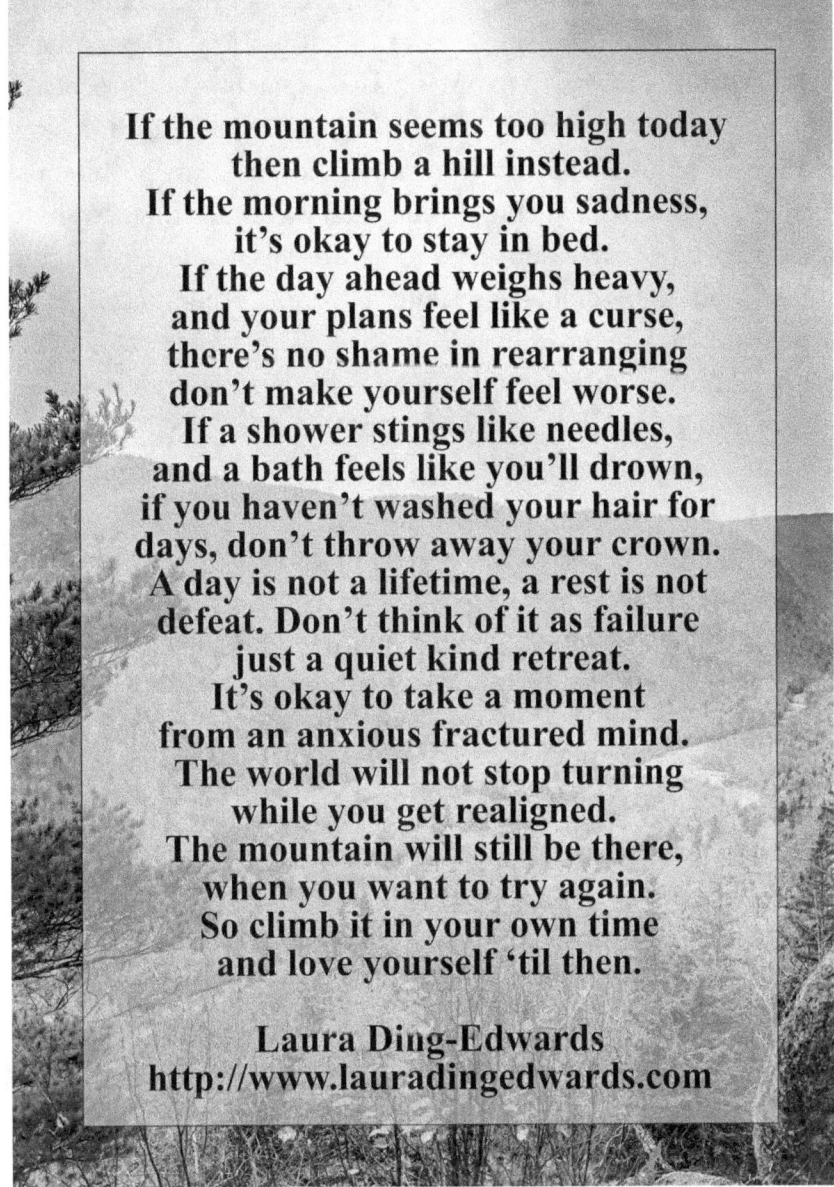

If the mountain seems too high today
then climb a hill instead.
If the morning brings you sadness,
it's okay to stay in bed.
If the day ahead weighs heavy,
and your plans feel like a curse,
there's no shame in rearranging
don't make yourself feel worse.
If a shower stings like needles,
and a bath feels like you'll drown,
if you haven't washed your hair for
days, don't throw away your crown.
A day is not a lifetime, a rest is not
defeat. Don't think of it as failure
just a quiet kind retreat.
It's okay to take a moment
from an anxious fractured mind.
The world will not stop turning
while you get realigned.
The mountain will still be there,
when you want to try again.
So climb it in your own time
and love yourself 'til then.

Laura Ding-Edwards
http://www.lauradingedwards.com

A massive U-shaped tree with no leaves catches my attention. I marvel at the twisting lines, prudence within unique spirals, turns, and bends, reminding me that not all trees grow straight to the sky; some dominant branches go sideways to form a "u." Maybe I am one of them. When I struggle to find myself, getting out of my head helps. Walking outside is an excellent reprieve from momentary hardship. I return to nature's kisses—sparrows and grosbeaks singing, peepers chirping, chimes swaying, hummingbird in slow motion drinking nectar, fresh strawberries, salt air, buttercups, pansies, fir boughs, dancing wildflowers, waves cresting. To share with others, we have sunsets, gentle breezes, waterfalls, hiking trails, look-offs, robin eggs, plus a trillion other possibilities depending on where we live. Cities have a host of secret sanctuaries waiting for discovery. My plan is to redefine myself, gather pieces, design a vibrant new mosaic. When too tired, my faith, as it has many times in the past, will pick me up, help me face the unknown.

Metaphorically, climbing over fallen trees and debris, I veer off my mountain road.

The freshness of spruce and fir pull me in. Under canopies of evergreens, I step on a spongy, moss floor. Beauty has me wandering into and onto unmarked, sheltered wood roads and paths. I turn, comfort beckons from the ocean below. Must find the route, see the view from the summit. Rushing is foolhardy. Major meltdown. Best climb, steady as she goes, take the rests and enjoy the sea from look-offs until I gain the stamina and endurance to reach the peak.

What is with my emotions? Fine one minute, the next the world is ending! What is with the caustic self-criticism, aloneness, overwhelming feelings of alienation? Are these the aftermath of head injury? Can I control words or events that trigger, make me anxious, turn me into a wacko or child sobbing her heart out? My threshold is fluid. I need to send someone a photograph—I thought of you today—nature's kiss.

"If you focus on the hurt, you will continue to suffer. If you focus on the lesson, you will continue to grow."

— ONE Family aiming ONE GOAL, Nov. 2023, YouTube

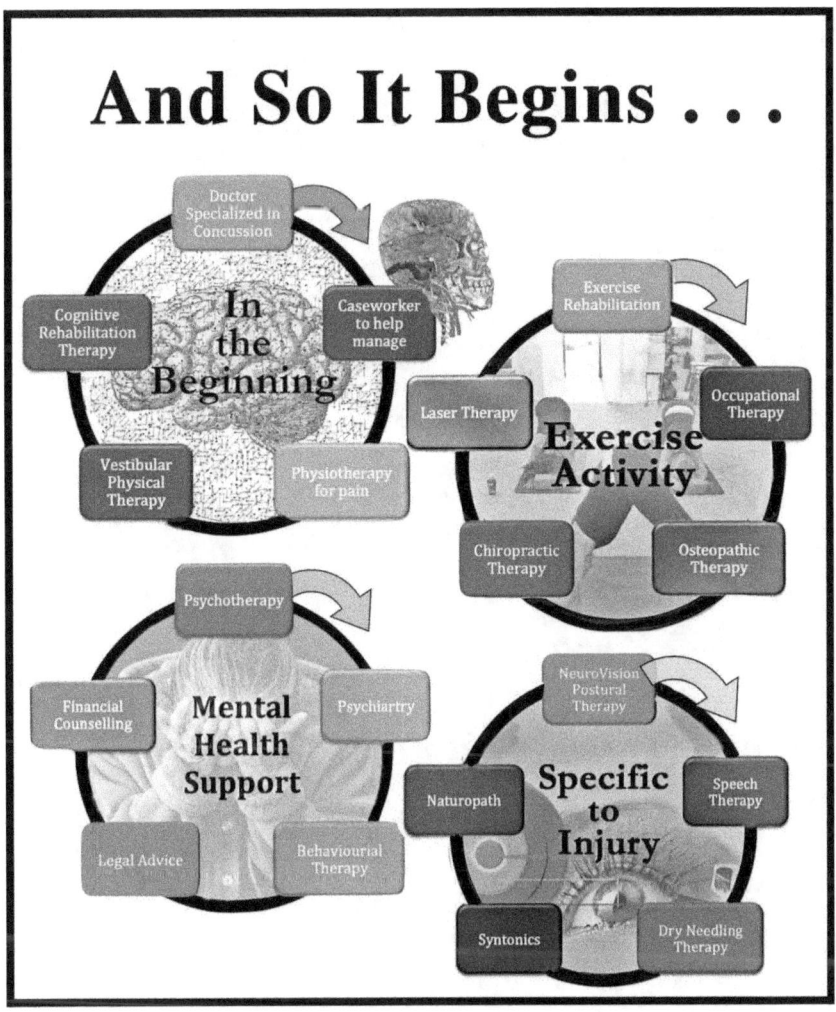

Hateful Forms

"Life appears to be too short to be spent in nursing animosity, or registering wrongs."

— Charlotte Brontë, Jane Eyre

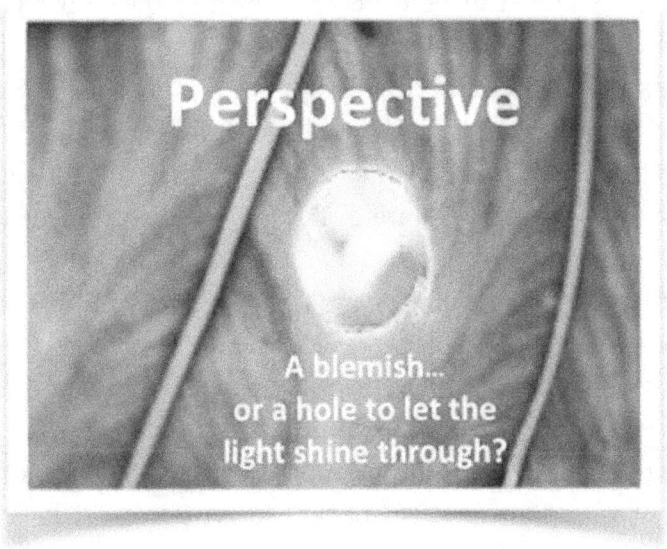

*O*ff work since February 2, 2016, I am unaware of procedure and process, have no guidance, feel isolated and lost, a freezing puppy whimpering alone on the side of a cold, deserted road. I draft several emails of appeal, desperately searching for the right help. If there is anyone who wants me back to work as much as I do, I assume it is my employer. No directives. No suggestions. No recommendations. My principal and staff reach out within the first month, but after that there is little connection. I spiral, questioning my value to the school, thoughts churning from the beast that crawled into my head while I was on the ground. I feel dropped like a burning potato, disowned. There is nothing from my school board, my boss . . . except forms and several requests for a return-to-work date.

My boss requires me to complete a "Request for Functional Information of Presenting Illness/Injury" form. I am willing but need help. When I receive the scanned papers, I go ballistic. Tears roll down my cheeks. Stunned, I stare, try to read the queries, centering on physical limitations, nothing applicable to people who suffered a head injury. Does our disability count? I detest that "d" word. The forms leave out executive and cognitive issues and symptoms, inability to sift senses, focus. Tears stream down my face, as I stare at the emotional grids and tiny spaces, based on physical symptoms. My brain trips to overload. Waves of anger and frustration consume. The paper blares the potential end to my teaching career. I cannot do this, am not ready, will be back. I drop in a ball to the floor, hate every aspect of this injury. Damn fall, damn crazy-ass symptoms. Papers and more papers. Documents, forms, pensions, assessments, medical reports, finances, insurance, compensation. The avalanche threatens to bury me! I would not survive without my sisters. Plopped in a triggered puddle, crying in fear, denial, and desperation, I send out another SOS.

My first struggle with paperwork is the word DISABILITY. I have tremendous difficulty accepting it. Advocates against the terminology claim it has a negative connotation. I agree. Many prefer different-abled. My sister helps me put it into perspective. I cannot do the work I once did; therefore, I am disabled. I refuse to let that define me, or anyone who is different-abled. When I get better, I will remove the harsh diction from my vocabulary, advocate for those who feel inadequate or "LESS THAN."

Second problem is figuring out a return-to-work date. Questions like bricks fly at me as I have absolutely no idea when I will be well enough; I cannot even function in my house, let alone a classroom with thirty teens. When asked to state a date my family physician writes, "undetermined," because I struggle to get to appointments, and that puts me in a major tailspin. It is not good enough. My therapists tell me I am not ready. I sink like a rock to the bottom of my precious ocean, gasping for air. It is dark under the surface. Desperate, I try to swim, but the current keeps pulling me under. For now, I tread water until I can swim.

My employer wants a definite date. I cannot provide one; I throw out hopefuls, thinking it will be okay. It is not. Why does it keep changing? They become suspicious. Of what? Why? If I could control my symptoms, I would. After family, teaching means everything to me. Complications boost anxiety. I cannot sleep. When I do, I have strange dreams and nightmares. I am falling, falling, not able to reach or teach. Tsunamis engulf the house. Am I a pupil or a teacher? Scary officials grill and attack. I wake and realize it is not a dream. I am off work, unable to function as I did before, my pockets stuffed with anger. My husband tries to comfort me, but he does not know what to do.

Give me a break. Bam! The forms sit on my desk waiting for me to complete questions about physical limitations. I ask again . . . What about fatigue, or head injuries? Which questions deal with cognition, memory, speech, inability to filter? I try to "calm" down, hate the word "calm". It implies I am upset. Not fair. I hold my breath—a foreign misuse of breath—an X-ray technician would say that before taking the film. Hold your breath. I swear, am livid. Their total disregard stresses me out, puts me back in bed, spiralling. I wish they could follow me for a day, see me struggle, realize I am not just employee #2424.

My spirit is crushed by belittling papers, essential to revamp those obnoxious forms to include invisible injuries. I cry, call my school board, give the representative hell. He only pulled the forms from a drawer as procedure dictated. Not his jurisdiction, new to the position. I spew anger and resentment. Sorry for the rant, did not know what I was up against.

Where are the questions relating to my debilitating symptoms, brain function, speech, immense fatigue, eye pressure, headaches, inability to concentrate, lack of focus, hypersensitivity to lights, noise, mental drain, nausea, slowed cognition, memory loss? These are the symptoms that apply to the concussed, a whiplash, or mTBI. The distress causes a great deal of harm. I ask for a better form that measures my disability. Nothing. I sense doubt, which stings as I pride myself on my integrity. Education on the consequences of brain injuries is necessary for employers, administrators, corporations, and government sectors.

For a functional assessment, documents should match the injury. Mine should have been pertinent to what held me back from my employment. The mind plays a bigger role in teaching than the body does. There needs to be a form so that those with brain injuries or invisible illness do not feel as demoralized or discredited as I did by a misaligned piece of paper, deceptive in its approach. I never followed up on whether they took my advice of creating an alternate form, too taxing. Surely, he passed on my suggestions!

Those erroneous forms catapult my stress levels into record-breaking heights, set me back months. Desperate, I juggle red tape, escalating symptoms, and increased pressure from their lack of knowledge about concussions. Fallacious papers defeat me, add insult to injury, dropped on my lap a second time. Did anyone even listen to my initial concerns? Fill them out—take two. I need union help. Administrators issuing insurance documents need education on head injury, and empathy for those who need financial aid. Filling out forms creates a humbling sense of reliance most try to avoid. Why make the injured feel guilty? Why base the process on potential abusers? Why? Honest claimants suffer.

And the poor doctors and therapists, overwhelmed by insurance lawyers demanding medical records, using the words on a report against clients, when doctors with the best interest of their patients at heart just want to report on the tiniest of progress for patient encouragement, and with mountains of paperwork on top of patient visits, it becomes too much. Is that why we have few concussion or brain injury clinics especially in Nova Scotia? They too need more government support, financially and legally. Head injuries belong in a different camp, need different criteria when it comes to accidents. My rant!

I wish we were a more compassionate people. In relation to my own work, with over twenty years of loyalty, I expected support during the first months, whether a check-in call, or visit. No follow-up at the board level, although staff at my school ask about me. It saddens me that people do not feel my absence. I gave my career everything. In retrospect, I should have had a better balance. Does it even matter that I invested and dedicated myself wholeheartedly? Did anyone notice the extras I did beyond the expected day in and day out with students, or did I just fade into the background? A workaholic, I gave everything, and most appreciated it. God, I miss my students. To this day many show appreciation for me as a teacher. That motivates me, everything clearer in the rear-view mirror. Yup, I stew. Need to let it go . . .

Despite doctors being unable to forecast my recovery, my employer continued to insist on a specific return-to-work date. I refused to write, "indefinite." My original, self-determined, optimistic dates fell by the wayside and got me into trouble because

I would give one answer then extend it. My brain was not where I wanted it to be. Not my fault. Doctors are evasive when I ask, I suspect because they do not want to dash my hopes. The brain heals at its own rate. Willpower a strong battle weapon, but a funeral marches in my brain.

My wish—the Nova Scotia Department of Education or the Nova Scotia Department of Health create a more comprehensive brain injury form or TBI functional assessment form, or whatever branch of government is concerned with invisible illnesses and brain injuries. Those wanting documentation should help with completion, be empathetic, and knowledgeable. In a distancing world, affirmations are needed more than ever. It's time we reassure and encourage.

"When you judge another, you do not define them.
You define yourself."

— Charles Dyer

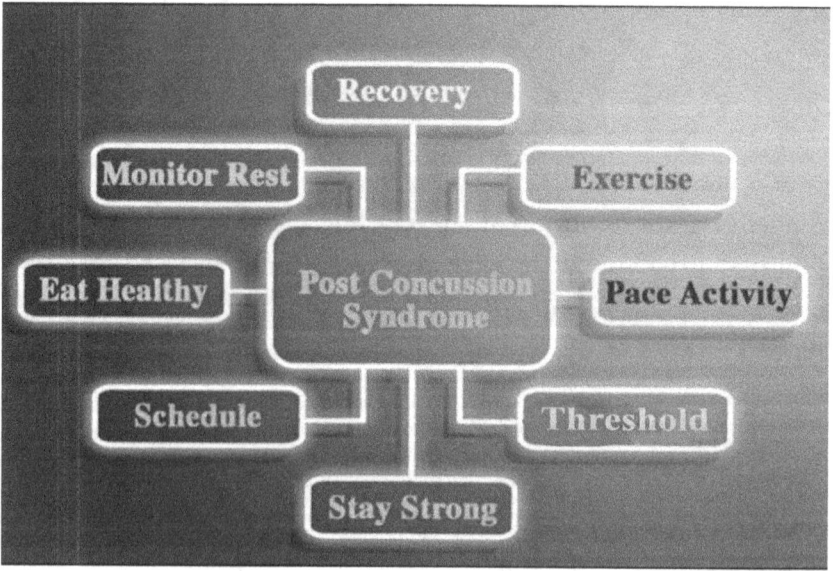

The Slow Road to Recovery

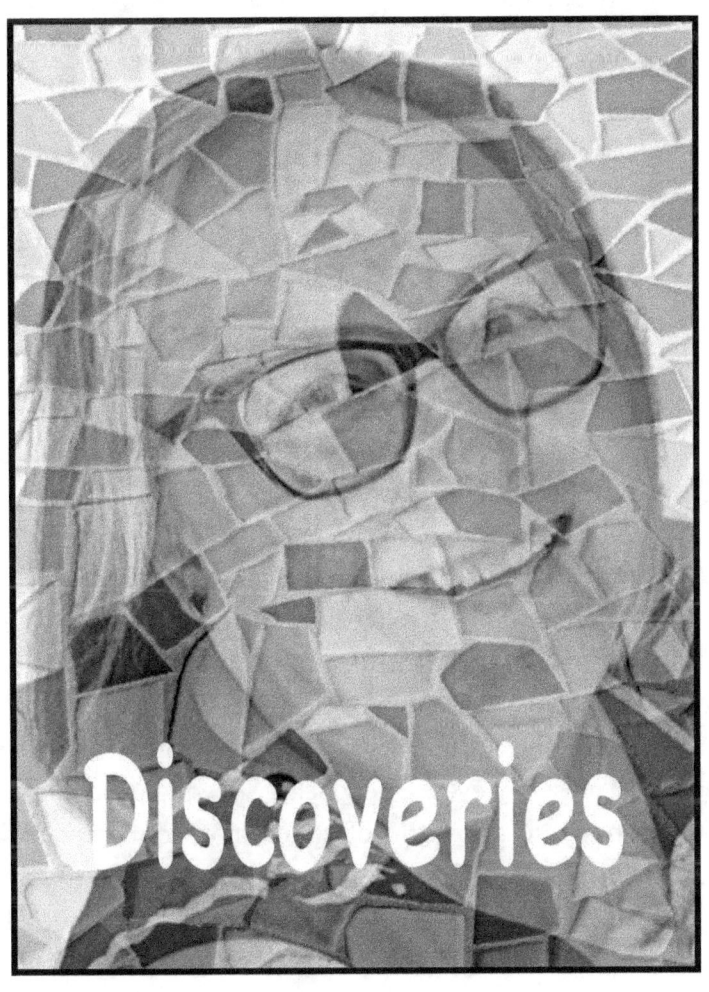

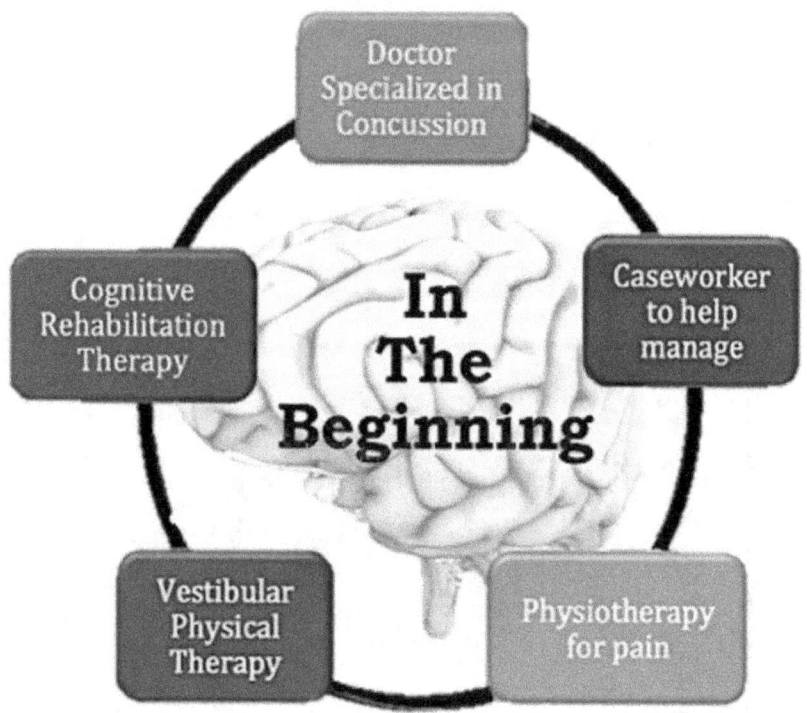

February 2016

My house overlooks the Atlantic Ocean and picturesque Port Hood Island, the back deck my favourite place in the entire world. During the winter months guilt, shame, and blame add to the complexity of healing. How do we measure emotional torment? My brain must relearn, categorize, juggle messages received from five senses. I close my eyes, a new beast showing upset. My unexpected journey into the world of concussion continues. Finding specialists is critical. Not going to trained professionals can add years of symptoms and duress. I know that now. Not content surviving, trying to avoid triggers, after a flurry of exasperating dead ends, and a distress call, May 2016, my sister (a.k.a. Sherlock

Holmes) digs up help. Because of my headaches and mental fatigue, she becomes an amateur sleuth, researching and—BINGO! She discovers a doctor and occupational therapist an hour away. Dr. Lok refers me to Jeniffer Hilling and to the concussion clinic run by Dr. David Cudmore, MD, CCFP (SEM), FCFP, Dip Sport Med, in Antigonish, Nova Scotia. My concussion presents daily challenges with self-regulation, memory, executive functions such as planning, organizing, strategizing, time management. Writing is essential for me; without it everything fades into nothingness, unable to retrieve anything without a cue. My husband remarks, "Just in that area?" Joking is his way of coping. Although not easy, laughing at ourselves helps to not take emotionally charged comments to heart. Forgiveness and understanding come into play. Brain injury is a beast, difficult on the person's family. Without proper tools, techniques, and strategies, exasperation and family upset occur. With my family on board, I keep a record in case someone else suffers a similar injury.

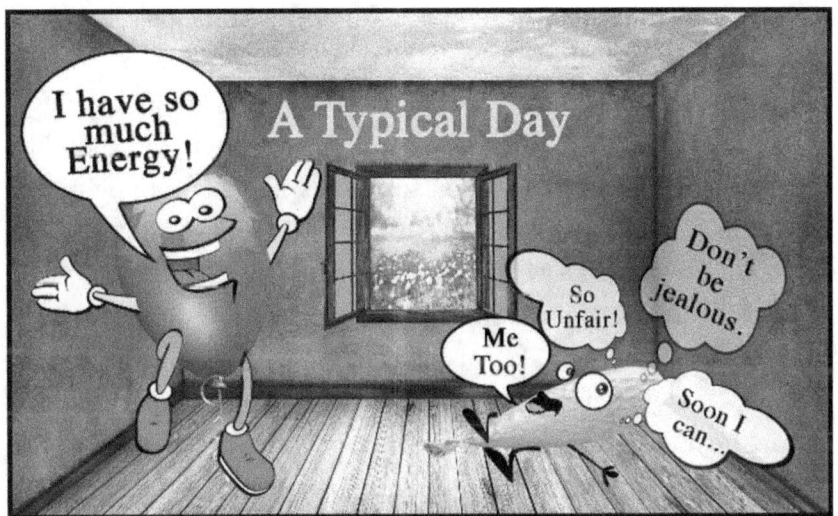

Fatigue

Exhaustion, so draining I cry. Everything, too much effort. Pressure and pain centre of my forehead. I am confused by frightening cognitive, vestibular, and ocular shortfalls. Mental fatigue depletes. Why is it so hard to focus, do things? I try to understand, can't.

After my ten-day February stay in hospital, Dr. Lok, refers me for physiotherapy. On March 10, 2016, I meet PT, Tanya Feehan and assistant, Liam O'Neill—a dynamo duo, she with her laugh, Liam with a last name he spells correctly with two l's. He teases me. I dish it back. Now if I put on a Montreal Canadian jersey, he would be happy, but in good conscience to diehard Toronto Maple Leaf fans—husband included, I cannot.

Tanya concentrates on my neck and mobility issues. My husband drives me every week, although I sometimes cancel because of symptoms. Pain radiates, a heating pad, my new best friend, plus its cold cousin, the ice pack. With them, I gain a sense of comfort. The team at the Inverness Consolidated Memorial Hospital, including Jimmy and Brenda Rankin, provide safety, create a relaxed, healing atmosphere, and make little of my stuttering. Their constant encouragement and Tanya's contagious giggle brighten everyone's spirit. She works on my neck and mobility, tapes my back and left shoulder, injured when I fell, to help with pain. I sustained both a whiplash and mTBI, making it difficult to figure out which is the culprit causing my symptoms. Neck pain, tight muscles, and strain cause headaches. A safe environment where you can make mistakes and sound weird is crucial to recovery. I am excited to begin my journey to wellness, but what about those less fortunate, unable to go for physiotherapy, who cannot receive treatment because of outside circumstances? Those who do not want to see a doctor, try to hide their injury, or those without transportation? Many individuals cannot access the care they need and give up, tired of being "a bother." Years later, they are still caged in a shrunken world, unaware their symptoms stem from a concussion.

As I said before, I turn to quotations to provide comfort. As my world shrinks, danger looms, a difference between existing, surviving, living. I am stuck. The brain heals at its own rate. I miss being in my classroom. A broken record. Only when behind my desk, will the world appear vibrant and colourful. Fingerpaints will flow into and around each other, filled with glimmers of the best colours from the Crayola box, splashed in a radiant, rainbow tapestry.

Without my faith, I would be lost. Following is the first verse of a poem I wrote.

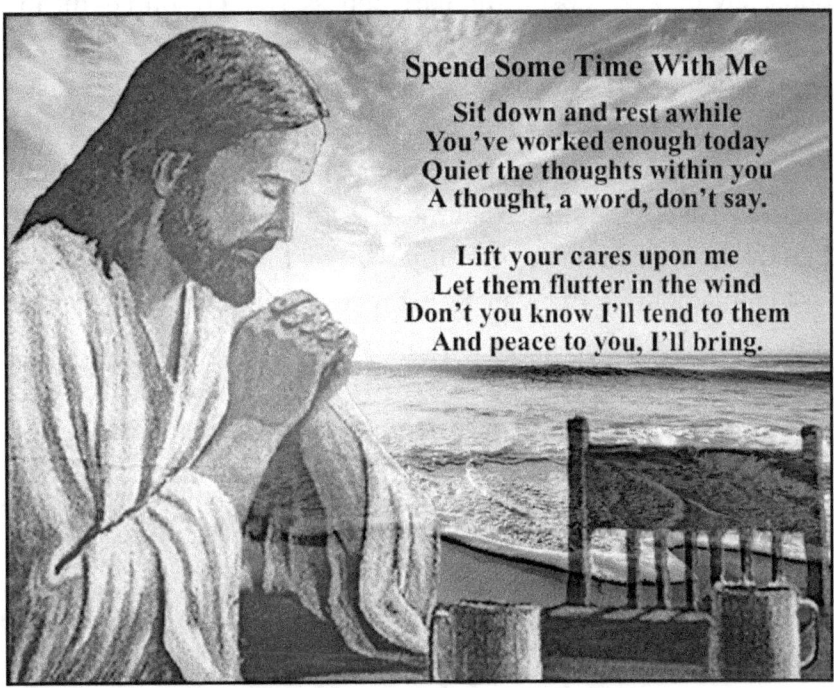

Spend Some Time With Me

Sit down and rest awhile
You've worked enough today
Quiet the thoughts within you
A thought, a word, don't say.

Lift your cares upon me
Let them flutter in the wind
Don't you know I'll tend to them
And peace to you, I'll bring.

Thank you, Peter Rankin, for the artwork. Bittersweet, I am thankful, but I should not be here. Too long off work already. My whiplash will require a substantial amount of therapy and work.

I hold myself tight because of swelling, pain, immobility. I learn with whiplash it is a slow crawl to recovery, important to stick with it, do the exercises therapists suggest. For my painful neck, extra-strength Tylenol and muscle relaxants help as do anti-inflammatories. I am at the end of my rope. Desperation escalates as I search to understand, reverse injury, return to work. My poor, dilapidated house cries for attention. Dust covers everything, can print my name on tabletops. Please do not judge me. Need Mr. Clean! Why are we, the concussed, left to our own limited resources? Does this lead to higher rates of misdiagnosis, unemployment, suicide?

My journey post-concussion is slow, frustrating. Many questions, few answers. Lost without a compass. Had I resources during those crucial first weeks—the period known as the critical window of vulnerability—I may have returned to the world quicker. That saddens me. We must be our own advocate.

The snowy winter over, we put sheer curtains on our outdoor enclosure to cut the sun's brightness. With sunglasses I sit outside. Cloudy days, I retreat to my corner, enjoy the whispering breeze, let my imagination fly. A snail, I stay in a shell, take breaks, pace, rest. I do a few things under a ball cap and wide-brimmed hat.

"The first step towards getting somewhere is to decide you're not going to stay where you are."

— John Pierpont "JP" Morgan, July 13, 2023

June 2016—The Yellow Brick Road

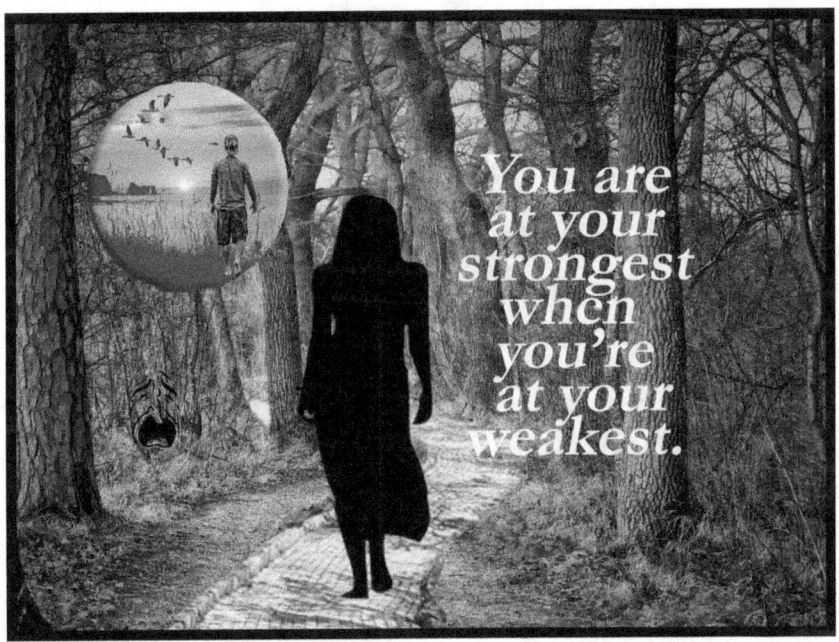

You are at your strongest when you're at your weakest.

"There were several roads nearby, but it did not take Dorothy long to find the one paved with yellow bricks. Within a fleeting time, she was walking briskly toward the Emerald City; her silver shoes tinkling merrily on the hard, yellow roadbed."

— The Wizard of Oz

Analogies soften a truth I cannot face. June 1, I travel the yellow brick road to Antigonish, meet a fiery redhead with a smile as bright as her personality, like Dorothy in *The Wizard of Oz*.

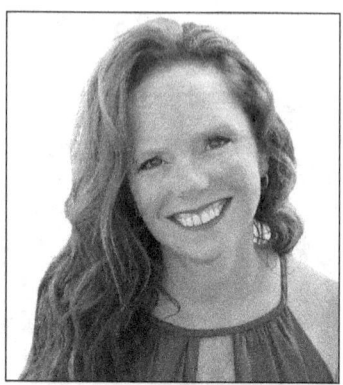

Jeniffer Hilling

Jeniffer Hilling B.Sc., O.T., Reg (NS), experience: fifty-one years of life, thirty years as an occupational therapist. Her own return to work after a concussion motivates. I am in expert hands. She teaches pacing, thresholds, boom and bust trap, tips and tricks to function. A clinician and educator for the Atlantic Region of the Canadian Brain Injury (CBI) Health Centre clinics, she specializes in post-concussion management, mental health, and persistent pain management. A keen advocate, she was director for the Antigonish Guysborough chapter of Brain Injury Nova Scotia.

She has appeared as a guest speaker at the Canadian Association of Sport and Exercise Medicine, Brain Injury Association of Nova Scotia, and the Nova Scotia Health Authority. A member of the multidisciplinary team mentioned earlier, Jeniffer helped develop psychosocial rehabilitation programming for adults living in the community with persistent mental health conditions. She works with CBI Health Centre professionals to create and deliver programming for individuals following mild traumatic brain injuries, dealing with persistent pain, or mental health disorders. Their aim is to create evidence-based treatment, and facilitate individual recovery so patients can return to their daily activities where they live, work, and play. Jeniffer empathizes with her patients, having climbed the mountain herself, and shares the following wise advice.

Occupation refers to all activities of daily living, NOT just work. It refers to how we occupy our day—including self-care, work-related activities, and hobbies.

Concussion Clinical Trajectories

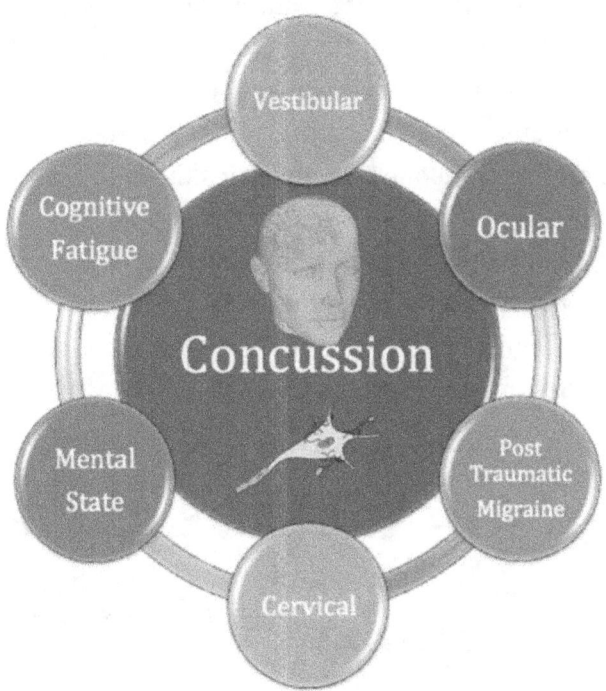

Pillars of Best Practice

"Early symptom management, education, support, reactivation into normal daily activity and routines are the pillars of best practice care after a concussion. Understanding the modifiers to recovery—fear of re-injury, medical history, a person's experience at the time of injury are vital factors. The therapist screens and addresses these to lessen negative effects. Occupational Therapy is one of the most diverse health professions focusing on enabling function. As a profession, the therapy aims to adapt, accommodate, teach skills needed for a person to do what they need or expect. What inspires me as an OT is making the right fit between the person, environment, and activity sought. Attentive, compassionate, exploratory questions and scientific-originated observations help me learn why a person cannot function to his or her potential, then find solutions to optimize abilities. Does personal experience make me more informed of the recovery process? I relate to the frustrations of functional challenges, unknown recovery times, persistent fatigue. I provide the science, evidence, strategies for management. As someone who struggles through functional challenge, I learned to adapt and resist, while applying the principles of pacing through the stages of function. Our job is as unique as is any activity, person, injury, or environmental combination. Therapists become experts in knowing what physical, emotional, cognitive skills are involved in an activity."

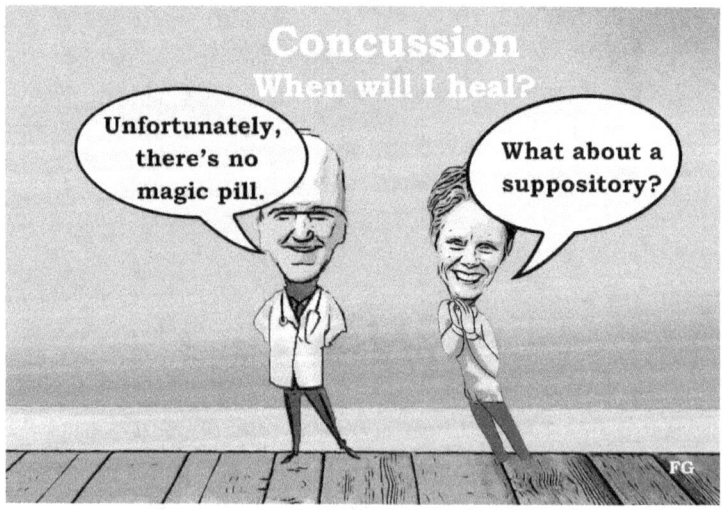

Wise words, Jeniffer. I plan to return to my teacher's desk, with clues painted on the walls to help young minds, shelves filled with pens, paper, books, when the world looks more colourful. Students will welcome me back, ask about my welfare, and I, theirs. A coherent entity, we will learn together. But my days are not the same. I miss them, colleagues, conversations, lessons, lightbulb moments. I am a sad clown. Every day I watch the big yellow bus pull up, kids laughing as they climb the steps. I wish I were going with them. And passing by Dalbrae Academy while driving to appointments at the hospital in Inverness is brutal. What lesson are students learning in my classroom? I gaze up at my window on the far end, facing the road and mountain, long to return. They are moving on without me. Soon, I will know none of them. Time closes in on me. This cannot be. Help me, Aunt Em, help! I dislike the road I am on, a myriad of fallen trees, potholes, missteps, flying insects ready to eat me. Please, Jeniffer, let us learn, so I can boot this stranger I have become out of rehab, regain my identity! I must find a purpose. That sums me up!

Antigonish Concussion Clinic—2007-2021

"I have learned something new from every one of my patients. It has been an amazing experience working with professionals who are a part of our team. Most patients get better in an abbreviated period, yet some suffer significant long-term trauma and symptoms. It is challenging yet rewarding to work with these individuals." Tara Sutherland, CAT Dip, SIM, BA, BPHEd, M. Kin, (coach, concussion rehab.)

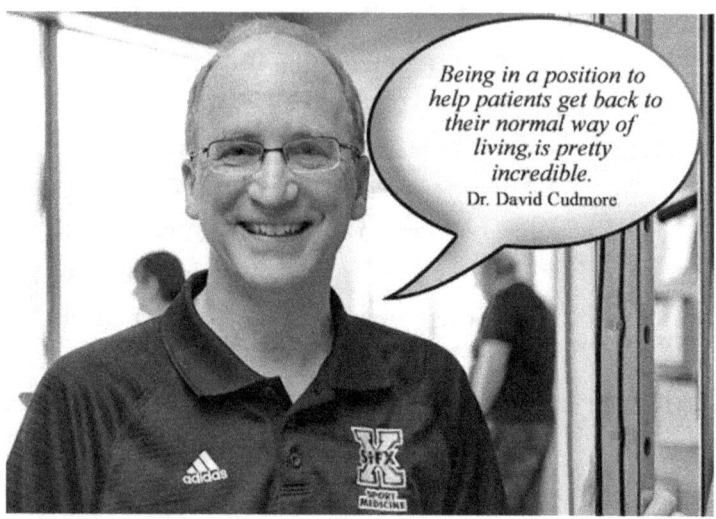

Being in a position to help patients get back to their normal way of living, is pretty incredible.
Dr. David Cudmore

For successful recovery, we need a knowledgeable support system to deal with shortfalls that occur after a head injury. The teamwork approach works best. Spokes on a wheel work through a strong fulcrum, bringing various therapies and assessments together for better patient success. I am fortunate to find multiple therapies through Dr. David Cudmore's concussion clinic and his trained concussion coaches. Cudmore and Sutherland opened the clinic in 2007, developing a diverse team of practitioners to work with clients, as a system of referrals for those needing specialized services. Here my snail-like recovery began, four months after my fall. With my type of injury, if seen within a month, chances of a full recovery increase. I reiterate . . . We must be our own advocates.

A Concussion Clinic: The Antigonish Model

(Tara Sutherland CAT (C), and Dr. Cudmore, MD; Dip Sports Med; CATA)

1. In the Antigonish clinic, serving northeastern Nova Scotia, referred patients are seen by an athletic therapist who completes a comprehensive history of injury, performs a concussion assessment using a modified Sport Concussion Assessment Tool (SCAT2) (McCrory et al., 2009), including an assessment of mental status, cognitive functioning, balance. The athletic therapist explains how recovery occurs, what the brain needs.

2. After this initial assessment the patient meets with both the athletic therapist and physician and an individualized plan is designed. This will include advice regarding physical and cognitive rest, modifications to work or school schedules, expert referrals if needed.

3. As a general rule the physician does not send patients for diagnostic imaging such as MRI or CT scans since imaging is usually normal as reported by McCrory et al., 2009.

4. Patients are evaluated for neck pain, a common coexisting injury which may require specific treatment. Expert referrals are often made for physiotherapy or massage therapy.

5. The patient is sent home with instruction, and a follow-up appointment.

6. The physician writes notes for modified work or school. Medication may be prescribed.

7. A consultation letter is sent to the referring physician or nurse practitioner, and a copy to the patient's primary health care provider.

8. Worker Compensation Board (WCB) forms are completed when necessary.

9. Generally the patient will be seen at the clinic regularly until he or she has fully recovered.

10. Athletic therapists followup via phone and email between clinic visits when necessary.

11. Progress notes are sent to the primary health care provider (WCB when necessary).

12. When the individual becomes asymptomatic at rest and is ready to return to a sport or activity the athletic therapists will do a standardized bike test at the Athletic Therapy Clinic at STFXU. If the patient completes this bike test satisfactorily then they are returned to activity according to the return to play guidelines set forth by McCrory et al., 2009.

Post-concussion Syndrome

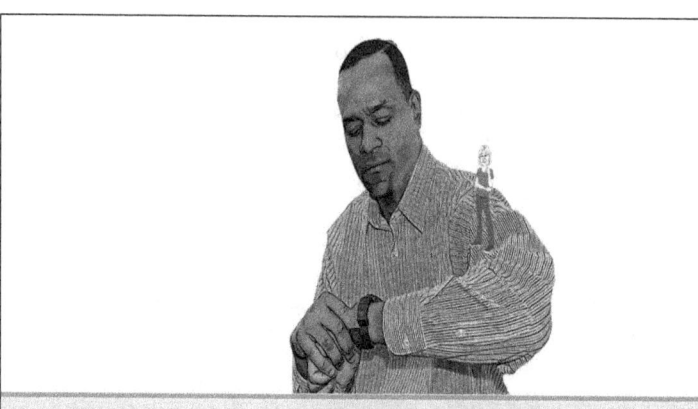

So What Causes Post-concussion Syndrome?

"After experiencing a [head] injury, 'volume knobs' and pathways in the nervous system become turned up. These include pain pathways, as well as sensory pathways involved in symptoms like dizziness. The brain is usually very good at filtering out sensations so that we can concentrate on the ones that we need. After a bang on the head this process can go wrong, for variety of reasons, additional pain signals and sensory signals can get through. Normally those 'volume knobs' get turned down again and the brain filters are restored as you slowly recover, but in post-concussion syndrome they stay tuned up, or even become increased further overtime."   —Dr. Jon Stone, 2009

It is reassuring Dr. Stone considers functional aspects of the brain, which seem to be missing in mainstream neurology. New on the horizon, functional neurologists concerned with the functioning of the brain rather than structure. A comfort for those with invisible injuries.

Not knowing where to find information, understanding, and

proper care should not take months. No wonder I keep falling down the rabbit hole. When injured, we blindly enter that ambiguous world of concussion, with so many curveballs. Oracles and riddles are too hard on the brain.

"A concussion can cause serious consequences if not treated immediately with a risk for mental health issues and delayed mental and physical processes, which keeps the patient from returning to a normal way of life. It is imperative we see those patients early on at our clinic and do what we can to get them back to a healthy, functioning state." (*Doctors Nova Scotia* magazine, 2015).

All the receptionists at the clinics greet me by name, making me smile, feel like a person again. Courteous and friendly they become my only social group. Travelling to and from appointments is gruelling. Embarrassing moments—I arrive for appointments on the wrong day, mix up times, find it difficult to trust myself.

Sunlight in its attempt to cheer peeks under my eye mask. Branches lining the narrow roads of Route 19 flash, create a sickening, strobe effect. I become a prisoner curled in protective custody—that is how I travel, having to stop because of nausea as the strobe invades my mask. The duration of symptoms is beyond control. The older the person, the greater the risk of potential issues arising. I was fifty-seven when I fell. With head injury, people urge, "Suck it up!" Old mentality. End of story. "Nothing's wrong with you." Wish they were right. New research encourages exercise and gentle exposure.

July 2016

We need to educate ourselves on what is available so we can create a plan with our doctor or nurse practitioner. Before my appointments with Dr. Cudmore, I write or print what I want to ask or tell him, so I do not forget.

Lists maximize doctor visits:

1. Write and share stressors and symptoms, including any that may seem unrelated.
2. Write personal contact information.
3. Bring a list of medicines, vitamins, supplements.
4. Have someone go with you to help remember what the doctor says.
5. Ask for a copy of your medical report for future reference.

One appointment is a daylong affair—washing, drying my hair (so hard), dressing, travelling, waiting, eating, bathroom stops—with two exhausted travellers crashing when finally home. Skip a day, same routine. You get the picture. I walk through a dreary, revolving door, no end in sight. I am thankful for access to therapy, and a supportive husband who carts me all over, as I battle over-stimulation, and an inability to function. Patience eludes me, my emotions, the trigger switch on a bomb.

Appointments consume our lives. Motion prevents me from driving because of problems with depth perception and peripheral vision. I need to close my eyes or have them covered. Willing to do anything, without knowing it, I work against myself. I want to resume teaching, with a clear mind, not one coated in Jell-O. Even cooking has me crying in fatigue. Raw with emotion, I cry far too often from frustration. It is not depression, but a profound sadness. Are they the same? I left my brain in my classroom. Before—my mind would travel ninety miles an hour, soak infor-mation, syphon and organize. Now information and stimuli flood, no partitions, screaming, "Hear me! Hear me!" "No! Me!" "Watch, me!" Befuddled grey matter gets trapped.

In a perfect world, I would be in my classroom, spouting quota-tions, challenging energetic minds through critical analysis, read-ing, researching. But I am not well enough *yet*. Safe to place that qualifier? A question or a statement? Must be a statement. If not, I will lose hope, spiral down into a dark, pitiful place. Anyone with a chronic illness or injury can relate. Imperative we hang onto that four-letter word—hope! Keeps us going. I need to become self-sufficient, understand the conundrum of losing my identity through no fault of my own. I am a dartboard, symptoms cascading in direct correlation to overstimulation, doing too much. I remind myself to be thankful for my increasing multidisciplinary team.

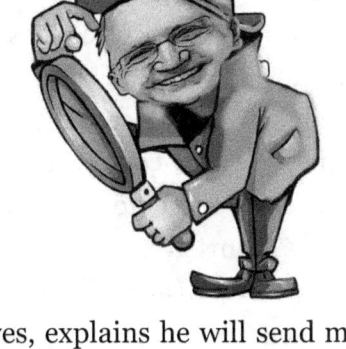

Dr. Cudmore navigates my program and progress, identifies short-falls needing further attention. He asks how I am doing, gives a gentle, genuine smile every time I visit. His assistants (Tara and Diane) after consultation regarding my symptoms, share my progress and concerns since my prior visit. Dr. Cudmore validates both by words and kind eyes, explains he will send me to experts to verify suspicions. His team management approach makes sense. He keeps his finger on the pulse on the condition and changes of his patients. Each time I visit, he notes speech improvement, helps reduce my awkwardness and discomfort.

When my husband and I eat at a restaurant, I sit with my back against a wall to block too many signals, avoid surrounding conversation. My occupational therapist gives me a pair of earplugs to cut down on noise. I later discover musician earplugs, see an audiologist, who fits my ears for molds. They cost shy of a hundred dollars. They filter, soften the sound; help expand my social circumference. With too much exposure, my head whirls, whizzes, takes hours to settle. Fifteen percent of people with mTBI suffer symptoms lasting one year or more. Panic! The idea is absurd. Not me. No way. Guilt lunges. Although enough to stop me in my tracks, my injury is nothing compared to people left with paralysis. Those heroes fuel me to push ahead.

August 7, 2016

Every year, my pastoral community celebrates a week-long summer festival known as Chestico Days. Sunday involves a boat parade. Hundreds of boats putter the harbour as onlookers cheer. To close the festivities, a firework display lights up the night sky. Tradition, my husband and I invite extended family to come watch from our backyard, but how do you deal with thirty people when you suffer from post-concussion syndrome? I want to take part in the closing down of summer, my world, small for six months. I need the warmth, support, and caring of family. My husband welcomes the first couple. Their discussion is animated; they speak over each other, too fast. While everyone catches up, mingles, enjoys themselves on the deck outside my window, I curl alone on my bed, door closed, lights off. I am not anti-social, feel like cow dung on the bottom of my shoe.

While family parties, on the inside of a gigantic transparent bubble, I chastise myself for three excruciating hours. Smidgens of conversation drift inside when the more boisterous speak or laugh. Everyone has fun under the stars, juxtaposed against brilliant fireworks lighting up the darkness, floating coloured-showers to the earth. Happiness outside, a pity party inside. Back and forth, my mind races. Can I join them? Too much talking, noise. A melancholy Charlie Brown, I cry into my pillow, need to learn how to manage my symptoms, work within my range, match abilities with environmental demands. I do a horrendous job, hide my emotions, crash into meltdowns that last hours, days, weeks. No one knows except my husband and me. We invisible suffer in silence.

"The music of hope is everywhere, but to hear it, you need to ignore the muddy jangle of life's hassles."

— Christine M Knight, Life Song, 2013

August 18, 2016

I visit my doctor for a follow-up appointment eager to find out when symptoms will dissipate and allow me to teach. Nervous, entering the office, I am hopeful. Soon, please say soon. He takes my vitals, sits, makes a note, muses at his desk. Braving what he might say, I find the words. "Dr. Lok, when can I go back to school?"

He does not answer right away, shuffles papers on his desk adding tension to a room closing in on me. We are the only two caricatures in the entire universe. Nothing but his concerned face, eyes squinting up and over his glasses to stare into my own as my stomach turns. His mouth moves, his voice, low, deliberate, strikes like a bullet, killer words ricocheting off the desk, walls, ceiling, mountaintop.

"You will never teach again."

He did not say that. How could he? He knows how upset I have been. I cannot muster a reply. Eyes filling, unable to counter, I bolt from the harsh office, him hardly getting the cruddy words out. Unable to hold the waterworks back, I rush through the narrow hallway, tears streaming as I run out of the building into the evening air, to the sanctuary of my car. My husband is taken aback. What gives Lok the right to make such a bold condemnation? Was he trying to shock me into realizing the extent of my injuries? I bawl, pound the dashboard and seat, curse, swear, scream at the windshield. So effing unfair. He is wrong! He cannot make such an outrageous proclamation. He is so very wrong, and yet, he is my doctor.

I am not ready to end my career, my passion. I need young people, socialization, satisfaction of teaching valuable lessons. No way is he correct. My husband sits in silence, knows I need to vent. When I calm, he gives me a hug. He knows how devastating the prognosis. Later at home, as I fitfully doze off, I yell out in nightmares, scream, wail, falling, falling, falling as the memory of, "I will never teach" cuts, slices, stabs. A tsunami pulls me under.

August 2016—Speech Language Pathology

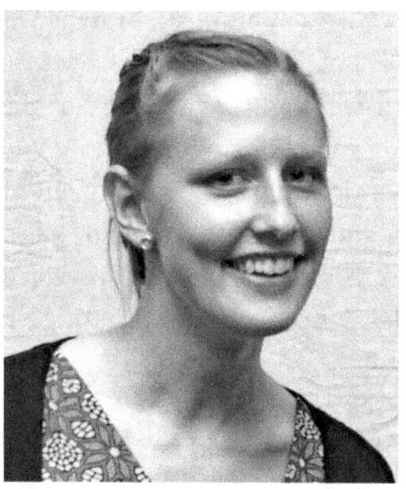

Marlee Mousek

Another beast I avoid, makes me self-conscious and bumfuzzled—my weird stuttering, driving me over the edge. Words come out twisted, leaving me perplexed. There is little written on neurogenic stuttering. When anxious or mentally fatigued, it worsens. I am not comfortable speaking outside my family or medical circle, must learn to laugh at myself or else curl inside my shell and never come out. Believe me, it is a consideration. A snail can sleep for up to three years. Oh my! I hope I look back on this journey through a different lens. Rather than time taken, lessons learned.

I meet my speech therapist Marlee Mousek, M.Sc., S-LP-Reg, in late August.

"The field of Speech-Language Pathology is broad, with many areas of specialty. I chose this profession to work with children, but found I am equally fond of working with adults. As we work towards our client's speech-language goals, I enjoy building relationships. Therapy is not only for individuals with speech impediments or kids late to talk. People can consult us for a range of challenges, including stuttering, stroke, brain injuries, social communication, hiccups, swallowing difficulties," says Marlee.

I learn about stuttering relating to head injuries. Speech-Language and Audiology Canada certified, Marlee is patient and creative with my treatment, teaches me much about the elements of speech. A Master of Science in Speech-Language Pathology from Dalhousie University (Halifax, NS), her knowledge and sincere regard for patients impresses. Speech disfluency is a disruption in the flow of spoken language. Types of disfluencies include stuttering, hesitations, fillers, and repetitions people insert.

Marlee is a constant backbone of support on this tedious journey. I feel lame sounding out words, learning to breathe so I can incorporate easy onset—starting each word softly and easily by letting a little air out. Then, using a relaxed mouth, trying not to let vocal cords tense, the sounds come out hard, or forced. From the beginning, we remove seriousness from the equation. She has me practising sounds and syllables using a slow, gentle, robotic, flat pitch or tone, without expression approach. I struggle to come to terms with the nagging fear I will never improve. Beyond difficult to read a tiny passage aloud; two forces, reading and speaking, too much. Everything about stuttering upsets me, a three-year-old learning to pronounce GAW, BAW, SAW, and derivatives thereof.

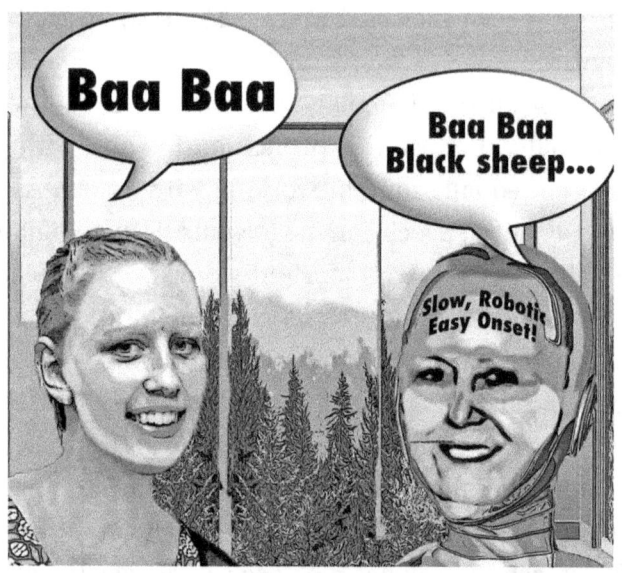

Ashamed, excruciatingly inadequate, I try to elongate syllables, speak without repetition. Painful! Every appointment exhausts. I want to go back down that rabbit hole, back to before—my classroom filled with abundance—unabashed teenagers, mystical bonds made. I panic. Symptoms for years. No way! Not me!

Marlee is always excited to hear the progress in my speech with each new strategy practised. Through monthly sessions, she challenges me, syllable arrangements difficult. My responses are hilarious; we make a game, laugh, work on sounds, syllables, pacing. The sessions require tremendous concentration and effort. At home I wear earplugs, dim the lights, rest, follow her advice. I use a robotic approach, speak with easy unset (speaking and going into syllables slowly) to help when tripping up on words. Rehabilitation creeps turtle-slow; remember the famous tortoise and hare?

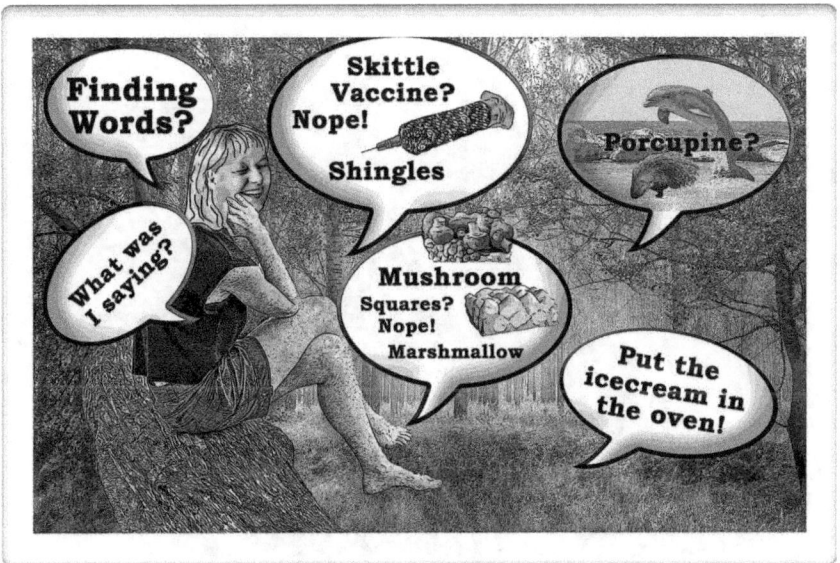

A companion on my journey, she helps with shattered areas of my life. Her appointments are enjoyable. Some treat me as if stuttering reduces my intelligence. I feel inferior speaking to people who know me. Desperate, I implement strategies. Words require effort, come slow, awkward. Mentally fatigued, it is worse. Marlee can tell I am exhausted near the end of our appointments. I am anxious as the calendar turns.

My discarded clothes sleep in mounds on the closet or bedroom floor; by day's end, 6 p.m., too exhausted to pick them up. "Stupid clothes!" Wish I had a magical nose. Too tired to sort items out, they remain. Half do not fit. They shrunk. I need to charge my batteries. I drop my food and utensils. Why? A big baby I use a bib because my food falls and stains. A terribly revealing fact, makes me laughable, but I would never think that of anyone. So, why do I rip myself apart? I am hopeful a therapist will figure this out. The lighthearted sound of sparrows singing, waves crashing to shore remind me when waters are murky, beauty is a few steps away. When the clouds obscure the sun, we can close our eyes, imagine a better place.

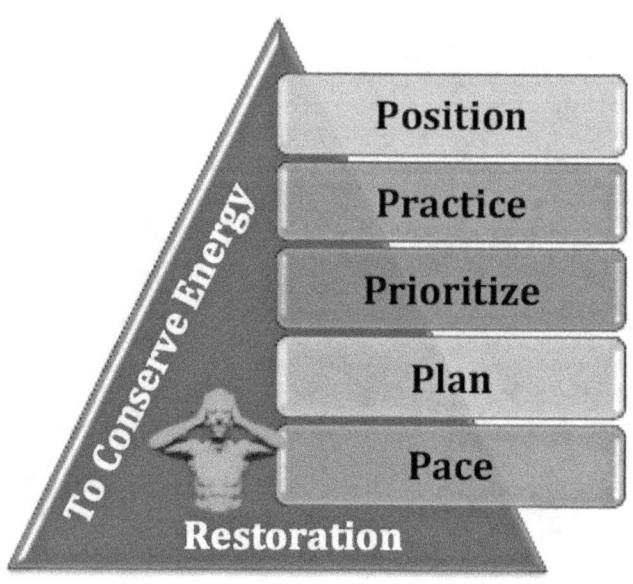

Because I have a deep-rooted compulsion to finish what I start, I overdo it, pay the hefty price of, "Lions, Tigers, and Bears," like the theme song in *The Wizard of Oz*, of the frightened Tin Man, Cowardly Lion, and Scarecrow as they search for answers. I am stuck in survival mode. During my trek along twists and turns, hills, and valleys of the yellow brick road, I stumble and fall. Powerful will, slow body. Running on fumes is risky, leaves me depleted, overwrought, stuck on a barren road of broken bricks. The more complex an activity, the more gas I burn. If the tank hits empty, symptoms bombard—Bye, bye, Dr. Jekyll; hello, Mr. Hyde! I perilously step forward, back, forward, back . . . Need to keep myself in check. Overdo it and nasty things happen.

Conserving Energy

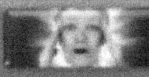

Pace

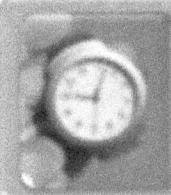

- Place time limits on an activity
- Break large tasks into smaller, manageable chunks
- Work within your tolerance level
- Take a break before onset of fatigue, pain, or emotional upset

Plan

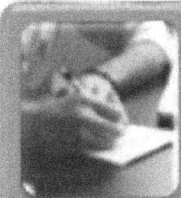

- Organize your time effectively by using a schedule
- Consider what needs to be done, how, and when
- Analyze each activity's energy requirements, and your own
- Leave time for the unexpected

Prioritize

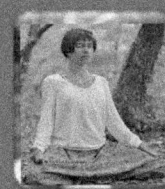

- Choose which activities are essential, which less so
- Avoid the push-through and have-to finish mentality
- Delegate tasks to others when possible
- Build in time for rest and recovery

Practice

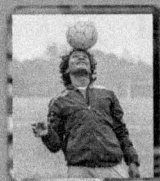

- Incorporate energy restoration into your daily life
- Replenish your energy bank when symptoms occur
- Take in a variety of activities, physical, mental, creative
- Eat balanced meals; get enough rest; nurture your body

Position

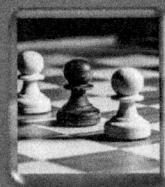

- Be aware of your body, do mental checks
- Sit if feeling fatigued or reactive
- Change position every fifteen minutes
- Organize workspace if working for long periods

On the yellow brick road to recovery, will the Great Oz answer my questions, cure me? With my muddled brain, I would yank off Dorothy's clinking, clanking shoes. Like her companions, I get down on myself. Is there a light on the horizon? I must believe that. Do I see flickers? Is it the snail timeline that drags me down? I am angry whenever I think of what I cannot do. A chorus of voices tells me to be optimistic, guard self-talk. I know but putting it into practice is insanely difficult. My mind is tired of crap . . . sick and tired.

In survival mode, I establish a routine. Threshold set. Allotments of gas are crucial to success. Increments of days, hours, minutes. Faces emerge as I tackle the day. My primary culprit besides symptoms, abhorrent frustration. I NEED my independence back! Our Rogue calls my name, far too early to try taking it for a spin. My therapists harp on pacing, scheduling, thresholds, difficult to master. It drives me bonkers to not finish what I start. I keep going further, stick with it another ten minutes, twenty minutes later, head pounding, claw clutching, vice grip, I crash. Constant tinnitus drives me bananas. Noises louder at night. Thoughts entangle and permeate. Travelling a thousand miles a second, I fall behind. When you hit the wall, you hit the wall. STOP! REST! DO NOT PASS GO!

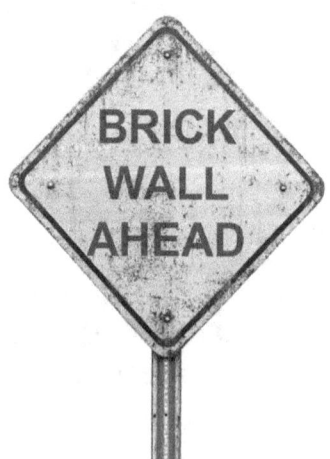

Boom, Bust, Calm

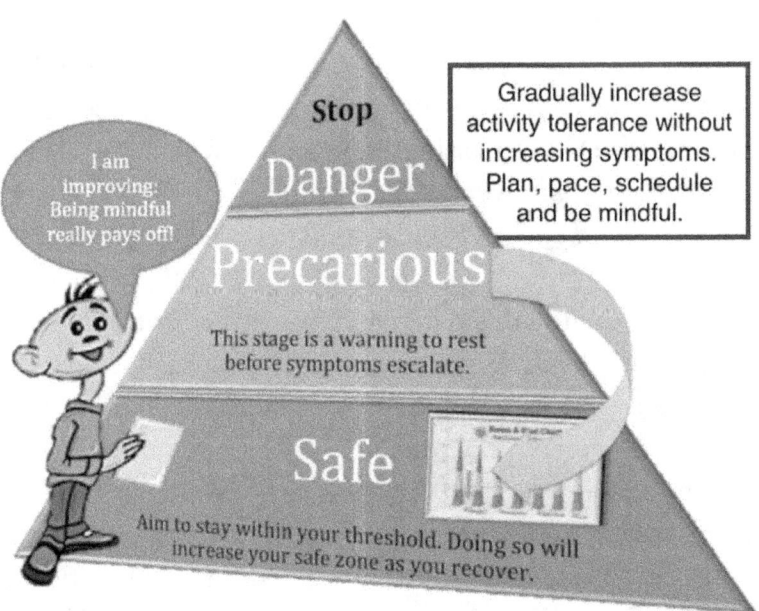

My Type A personality prior to injury—push through no matter how tired, goes counter to concussion, my work philosophy, and constitution. I must challenge one by one, rather than overwhelming the brain. In the eye of a hurricane, calm one moment, wild winds whipping me the next. A nor'easter. Troubled thoughts fly. Self-judgment percolates pent-up energy until it cascades into a grave of white foam. One moment I float away, next, squeezed, squashed, sandwiched between bluffs with deep, dramatic slopes and rugged cliffs. I am on the edge of the world with the ocean below. Gingerly, I tread up the mountain, traumatized by my fall. When frustration mounts, I turn to what brings comfort—prayer. Does post-concussion syndrome for dummies exist? I get upset, angry, beyond frustrated, sidestepping dark black borders of depression and anxiety that rear like trolls when optimism disappears, fortitude mocked by a fire-breathing dragon. Exhausted, my heart rate climbs, scares me. Dr. Cudmore suggests my body has trouble regulating various systems, thus fast pulse, and other physiological symptoms. Headaches, foreign prior to my fall, cause crippling ice picks above my eye, radiating from my neck, or into it. When my willpower and brain clash, my bully brain wins. When symptoms intensify, my brain broadcasts, *I told you so.* I succumb to the need for rest and deep breathing. I work towards exposure.

Exposure—state of having no protection from something harmful. With PCS, it involves exposing ourselves gradually to more senses—lesser to greater in intensity. I expose myself to triggers to increase my tolerance to the point of bringing on symptoms, then back off, like starting with a waltz, moving to the foxtrot, working to the tango, finishing with the sassy East Coast swing better known as the jitterbug or Mull River shuffle made famous by Jimmy Rankin. Gradual, steady exposure increases tolerance.

I get frustrated when I must search to find what should be easy. Tears flow. Help! Mystical folk run away with my clip-on glasses. My husband after hours of searching rescues my prescription eyeglasses from the garbage in our kitchen. Sound familiar? He finds my specialized earplugs with miscellaneous junk. Oh, my! My OT tells me depleting my energy puts me at risk of triggers where a word or sound has me reacting and reliving trauma. Not my fault, the brain's reaction. To gain control, I ground myself in the present, do as my therapists advise. Smack. That is me trying to knock sense into my skull. She suggests I make a list of what nurtures. With proper tools, I adapt, watch/listen to television; nothing with motion or complexity. I mute commercials. My husband teases me for watching *The Bachelor* or *Say Yes to the Dress*; they do not tax my brain. Keep it straightforward—should become my mantra! My wish is to return to my students and colleagues, do not want my career to end with an accident.

I pick at writing. One of the few resources left because I can control my environment, that network in the brain deeply embedded. Jeniffer encourages me to write in fifteen-minute increments in silence, lights dimmed, breaks in between; my words jumble and jump. I try to solve the world's problems; ideas spill faster than I can pen them. Although laborious, expressing myself on paper becomes my life jacket. I refuse to give up. Pacing becomes my new norm to prevent symptom escalation. Two steps forward, one back. Hope lingers as I stumble over rough terrain.

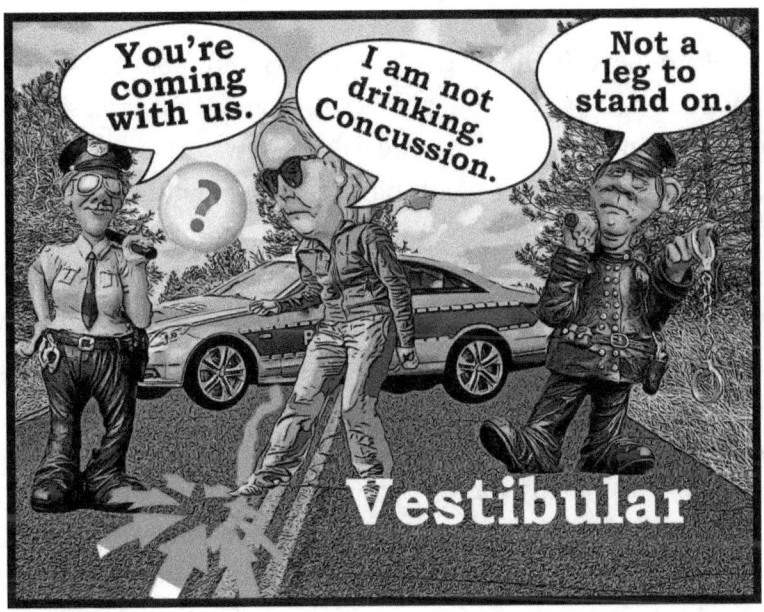

Vestibular Issues, Shannon Estabrooks

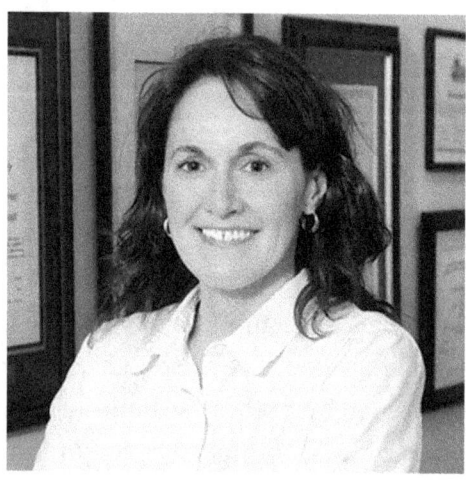

Shannon Estabrooks

I am off to meet Shannon Estabrooks, BScBio, BScPT, Dip Sport PT, Active Life Physiotherapy in New Glasgow. Once assessed, she works on concussion rehab, specialized physiotherapy, vestibular equilibrium function, gait, balance, coordination, ocular/eye movement. I had balance issues prior to my fall because of a loss of hearing in my left ear, but this is different, more pronounced. She recommends a weighted vest for stability. A crucial catalyst to healing, Shannon affirms my efforts, acknowledges how hard I work. With her expert guidance, I do what she prescribes and more. It is the "more" that kicks me in the butt, leaving bruises I kicked myself so many times.

New vocabulary enters my world with each therapy; I build a tool kit. Experts recommend a gradual return to cognitive and physical activity, with a focus on activities of daily living. Back In Action Physiotherapy offers resources on their website and a terrific downloadable PDF: "Reconnecting the Pieces: A Guide to Understanding Symptoms and Recovery Strategies for Patients and Families," 2014. It provides five steps to recovery, including educating on limitations. I am pumped to receive validation.

Shannon proves to be a skilled physiotherapist and vestibular specialist. My husband drives me to see her every two weeks. On Shannon's suggestion, Dr. Cudmore refers me to Dr. Toby Mandelman, Doctor of Optometry (OD). People do not realize a difficulty with vision may be the source of symptoms. There is a wait.

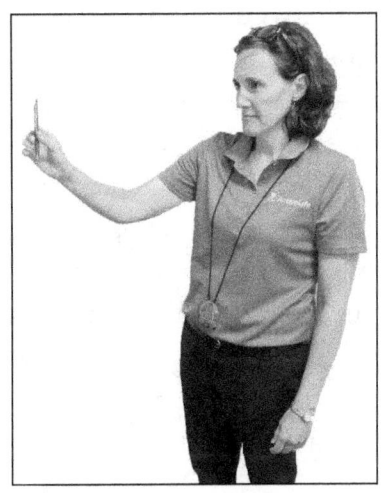

My husband drives me to three weekly appointments, never a word of complaint. I respond better when he, and those around me speak gently. He supports me dimming lights, turning down volume. Without hesitation, he takes over household responsibilities becomes an awesome cook. We do, however, have challenges with communication, thus a section further on to help with what can be deal breakers. I learn head injuries increase the risk of divorce. Important to give the concussed respite, not blame. Close relationships change, patience needed.

What does a concussed person do without family support? I include a section to acknowledge families. Many of the suggestions come because I lived them. It helps an incredible amount when loved ones know the dos and don'ts of head injuries. For example, please do not bombard me with questions. Give me time to speak and to receive your words. Lower expectations, decrease my responsibilities until I can handle more.

The wide band around my forehead squeezes and creates pressure when I do too much. I have no control over pain. Take it away. Music, loud noises, fast talking, and lights compete for my attention, have me dissolving into a jelly puddle. "See me! No, me. Hear me! No, me." Overwhelmed. One person at a time! One sense. My damaged microscopic neurons and circuits malfunction, looking for . . . what was I saying? Too many lights. Boom! Set fries. Gas tank empty. I never knew fatigue could be debilitating, mushed applesauce.

Tranquility does not come, my mind a clanking casino of noisy slots refuses to stop at red lights or recognize universal DANGER signs. Overstimulation marches like the Energizer Bunny—beating, banging, pounding his vexatious drum. Thoughts race ninety miles an hour, collide, tangle like multicoloured silly string bursting from a tin can. I need help to put them back in, but organization and structure are enemies.

Mental Health

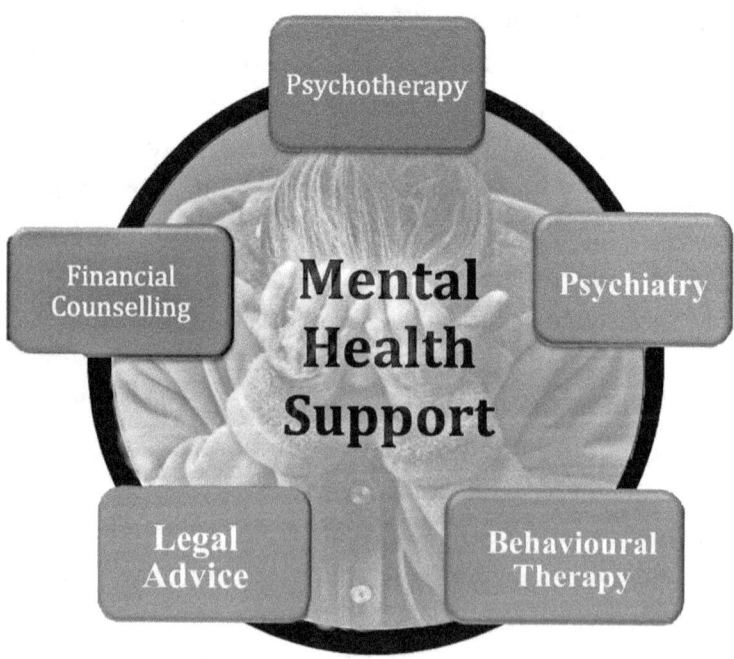

September 2016

Dr. Cudmore refers me to a psychologist. I agonize. Plans lofty, spirit driven, but my body languishes in bed too much. I can regulate the temperature with my air conditioner, always too hot in other areas of the house. I close the door, drown out sound, control lights and blinds. My bed provides less pressure on my back and neck. I use a hot pad or cold press or transcutaneous electrical nerve stimulation (TENS) machine. It is my safe space.

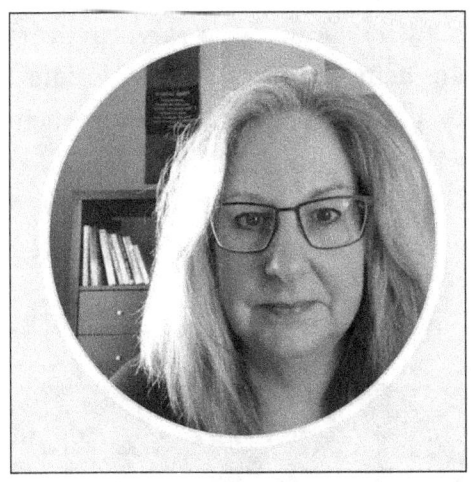

Wendy Digout

To help with a life turned upside down, I go kicking and screaming to Wendy Digout in September 2016 for cognitive behavioural therapy. She, too, had a concussion. I feel safe. Wendy says it is normal for someone with my injury to take two steps forward, one step back, and experience heightened emotions. Again, professional perspective from someone who understands helps. She explains that a concussed brain can be hyperactive—easily agitated and hypersensitive. Or hypoactive—shuts down because the body is tired of fighting, leading to extreme fatigue, the kind I experience. My goal is to realign emotional irregularity, balance hyper and hypo.

Wendy notices how hard I am on myself, speaks about being more compassionate and less judgmental. Throughout the consultation, three times, if not more, I lose my . . . In the middle of a sentence or question, I lose . . . my train . . . of thought. Gone— Nothing! With prompting, I retrieve it, another sign of inadequacy. Too much on my mind, too emotional, too everything. Forgetting scares the crap out of me and I fear a connection to dementia. Is there? We go through analysis, a Ping-Pong game, scrutinizing symptoms, activities, searching for answers. What was I saying?

Seeing experts who allow me to raise my fears and concerns with no judgment helps me lift the heavy weight from my chest. Okay to be angry, bitter, sad, frustrated, overwhelmed. The initial step in handling the mental trauma faced in child and adulthood is being aware. Psychologists are part of the package, denying their help means slower advancement. We assume we have dealt with trauma and triggering past events, but if they continue to haunt and show up . . . then not enough.

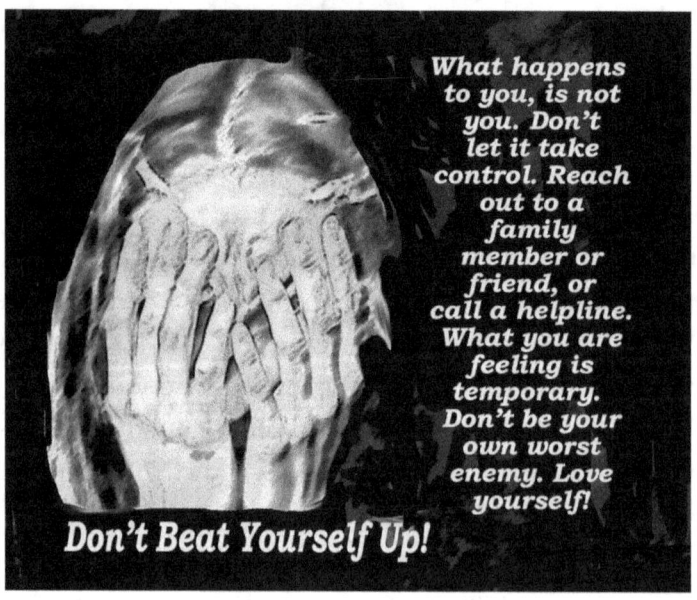

What happens to you, is not you. Don't let it take control. Reach out to a family member or friend, or call a helpline. What you are feeling is temporary. Don't be your own worst enemy. Love yourself!

Don't Beat Yourself Up!

Those visits guide, help me analyze my feelings toward my injury, gain clarity. My family respects my efforts. If they have negative or critical opinions about me, they keep them to themselves, which I appreciate. I am sure they wonder at my behaviour, brain fog, forgetfulness, dense responses, but they let them go into the wind where they belong.

Why fight mental health help? It is not a sign of weakness. The idea of sharing what is personal is not repugnant. No one enjoys sharing dirty laundry, being vulnerable, stripped naked. Mental health impacts the physical. What do we do when we feel we have no one, are a failure or unable to secure one friend? We reach out, not judge with the harshness of a bristle brush. Shaming has no place in recovery. Reading inspirational stories helps. Prior to my fall, I was ignorant. Like most other injuries or diseases, we only learn when affected, then we want to learn all we can to spearhead recovery. Reading post-concussion stories offers a much-needed life preserver. The brain is a unique vessel, a complex marvel, undoubtedly among the world's top wonders. An uncanny similarity I find in the following story. I cry the entire way through.

Julia Nunes is a writer who suffered a concussion and post-concussion syndrome.

"On good days, I fight through the brain fog and write in spurts at the computer. I run around a bit with my kid. On bad days, the fatigue is crushing. There is this pressure in my head as if a blunt object is expanding inside my cranium, straining to get out. If I do too much—walk too far, read for too long, forget to pace myself—a piercing headache erupts. Every day is a calculation: how much will be too much?" (Nunes, *The Toronto Star* 2016).

She is writing about me. My heart goes out to her and all suffering from a brain injury. She continues . . . "I'm in the kitchen pouring rice into a cup when my husband asks a question. I look towards him, but my brain can't do two things at once. The rice hits the floor. Thousands of grains scatter under the counter, the oven, the fridge. I grab a broom but can't focus. My neurons are in overdrive: dinner is late, I must get downtown, but I can't drive that far, and the 45-minute streetcar ride seems daunting. This is the new me. The old me ran a half-marathon and researched a book while working towards a master's degree and writing TV scripts to pay the bills. The new me gets flustered cooking rice. This is what concussion has made of me. And I hate every second." (Ibid).

Encouraged, I am "normal," I begin activities, challenge my brain, play memory, and word games, start meditating, exposing myself to new things. I try listening to soft, instrumental music, add more writing. Instead of burying myself, I embrace a new mantra—concentrate on what I can do, rather than what I can't, grateful I can access resources.

Guess what? I planted a cactus garden. Why cacti? They survive in harsh, dry conditions, are slow growing, require little water, connect to my slow recovery. They will stand for what was, rather than what is. Here's hoping. My parents had a green thumb, so I expect the best. My cacti, all but one, turn yellow. Did I over or underwater? Difficult to get the right balance. I overwatered. Too much care. I turn to writing. Finding light in darkness leads to a happier, more fulfilled life than succumbing to darkness and endless questioning. My thoughts spill, fall onto the page, an ideal outlet for releasing emotions.

January 2017—The Beast

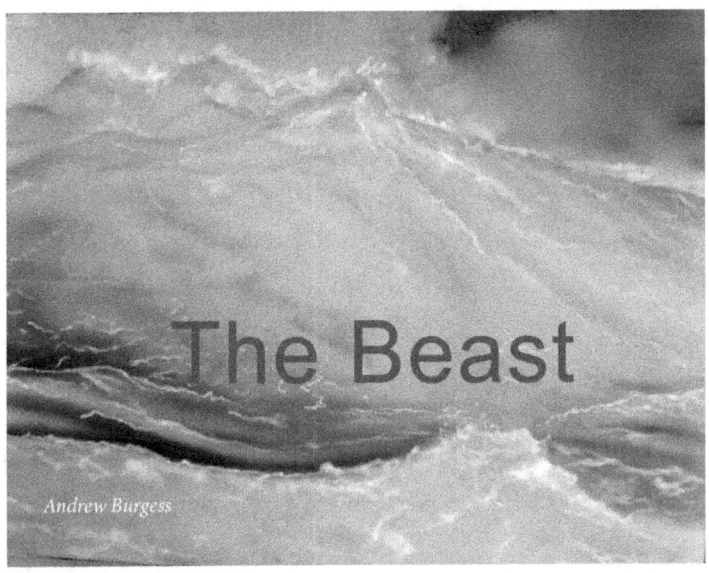

A year after my fall, I can do more, but severe fatigue is still an issue; my forehead squeezes, screws tightening as I struggle to keep up. Recovery is arduous, memory tenuous. I attend therapy sessions, work with Jeniffer. By managing my environment and pacing, symptoms stabilize. I am in a movie, tense moment. A bomb is about to go off. White? Blue? Green? Yellow? As the clock ticks down. Which is it? Hurry. BOOM!

I struggle adding appointments to my phone, get confused, forget, buttons too tiny. Do not give me complicated rigmarole, I will run for the hills. I search for apps to help with challenges, like a calendar to avoid double-booking. No time limits. On-the-spot stuff kills me. Colouring apps relax as does instrumental music like Dan Gibson's *Solitudes*. My husband and I compile a list of the things I require.

I can't stop thinking about school. I am out of sorts, desperate to drill lessons into bright minds, chant subject-verb agreement rules, listen as they discuss the story or poem recited. My routine for twenty-plus years. This is the inordinate difficulty and challenge—my lost job where I strived to make a difference for each student. Forever proud of each one, I do not want my career to end with a fall, a hospital stay, no goodbye. Dangerous steep slope—when you cannot perform, be productive your self-esteem tanks. Down, down, down we go, back into the black bunny hole.

Persistent post-concussion syndrome (PPCS) is real. Bingo! Not sure if I win or lose. As I step into a new year, I appreciate, minus dastardly forms, my employer and union. The forms triggered a violent reaction that brought home my insecurities. If my boss had been more aware of the impact, I might not have suffered. Knowing my job awaits allows me to concentrate on rehabilitation. Even though Dr. Lok told me I'd never teach again, I did not believe him, refused to listen. I still couldn't provide any permanent dates for return to work as Dr. Cudmore stretched my return dates. I needed to hang onto hope and was determined to get back to the classroom. I would not give up without a fight.

Employers need to know a return date with an mTBI is near impossible in jobs that are in a loud, busy, multi-sensory workplace.

I start an individualized care plan, in Antigonish, two days a week. My one-year anniversary! Breathe in, breathe out, deep belly breaths. Settle the parasympathetic system using suggested techniques.

Steps

To help me regain abilities Jeniffer breaks my basic care into steps. At first, I do not understand why showering became difficult after my injury. She explained why—too many steps involved—a fact to which the uninjured are oblivious.

To take a shower: 1) Gather toiletries; 2) Collect clothes; 3) Undress; 4) Turn on faucet, regulate water; 5) Shampoo hair; 6) Rinse hair; 7) Condition hair; 8) Rinse hair; 9) Wash body; 10) Wash face; 11) Towel dry; 12) Brush teeth; 13) Dry hair; 14) Apply deodorant, moisturizer; 15) Put pre-selected clothes on; 16) Put away night clothes; 17) Clean up.

Seventeen steps. No wonder exhaustion taxes. If I compartmentalize, I no longer perceive myself as inadequate. Four steps create my magic number before I hit fatigue, the steps will increase over time. I understand. We should not beat ourselves up if we cannot do things. Instead, we should break activities down, do at separate times, rest between each stage. Once I grasp the concept, break the steps up, I enjoy more relaxed showers without as much fatigue. This is huge! Progress baby!

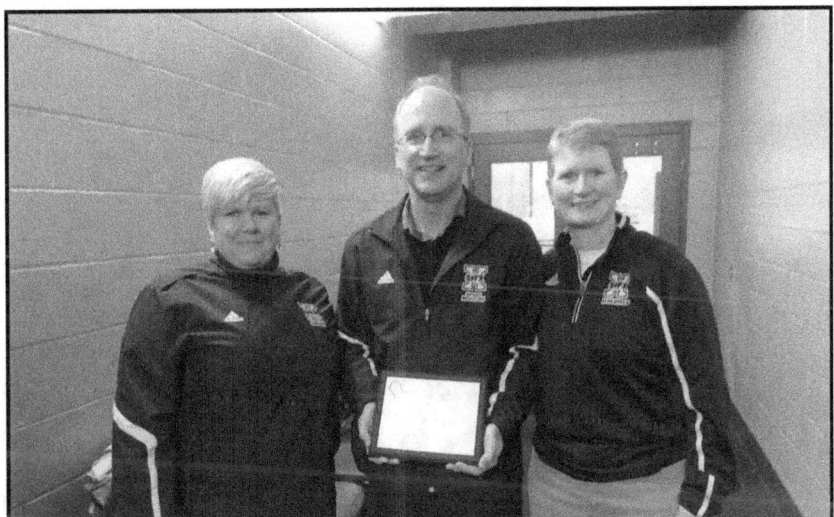

Dr. Cudmore Receives Brain Injury Canada Special Recognition Award
February 11, 2016, Center Dr. Cudmore
Ange Wylie and Tara Sutherland, athletic therapists, Photo Credit: StFX Athletics

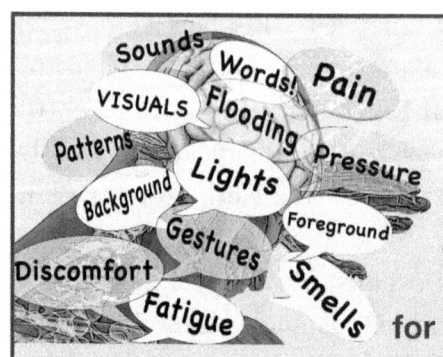

A Simple Task with a Brain Injury? Or is It?

Conversing requires the following steps taken for granted by the uninjured.

1. Pay attention to the face
2. Not get lost in physical appearance
3. Focus on the voice and words
4. Block facial expressions
5. Block pattern of clothing
6. Block flooding background visuals
7. Block flooding environmental sounds
8. Block distracting gestures
9. Block flooding lights
10. Block flooding senses
11. Block body language
12. Hear inflections and tone
13. Concentrate on the words
14. Focus on the meaning
15. Try to get the message
16. Keep up with the speed
17. Filter extra details
18. Absorb what is being said
19. Slow racing thoughts
20. Speak up if unable to process words

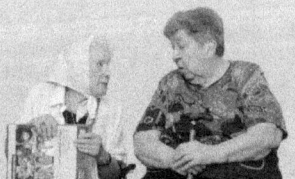

No wonder we get tired. I close my eyes, ask people to slow down, raise or lower their voice, use fewer details and gestures. I have trouble filtering. It creates a massive struggle with hearing, listening, and absorbing what is said. Too often I simply nod, or say yes, even though I retained nothing.

Prior to leaving for appointments, I try mindfulness exercises. Impossible to settle. I curse! Swearing ricocheting into my vocabulary post-concussion. Even poor Alexa, Amazon's cloud-based voice service, gets an earful when she mixes my words. Not her fault. One full year of recovery. Am I an anomaly? Why does my mule-eyed brain create a fog so thick I cannot slice it? The monumental, heart-wrenching three letter word, "WHY?" haunts. Wearing my weighted vest, I leave home. Show of defiance! I make my own decisions. Hubby is scared I will bite his head off. I am thinking about teaching, grieve my students. Grief (of persons, pets, career, place) a process. I need company.

I arrive at physiotherapy and Liz reads my frustration. With professionalism, she talks me down, recognizes my deadlock, assures me I am not alone in my reactions, praises me for not cancelling. Using psychology, she shares words, gets on with rehab. I discover, as much as I wanted to toss my weighted vest, I am not ready. Jeniffer also knew I would be emotional. Instead of doing cognitive exercises, we talk about what to do to lessen hyperactivity and hypersensitivity. She explains why my body reacted, confirms my feelings, poses no judgment, laughs with me as I share I am as headstrong as Wile E. Coyote. We scour my individualized program, look at my scheduling, which is hard on my head. She sets up my appointments for the next two months, eases stress related to booking. I leave in better shape. Hopefully, it is enough to get me through.

"We have only this moment, sparkling like a star in our hand. And melting like a snowflake."

— Marie B. Ray, prolific writer, editor

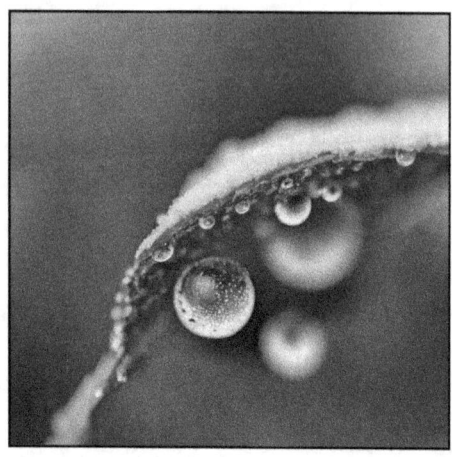

Are those dewdrops, raindrops, tears, or melting snow? I am wound up. Why do anniversary dates hold such power? My therapists say I suffered trauma; my injury turned my entire universe upside down—robbed me of a job I loved, a major part of my identity. Nothing is as it seems, eh, Macbeth? It took away my ability to drive, shrunk my world, saran-wrapped it. My bedroom is my place of sanctuary. Sometimes I sleep for hours. In a week, I speak to my husband, sister, rehab team. Honey, I shrunk your cosmos. My girls live away, have busy lives of their own. Isolation, loneliness . . . formidable. One year after my fall, still off work. I would have said you were crazy, the idea preposterous—a conclusion from someone ignorant of the impact of head injuries.

I decide to paint my fingernails. First sitting—remove old polish, a hard task with spatial issues and small fingernail surface. Next day—clip and file, concerted effort to keep my focus but good for my brain to practise. Third day—polish two thumbs. Shaky, more polish goes on my hand. I give up. Fourth day—mad at myself, I try my index fingers. The concentration causes the achy-breaky forehead claw. I stop, need a day off, aim for the middle fingers on Saturday. Two fingers a day until I finish and scrub the skin so the nails look decent; they don't. I feel inept, a clear snapshot of fatigue. If I could drive, I would go to a salon. Argh! What do I do when the *bleep-bleep* polish needs to come off?

It is challenging to stay in the present. The teacher in me grieves. Eyes watery, I shake my head. What was ludicrous is my reality. I have never been a crybaby. Am I now? I am sick of managing. Sick of scheduling. Sick of plotting, planning . . . 365 days later. Why so slow? Age? Health? I should have been teaching, drafting stories, editing chapters started decades ago, exercising, walking, losing weight. Instead, I am on the road three days a week travelling to medical appointments, wanting, needing rest. I want my life back! Can anybody hear? Am I screaming into a vacuum? Where is everyone? Rescue me from this nightmare and return me to my former self. Squeeze hard. I do not care if it hurts. Grease and squeeze me like a squealing piglet through a keyhole, anything to put me back. Tears blur the keyboard. My head aches. I swear.

Topic must change! Get my mind off my anniversary. I imagine my dear, sweet grandson Aden—his face lighting up with a humongous grin, running toward me, arms opened wide to give me a loving hug and kiss. My only grandchild, in 2017, with blond hair, and sparkling blue eyes, he squeals as he recognizes Grammie Bear; seconds later, a tear slips down my cheek. My heart aches. He lives far away in Edmonton, Alberta. My attempt at mindfulness backfires; loneliness swarms. I miss him, try to enjoy the sun cascading through the window. I need my babies closer. I must be present in every moment, and make it count. I hate being slowed down. The bleepin' ice robbed me. February 1, 2017, I hate you, or should I say February 1, 2016? The date takes on too much significance. Should not be. I should see it as the beginning of a new year of steady progress, improvement, chance to return to my classroom. Instead, it blares what I lost.

Groundhog Day, I am ready for spring's fresh growth, soft twitter of finch and grosbeak. The rolling hills and valleys need a vivid green blanket to cover them, vibrant yellow crocus to push through winter's leftovers, determined to show brilliance after lying dormant. I want to witness a snowdrop—harbinger of the season, blooming with its characteristic curled stem, bursting alive in a white lantern teardrop, delicately peeking through snow. Will I see an early pansy, tiny face dressed in peekaboo colours, one shade catching the eye, then another poking through cracks in the sidewalk? Such a tenacious, mischievous flower. Can I, like them, come through the whiteness of spring?

Tenacity is a noteworthy characteristic. The secret is finding the right balance. My sincere hope for improvement is in unfolding beauty, vibrant, lush greens, dancing, laughing, healing colours. It is what I want my new year to be—alive in expanded capability. Quotations continue feeding my soul, a penchant for skinny, fat, short, or lengthy ones. In the words of others, I find comfort, solidarity, inspiration. I place them on my fridge or in my phone, a booster shot on onerous days. This is not the road I expected to be on a year ago. I struggle to get ready for physiotherapy. Cannot do it. Cancel. My favourite—Simon & Garfunkel, "The Sound of Silence"—plays sage advice. The irony in their lyrics, no one listens. Water drips, creates silent spirals of connection. I retrace my steps; that fateful morning before work, I knew my future. A year later, I do not.

Ask the person in your life who might be suffering what works for them.

February 2017—Post Traumatic Vision Syndrome

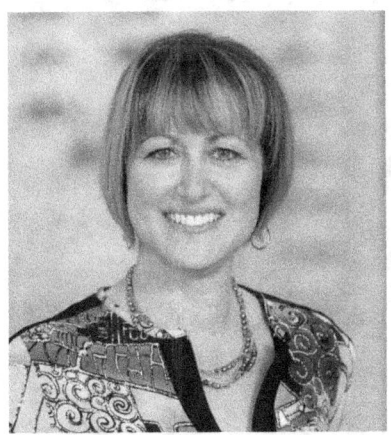

Dr. Toby Mandelman

For years, Dr. Toby Mandelman (Nova Scotia, Canada) studied prism glasses and their healing effects on the injured brain. My first appointment is in February 2017, one year after I fell. After a litany of preliminary tests, I step into her examining room. She has Shannon's copious notes. My impaired binocular vision is causing poor saccades, (rapid eye jumps, focusing from one object to another), weak pursuits (smooth eye movements tracking a moving target), and the compulsive need to blink. She diagnoses me with post-traumatic vision syndrome (PTVS) and a visual midline shift (VMS).

"Over 90 % of concussions and traumatic brain injuries (TBIs) result in some degree of visual dysfunction. Post traumatic vision syndrome (PTVS) is the clinical diagnosis for the visual symptoms that appear following a brain injury." www.optomitrists.org

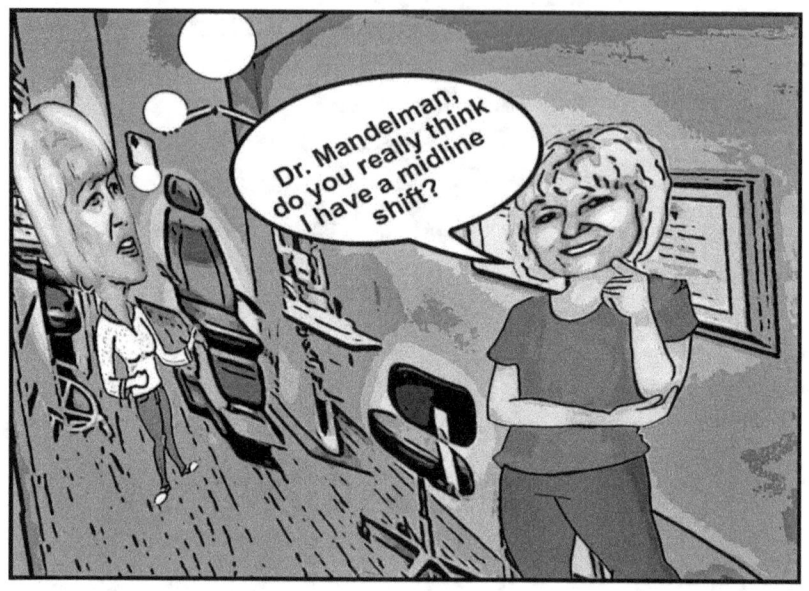

The VMS causes me to "List" to the left and posteriorly, affecting balance and spatial awareness. We discuss treatment: glasses with yoked, base-in prism, which stabilizes the ambient visual system, and allow me to read more comfortably. Dr. Mandelman tests combinations of lenses and prisms. The impact is immediate—I cannot believe the dramatic difference when she adds prisms to my prescription. Prior to that, I staggered down the hall, she observing me zigzag. Proper prisms added, like magic, straight as an arrow. She recommends Shannon continue neuro visual postural therapy (NVPT) to correct visual imbalances, bring the ocular-visual system back to normal. I learn unfamiliar words. Despite my eye problems, I see with greater clarity. I am getting a handle on this beast. Specs allow the sun to be my friend, lessen hypersensitivity.

Weeks later, Dr. Mandelman fits me with my first individualized glasses, forty percent tinted blue to block brightness and reduce eye strain. Prism therapy helps stabilize the ambient visual system (spatial awareness). Allows it to ground the focal system so perceptual reorientation can occur, so I know where I am in space.

I cannot depend on my auditory or visual systems to give me clues; they are not reliable. Armed, I feel steadier on my feet, do not have eye strain. Eureka! Joy. Joy. Every day, I do exercises to help with balance, speech, cognition, attention, and managing emotions.

Dr. Clark Elliott, *The Ghost in My Brain*, 2016, refers to them as brain glasses. He claims they talk to the brain and retrain it. I need to sit and let that concept marinate, a mysterious frontier, to go beyond where no man has gone before. So much to discover, learn, and share. With complex text and complicated ideas, I take baby steps, use the black background on my computer, set assistive details to larger font, have the computer read to me. I resize my font, print, on purple or blue paper (less contrast), read in dribs and drabs. The letters appear larger or smaller with shadows; font plays tricks, I stop.

The need to change glasses will be a good sign. Cause for excitement? There is something to the power of getting the proper treatment and prescription post-concussion. "The continuous, ambiguous misinformation and stimuli cause balance and visual issues, cognitive difficulties leading to extreme mental fatigue as the brain tries to sort multiple signals." (Dr. Mandelman, CTV News story, January 28, 2016).

For short periods I can peer out the windshield with prescription sunglasses, no longer buried in a blanket to obstruct the light and flashes.

Shock

Except for appointments and a restaurant when travelling, stuck at home for twelve months, I am eager and excited to seize the opportunity to shop at Dartmouth Crossing after seeing Dr. Mandelman. Individual shops are less noisy than a mall, so I plan to handle them one at a time. To say I am enthusiastic is an understatement, although I am conscious and worried about my stutter and fatigue.

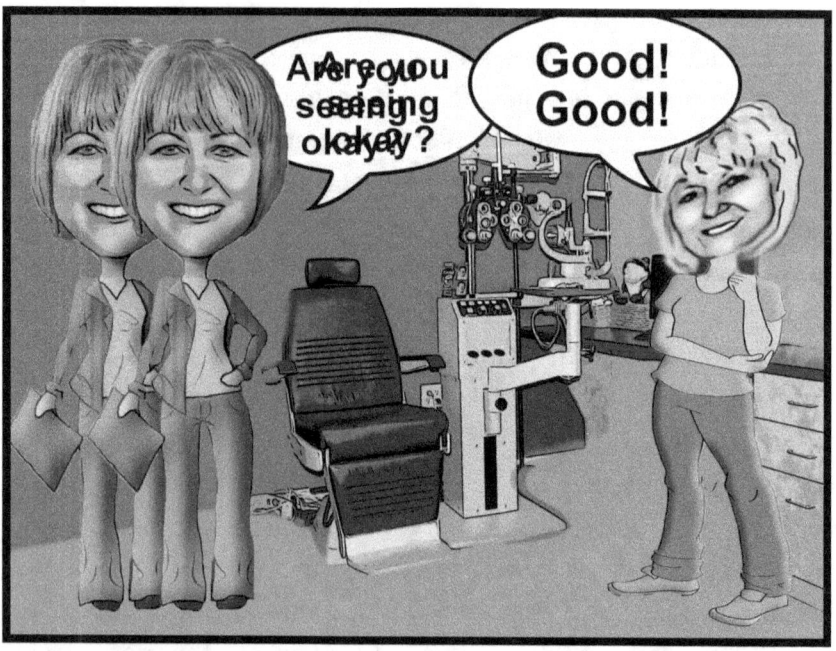

A strong coffee allows me to muster courage, dark glasses my shield. Anxiety consumes, but I want to prove I can do it. I need new clothes; the others shrunk. In person, I can try on an outfit. Ordering clothes online, a hit-and-miss. Good feelings bubble up, I am on a mission. Here goes . . . I open the door, case the joint, and take my time walking the periphery, to get a sense of the layout. The store is quiet, a saleslady watches me from behind a counter. Does my uneven gait give the wrong impression? Would she think I am drunk? Surely not. Bright colours come at me under fluo-rescent lights, but I take my time, feel the material on new styles, hopeful I will find something. I cannot wear anything scratchy or itchy, need smooth material. She watches me out the corner of her eye, folds items, making me uneasy.

Looking for something cozy for the winter and to feel better about myself, I think it best to go up and ask for help, forgetting my stutter in the delight of getting something new. I walk straight up so she can hear and ask, "Do, Dooo you, you, you, h-ha-h-aaa-ve swe-swe-ter d-d-dre-dre-sses?" I feel like the backside of a donkey, the words painstakingly difficult to get out. Does she understand me? The supercilious clerk responds, "Yes, yes, yes. We, we, we, ha-ha-have dresses."

Her words punch me in the gut. Emotions flood, cheeks burning, flushing a horrible, blazing red from a terrible sense of inadequacy. I need escape. Have to get out. Fancy dresses and gorgeous women's clothes line the racks but it is her face that comes at me, dripping with judgment in a bright store suddenly gone dark. Does she think I have something "wrong" with me? Shocked, I struggle to move. Well-dressed, there to please the customer, why did she parrot me? To make me feel better? Flabbergasted I remain frozen, eyes tearing, wretched rain welling from the bottom of my toes. Emotions cascade through every vein and artery. She did not do that. Make fun of me . . . did she? Blood rushes; my countenance crumbles. Trying to hold back waterworks, I cower, shuffle backwards toward the exit, wish I could put her in her place, instead, I spew something about a head injury, turn and run. She does not offer an apology, or ask if I need help. Outside, I hightail to the Rogue, tears flying in the wind as I drop onto the rust-coloured seat, bawl, sob, and rant. I am inconsolable. Did I look that bad? My husband, not knowing what to do, tries to console me. Upset I cannot listen. We sit in the vehicle, he trying to calm me, feeling bad, my shopping excursion turned to shambles.

Did I experience a glimpse of humanity's underbelly—people judging, dismissing, demeaning those who do not meet society's bogus standard? Did I not look, sound, or act right? Was that the saleslady's plan to get me to leave? My heart rips, a taste of the scathing humiliation and ridicule too many feel in daily encounters. The day ruined, my self-esteem tanks, I weep, bawl the entire three-and-a-half-hour drive home. We had gone to Bedford and Halifax for a medical appointment. We thought retail therapy would cheer me after being isolated. Instead, a saleslady destroyed my fledgling confidence. That cut stays with, steers me away from public exchange for an exceedingly long time.

I am back on my bed, trip taking its toll, fatigue, pain, and fibro flare-up. Understanding and accepting individuals who talk, walk, or exist differently is a challenge for society. We need to be kind, stop judging, show common decency.

April 2017

Two visits and months after receiving my new specs, I can read in thirty-minute increments. Yippee! And feel steadier on my feet.

May 2017—Excitement

My oldest daughter has a smile beaming across her face. She is getting married. Her news is bittersweet. Will I be able to go? I will push myself and make myself well, no matter what, forgetting that is the last strategy I should set. Over the moon, I am excited for her and the young man who came into our lives a few short years ago. He is a gem, and I feel a special connection because of our creative souls. He is a carpenter and artist, can do anything he sets his mind to, quite the impressive young man, and soon to be my son-in-law. She gives us more exciting news. A destination wedding in Croatia. I hug her, emphasize how happy I am for them, but my insides rip, gurgle, and spasm with the provocative question of will I be well enough? A dream of a lifetime to travel with my adult children for such a joyous occasion. Only a few invited. We skirt the idea of my being able. Verbally I am all in, but inside my guts have not stopped somersaulting and rolling down one of the steepest cliffs in the scenic country she chose. Fantasy versus reality on either end of a duel, a fight to the death. My husband's starlit, blue eyes pierce my own; he knows. He damn well knows. I look away, refuse to see a dream of a lifetime shatter. One way or the other, I will manage my symptoms. Family will help if I need it.

My dark glasses, ball hat, walking sticks, good shoes, no issues. Right? My thoughts I keep to myself so as not to upset anyone, but when safe and secluded by myself, I scream, sob, bawl, and curse my circumstance. A violent war pulls opposing forces to opposite ends between the logical part of my brain and my stirred-up emotions. My heart and soul frantically want to sail in a ship across the sky, fourteen hours in airplanes, languish high among the clouds where dizziness might hit. I will climb the steep mountains to spectacular inlets, alcoves, and the destiny spot itself. Heat and sun enemies; hotels, noise, not a problem. Superwoman! Who am I kidding? When fibromyalgia flares, I cannot sleep. It sets me over my threshold and PCS symptoms explode. No problem. Easy, breezy! God, I wish it were. I will balance activities in a foreign country, get up in the morning when everyone else does, ready to travel, order my headaches to disappear, throw the forehead claw in the cargo bay when we take off. Better to pack a bag and leave my PCS behind, absorb a sensational two-week trip with my husband and family to stunning Croatia, sink in the wonder as my daughter marries the love of her life. Life is grand! Do not even have a passport! Must order one.

I ask my therapists if they believe I can handle such a lofty excursion. They are cautious in their response, delicate in sending a message I do not want to hear, do not know the strength of my constitution. But where does that quality line up with recovery from an mTBI? With the biggest and most tender heartache, and a brain that is not where it was prior, logic like an earthworm, tunnels inside my head, refusing to stop munching my brain— Too much! Am I telling myself that, or is it the case? In silence, I scream. Agitated, a tsunami floods my room. Idiotic fall! I am Mount Garibaldi, ready to erupt. No, I am on Dinara, the highest mountain in Croatia, overlooking the Adriatic Sea. I wish. Crushed, my body speaks the truth. Anxiety surges. I need to calm myself. Emotions fire on all cylinders. What to do? Fitbit shows my resting pulse at 110. It is usually over 100, with little effort. Yup, worked up I am. I received the watch as a gift to track my pulse. I work my way up to a thousand steps, far from the recommended ten thousand, but must start somewhere. As I feel better, I plan to be more competitive, challenge myself, although it is hard, my symptoms flare. Truth is, I am heartbroken. If I tag along, I will pull everyone down when the trip should be all about my daughter and her soon-to-be husband. The travel beyond my capabilities, the unpredictability, a risk, the flight out of the country, inadvisable. I knew the minute she mentioned it. Had I not fallen, I would have been smiling and dancing on top of a mountain overlooking the Adriatic Sea, comparing it to my back door Atlantic Ocean.

On my daughter's big day, May 30, 2017, I cry, feel robbed of one of the most cherished moments a mother can have. I am bitter, sorry for myself, adding fuel to the fire of losing my career, my identity, my life. Good people surround me. Beyond believable, love flows over the continents as my other son-in-law and youngest daughter stream the ceremony, thoughtfulness alive across the globe so I can watch. Thanks to modern technology, I get to see the wedding ceremony and the backdrop of beautiful mountains falling into the sea. Love my babies all! It is difficult to face adversity when it mocks your ability to fight back. When less vulnerable, I will compose myself, dwell on the here and now, deal with pain, forgetfulness, and let go. An everyday challenge to search for the sunshine, but much better than a day that is dark.

Sleep, my nemesis, plays out of reach, a carousel of scattered thoughts refusing to re-enter the Crayola box. Ideas spin in a front-load dryer. Ideas bounce. Nightmares fall into dangerous, messed-up classrooms. Over and over, they fire me. A student and a teacher my simultaneous role. Reversal. I cannot breathe. Melatonin relaxes. Is that possible? Through self-awareness, I find myself clenching my fists, tensing my body even when trying to sleep. Some of us wind ourselves so tight, suspected leftover of the fight-or-flight response, necessary in case we have to run. PCS is a beast, and I am fighting to accept its hold over me, ready to move on and be done with it. If only it were my decision. Occasionally, I try to act as if nothing is wrong; it bites me in the ass.

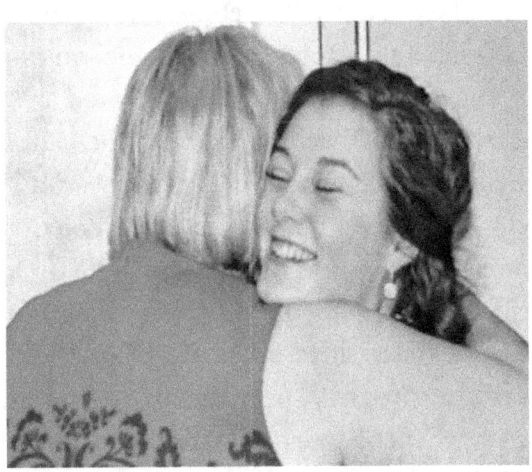

I receive my teaching assignment for the new school year, once again fall down the dark, rabbit hole because I know I am not ready. No matter how much I try, I aim high, give chunks of time, unrealistic dates, pray one will work out. It takes everything out of me for doctors to put off my return. My employer needs to plan for substitutes making my situation tenuous. It tears me apart; I still have trouble functioning at home.

June 2017—Assessments

On June 1, I have another speech assessment. "Francene has been seen for five sessions. Treatment goals include a constant voice in, easy onset and smooth start to, appropriate breathing and rate during speech. Exercises completed incorporate these strategies into the repetition of sentences of varying length and complexity.

Francene has been incorporating these strategies into conversations with familiar people. Initial part and whole word repetitions, avoidance, and revisions characterize her disfluency. Fatigue contributes to the severity of her speech." Marlee Mousek.

"Sixty percent of adults who stutter, experience social anxiety, which has a negative impact on the success of speech therapy for adults." (Wilder, Lisa; 2015). Self-conscious, I only talk to family and health professionals, avoid crowds, do not answer the phone. I investigate the Resiliency Program offered to school staff through the Nova Scotia Teachers Union, chock full of resources, opt for online counselling once a week, as my sessions with Wendy end. Matched with Carmen Burnaby from British Columbia, I am nervous, but we gel. She counsels me from June to October 2017. It's a comfort talking to someone who knows nothing about me. Carmen gives me strength to advocate in relation to appointments hindering my progress, provides emotional support on my solitary Robinson Crusoe journey, with only scarce, dim light. I have tremendous difficulty finding my brain's dimmer switch. Another analogy, my brain is a shaken snow globe. While on this mountain, I pass through four distinguishable Canadian seasons several times. At first, the precipitation gently falls, and I am okay. But when someone disturbs the dome, snow goes everywhere. The wind comes up until it's a blizzard and no one can see or function. Everything shuts down—overloaded. I need to find balance.

June 5, 2017

Dr. Mandelman is pleased with my progress. I continue to wear my yoked prisms and tinted lens while she checks into a suspicion I need syntonic treatment for my peripheral vision.

A turtle garden ornament represents my journey, its bobble

head symbolizing brain fog, inability to filter senses. Its huge smile reminds me of gratitude. The cheerful baby riding on its back reflects a willingness to carry others. That is my life's mantra. A butterfly on its nose, a bonus—we grow through metamorphosis. What will I become? Can I accept it?

A flashback . . .

In 1994, I published *A Rose in November* about individuals facing adversity. I had the privilege of meeting tremendous, salt-of-the-earth folks and discovering the inspirational stories hidden behind their smiling faces. In the ladies' section of a Woolco store I discovered a mother like no other; in town I found a strong lad battling leukemia; met a brave man in a wheelchair; spoke to individuals who never gave up, no matter how bad the storm. I cried, laughed, learned what is most important.

I had pluckiness back then. Imagine me as a visitor coming to your doorstep and saying, "I want to hear your story," although I did call ahead, setting up a good rapport, which is important from the get-go. We size others up in seconds and draw first impressions. Authentic to myself, that meant sharing a bit of me as well. I was gutsy, no one threw me out. Instead, they offered a Cape Breton scoff while we laughed, cried, paused, and talked the hours away. Strangers poured out their hearts like a watering jug over a gorgeous hydrangea with bright blue blossoms about to bloom, knowing I would honour and respect their words. I agree with Howie Mandel. We need to share our invisible monstrosities and spinoffs. In stories, insights, experiences we see ourselves, clarify our thoughts and feelings, learn we are not alone. Am I repeating myself? Did I say this before? Repetition helps. I am putting words to paper, a sign of hope. Hope floats, doesn't it? On stormy seas, waves cast me adrift. How long can a boat survive in an angry sea, bitter gales churning undertows and riptides? I do not know what to expect, how long this crazy blizzard will last.

October 3, 2017

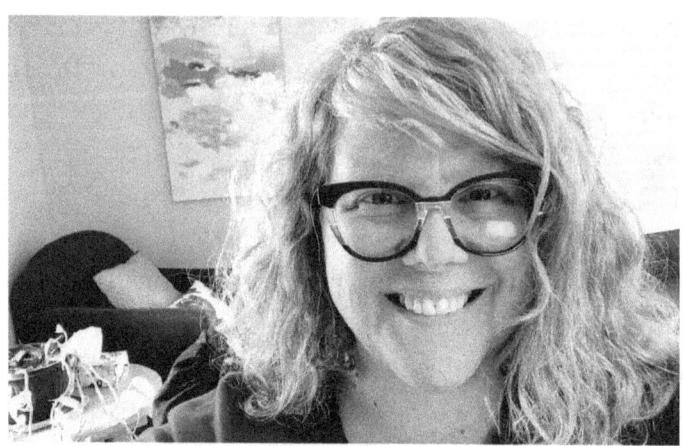

Cathrine Chambers

I begin seeing psychotherapist, Cathrine Chambers, biweekly, for concussion trauma and PTSD. I manage thirteen sessions before my hectic schedule results in symptom detonation. Driven to make myself better, I am making myself worse. Cathrine is an exceptional, down-to-earth, kind clinician. She helps me with PTSD symptom management, especially during hyperarousal of the autonomic nervous system. She shows me how to identify and manage triggers and affect regulation around feelings of frustration related to the physical and cognitive impairments associated with PCS. She knows her stuff. That is important. Clients must feel safe with their therapists. We work on intrusive thoughts, physical reactivity, and emotional distress after exposure to traumatic reminders, avoidance of trauma-related stimuli, hyper-vigilance, difficulty concentrating, and sleep disturbance. Cathrine explains that because of the presence of both PCS and PTSD, my physical and psychological symptoms get aggravated when I overexert myself physically, mentally, or emotionally. An intensification of post-concussion symptoms results in an increase of post-traumatic symptoms, and vice versa making for a vicious cycle.

We focus on improving my overall level of functioning as I struggle to complete activities of daily living, requiring an elevated level of support from my husband and family members. I recognize triggers, learn to relax the nervous system and access feelings of calm in the body. But it is an on-again, off-again success, reminding me of the importance of pacing. She adjusts my sessions based on how I am feeling, takes breaks during our conversations to ensure I do not get overwhelmed. My speech poses a challenge, requiring more time to express myself. I am scared I will lose more time from work. My gut tells me what I do not want to hear. How can I go back to teaching when I cannot filter or multi-task? Doctors steer me from recovery dates. I think of little else, am angry, replaying that day. I am more determined than ever to fight through the weird pains in my head, dizziness, fog. With short-term memory; and even instant recall, someone must cue me.

I need to set healthy boundaries, regulate the autonomic nervous system, rewire the brain to be less reactive to relational triggers. A central focus of our therapy is building on improving existing coping skills to improve daily functioning. I begin to feel a sense of control over PTSD symptoms, my ability to effectively respond to managed trauma triggers. It builds confidence. Cathrine helps me realize too many appointments during the week activates both my PTSD and post-concussion symptoms. Seems to me a fear of facing therapists is detrimental to our becoming the best we can be.

Christmas 2017

My husband and I need to pick up stocking stuffers, most of my gift shopping finished online. Overconfident, I slip into Lawtons Drugs in Antigonish after seeing Dr. Cudmore. The ladies in the gift department are kind, but the store is Christmas insanity. Get me out! My husband wanders off, not realizing the busyness cries overload. I reach down to grab a stocking stuffer, a package of Lindor chocolates, trying to keep my balance. The flimsy shelf gives way, I stumble, grab on. Mortified, my arms fly, cheeks flush redder than apples. Embarrassed to tears, I try not to show escalating distress. I must shift, and crouch to pick up what has fallen. I could ask a clerk for help, but they are running off their feet. The floor swallows me whole, water stabbing my eyes. To recover the chocolate, I must manoeuvre to my knees. Yup, get onto the floor and stay there until I pick up the candy.

People in line close by gawk. Really? With tremendous effort, one by haunting one, I replace each package of three. On both sides of me, customers wait, lost in their own worlds. On my knees on the floor, no one asks if I am okay. I feel like the dirt on the bottom of my shoe. Face as red as the Canadian flag, tears flow. I blink them back. It is Christmas time! Peace and joy and giving . . . why doesn't someone help? I know in my heart, if on the opposite side, without hesitation I would have bent over, picked up the chocolate, no question. In that, I find consolation. The candy now on the stand, how to get up? Balance is precarious. Through fog and overstimulation, I gingerly hold the larger shelf, pray it does not collapse, wish my husband would return. I unfurl. A dreadful execution, manage to stand. Back on my feet, head down, I stumble out, fall against a huge wood crate at the store entrance, sales flyers scattered on top. I grab one, pretend to read, take deep gulps, wipe falling tears, ground myself behind headlines until you-know-who comes looking. Back inside the car, I bawl as he tries his best to soothe me. He feels bad he left me. Not his fault. Impossible to be with the injured 24-7, and I thought I would be okay. Seems my willpower is ahead, mind working to catch up.

Shame and cruel inferiority shadow me for days as if I did catastrophic harm to the world. "Why" speaks of my insecurities. Why does this injury make me so emotional? I hate it! When injured, we lose a part of ourselves, judged by how we look, what we wear, how we act, how we handle ourselves. Our sense of self floats in fragments. We cannot control others, only ourselves. A keen realization—with PCS, trivial things become big, grow out of proportion. I take the difficult, see it as a challenge to overcome, a net in which to score, a finish line to pass. Do not lose hope. A map will improve things.

Christmas is a favourite time of year but even decorating the tree and the house takes tremendous effort and energy; I cannot take part as I used to. My husband, saint that he is, puts up the tree, garlands, angels, manger, and lights, has the house ready for the baby Jesus and the season we both love. I get to enjoy his hard work, pick at the tabletop, or light pine-scented candles hoping the new year will bring more progress.

2018—Which Way Do We Go?

"You must trust in something—your gut, destiny, life, karma, whatever. This approach has never let me down, and it has made all the difference in my life."

— Steve Jobs

I am aware of the direction to take . . . but I cannot reach it. My brain is now wired differently! February 1, 2018, approaching the two-year anniversary. Fixated, I fall into a tailspin, pray someone will pull a door open, release a lever, drop me into a dark cellar or return the years snuffed away. Our lives change following head injury. Instead of fixating on the past, I must plan, move forward, give my best, so shame, blame, and self-chastisement can disappear, allow me to be whole again. Sounds great on paper. Emotions ride high; I try to keep them in check, scared to reveal true feelings because others cannot handle them. Dark voices judge based on productivity, condemn, no matter how valiant. Not being in control deflates and disheartens. I need to find my value within. I spend my day moving in baby steps, terrified. Outsiders see improvements. One precept that rings true, takes time to recover . . . I skid into a funk as I did in 2017, petrified symptoms will linger forever.

BEWARE BLACK ICE! I fight, take one step in front of the other, even as I hit rock slides, fallen debris, and treacherous roadblocks. This injury does not decide who I am. Online, I search for local, regional, provincial interactive support groups, but most are in the US. Where are the ones geographically closer? I cannot find any. Do I know where to look?

"What I hear regularly from support group members is that the most valuable benefit of a support group is finding a place where you feel comfortable and can talk with people who get it, who truly understand your issues." (Webster, Barbara, 2017).

Pink Concussions—the non-profit group, developed for women over twenty-five who suffer with PCS states, "Women and girls have been documented to have a higher number, and more severe symptoms than males . . . One of our goals is for sport, academic, military, and medical communities to create female specific guidelines."

A stuck record, I cannot reiterate enough. Concussion is more than a head bump for 20–30 per cent of victims. The qualifiers of concussion are scary—*usually* caused by, *usually* temporary, *usually* recover, *most* are mild. "Usually" and "most" are loaded words. What sets us apart? Am I sabotaging recovery? Are too many variables involved? On February 6, 2018, I discover another physiotherapist living in New Glasgow, Liz van Zutphen; I recognize the name as I taught her younger siblings.

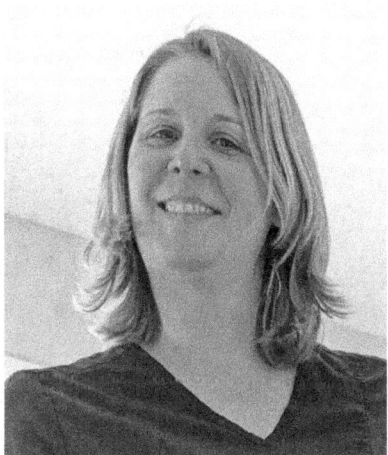

Liz van Zutphen

Since 2002, Liz has worked with the Canadian military and in private practice at Balance Physiotherapy. Her clinic is part of a network called Complete Concussion Management with locations throughout Canada and the US; their focus is on young athletes and training for professionals. Liz completed a Master of Clinical Science Manipulative Therapy from Western University and became a member of the Fellows of the Canadian Academy of Manipulative Physiotherapy (FCAMPT). In Nova Scotia to date, she is one of thirty-seven physiotherapists to achieve fellowship.

"On assessment, Mrs. Gillis had head forward posture with an increase kyphosis (curvature of the spine) in the cervicothoracic junction; she had downward rotated scapulas (shoulder blades) and her head was side bent to the left. The left rotation and right-side bend exhibited restricted range of motion, along with reduced extension at the cervicothoracic junction. Tightness was present in the retraction of the upper c-spine along with weakness in all muscle groups. The upper fibres of traps displayed tightness, with the left side being more pronounced than the right. This was accompanied by stiffness during rotation and extension through-out the thoracic spine, and fixation of rib 4 on the right. A decreased proprioception was observed for proper head posture and knowing midline. The shoulders exhibited a reduction in range of motion (ROM). Mrs. Gillis is presenting with upper cervical stiffness left greater than right, postural dysfunction—tight pecs, upper fibres of traps (trapezoid muscles), left greater than right, facet joint stiffness of L4/L5. An up slip of the left innominate and decreased post rotation of the left SIJ (Sacroiliac joint at the base of the back where the spine joins to the pelvis) is present due to spraining of the left SIJ. Her muscle groups are very weak due to deconditioning. She requires further vestibular and oculomotor testing. Rehab focuses on restoring proper joint and muscle movement, strength to the cervical, upper thoracic and lumbar spine and pelvis. Mrs. Gillis reports improvement, however, requires ongoing therapy to restore her ability to perform activities of daily living. Movement results in exacerbation of post-concussion symptoms. She is trying to increase her walking within a safe working heart rate; however, progress is slow." February 2018, Liz vanZutphen.

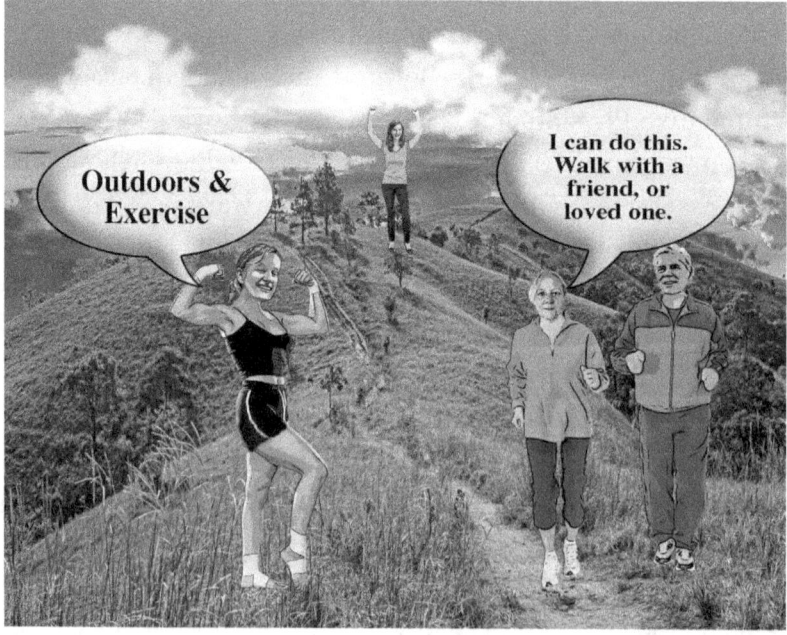

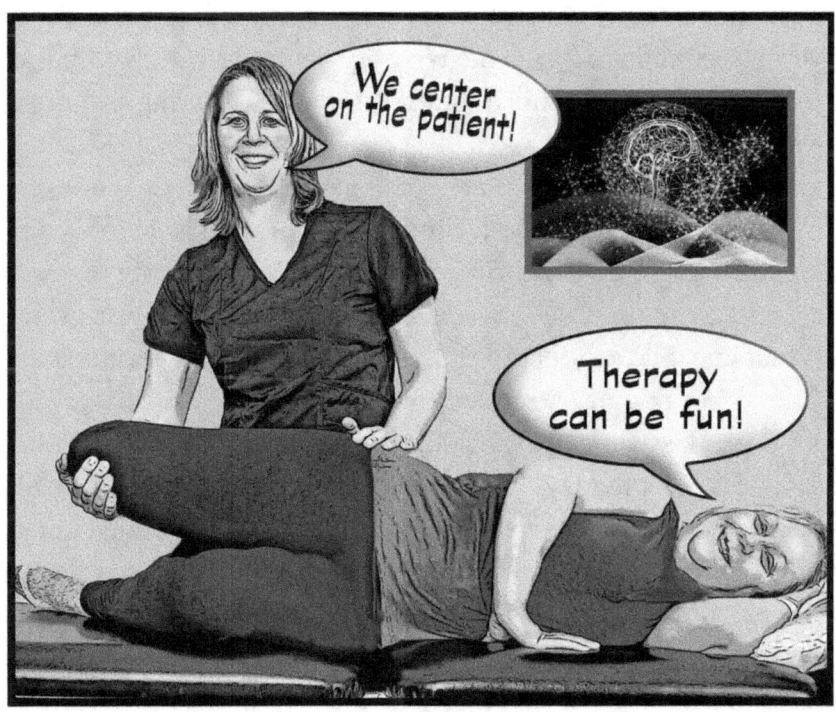

Over the months, Liz provides cranial sacral therapy to help straighten my posture, performs joint manipulations in my thoracic spine (mid-back), and mobilizations of my neck muscles. She performs strengthening exercises for the cervical spine and scapular stabilizers to strengthen my neck, gives me home exercises involving neck movements coordinating neck, eye, and head, to treat my vestibular system and dizziness. Chest out like a puppet on a string, the handler pulls tight, helping me know my centre. My range of motion is poor. Hurts. Stretch tall. Sit straight. Avoid slouching. Good advice! Plant your feet. Feel the toes, the heels. Find a target. Take a step. I push my soles tight into my footwear. One foot in front of the other climbing up the foreign ridge, I will someday reach the summit even if dense fog ahead. I arm myself, block out distractions. Balance suffers. Cannot filter. Too tired. Concussion—difficult to grasp this invisible miscreant marauder can stop me dead in my tracks, has no colour, although a definite grey. Stress and anxiety make recovery daunting, difficult finding balance between too much and too little, effort bringing a host of nasties.

Liz emphasizes another area of benefit is cardiovascular exercise, as this type of exercise facilitates good blood flow to the brain. The issue with PCS is figuring out the optimal heart rate that will not raise symptoms such as increased pulse, the notorious claw, and fatigue. She conducts a treadmill stress test to determine my optimal working heart rate, encourages me to buy a smartwatch and to exercise at my threshold heart rate daily. That means going for a walk. Cloudy days are best as the bright sun triggers headaches. Donning ball cap, shades, and collecting my walking poles, I am ready! Liz's comprehensive approach ensures I feel heard and taken care of. She pieces me back together, Humpty Dumpty style. I am fortunate to count on her guidance. These professionals understand the situation, make a difference. For those with unseen illness and injuries, self-advocacy is essential. It's the only way I found my care team.

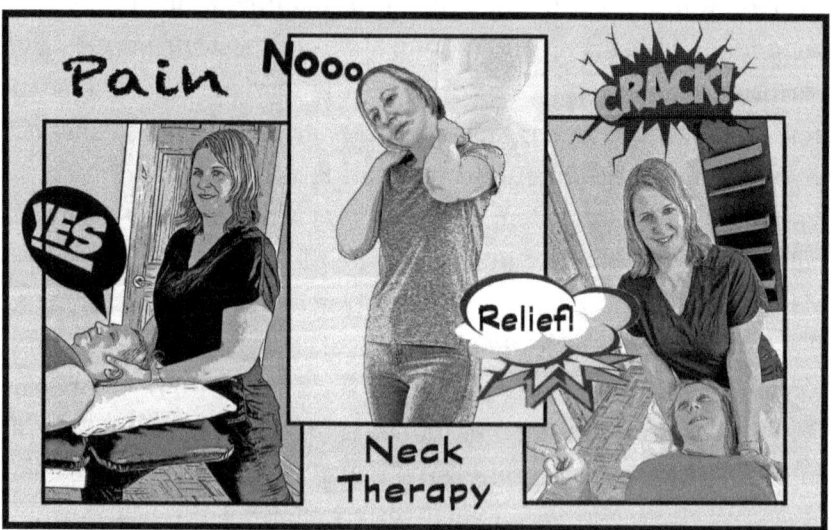

Two years after my accident, I discover dry needle therapy, so continual research and asking around is imperative.

"With post-concussion clients, trigger points of the trapezius and occipital muscles refer pain into the head, causing them to be symptomatic with headaches. A trigger point is an area of tight muscle that refers pain. Dry needling is an efficient, effective treatment which involves having acupuncture needles inserted into the trigger points, which are then pulsated to stimulate a twitch response that causes the muscle to relax." Liz van Zutphen, PT.

Dry needling is uncomfortable, but if the result is improvement, I will take it. Liz places needles near the base of my skull, top of my neck, along my spine, troublesome areas since my fall. The needles leave me achy, but I gain mobility.

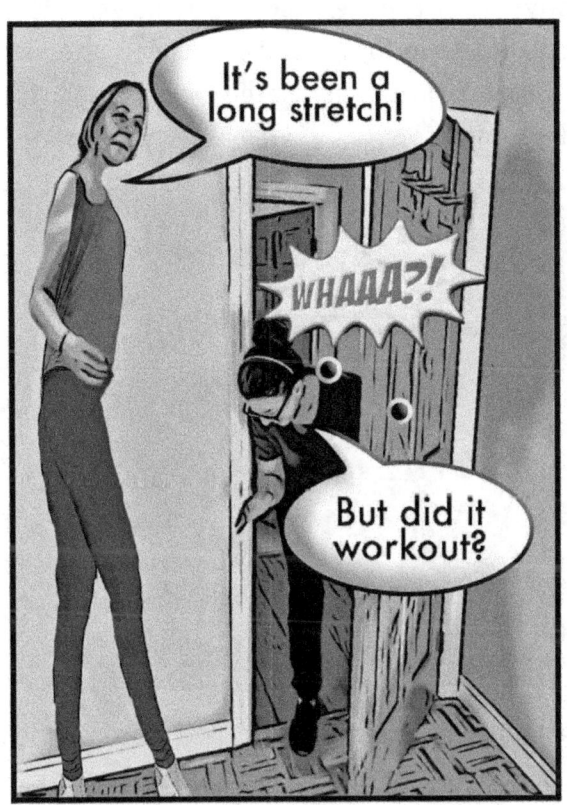

Massage Therapy

My shy, reserved, introverted self never thought she would enter-tain the idea of massage, but after hearing the benefits, it is worth a shot.

February 13, 2018

After weeks of internal argument, I swallow my pride, go for it. I shower and wash, scrubbing my body to prepare for whatever is to come. I avoid mirrors. First time in my life . . . drum roll, please . . . a massage! Yup! Shy, reserved me books a massage with Linda at Balance Physiotherapy. My nerves rattle. What to expect? A stranger is about to place her hands on my back, neck, shoulders. Can I run? My eyes sweep the table, white sheets, pillow. I keep my eyes down, want to run for the hills, consider a necessary step to recovering. Best take arms against the foe and rise to the occasion. Can I convince myself?

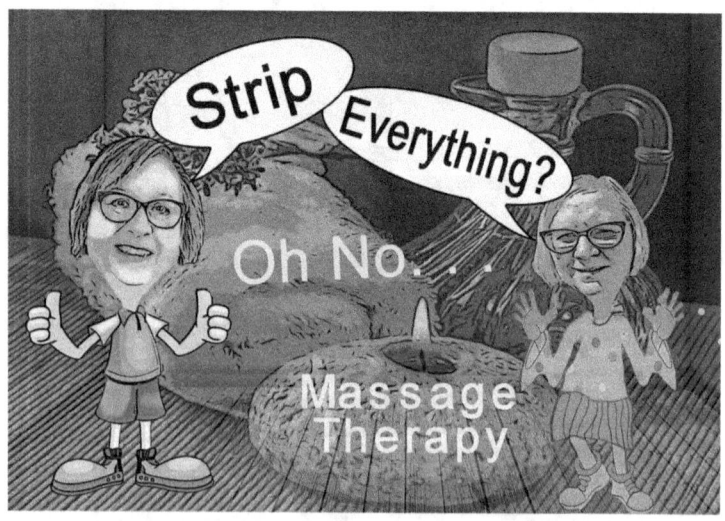

"Undress and slip under sheet." The words ricochet off the walls; my face blushes vermillion red. Linda leaves the room. Never have I ever. I lift, bend, squirrel under the sheet. My mind escapes to a beach, wind whispering, blowing my hair, I dive into fluid water, caressing my skin. Heart racing, I melt into the massage table, my eyes squeezed shut. The adventure begins. Linda has twenty-eight years of experience and knowledge. In our sessions, she takes charge of explaining massage therapy—the practice, its significance, and benefits it brings to clients. She wishes I saw her earlier—before my muscles healed improperly, formed scar tissue. Without referrals, I would not be here.

Within minutes of massage, I can dip my head down with less discomfort in my lower back. At that moment, she gains my trust. When she touches each knot, the pain radiates deep into connective tissues. Her fingers knead each one, screaming back in reluctance. Experiencing the pain, she explains, is beneficial. No pain—no gain. Whoever made up that *bleep-bleep* phrase? The discomfort is temporary as she loosens muscles. I control the intensity. The more she massages, more tension she releases. Because of fibro, I am more symptomatic than most.

"You must be in pain 24-7," she comments.

How can she know? My eyes fill, somebody GETS IT!

She explains. "A trigger point or knot in the muscle causes compression and irritation of the nerves exiting the spine. When irritated, nerves cause a protective spasm to the connected muscles, and trigger points develop with increased levels of biochemicals associated with inflammation and pain. You need lots of work. Many triggers and knots," she says.

Take it from a shy woman who stepped out of her comfort zone; people underestimate the benefits of massage.

Oh, the years of youth, my biggest challenge continues . . . getting through the claw.

February 14, 2018

Dr. Cudmore reassesses me in his clinic. He acknowledges my progress but says he cannot predict a return-to-work date, marks me off indefinitely. The hammer falls. I held off with Dr. Lok, fabricating hopeful dates. Now I have no choice. Despite my two-year battle, he assures me if things improve, I can return to teaching. It is a sad day, a major blow to my spirit. I cry for a week and then some, practise meditating to cope. I envision the twinkle of my deceased baby brother's brown eyes, a radiant smile cheering me as it did every day when I was a young girl and teenager. He wipes my tears. I will help others not feel alone in the world. Now more than ever, it is a mission, advocating for mental well-being, teaching mindfulness and self-realization. We must focus on mental health and suicide prevention if we are to win the battles related to an inability to cope and thrive, overcoming devastating mental and physical illness that lead to increased suicides.

Memory

"Out of suffering have emerged the strongest souls.
The most massive characters are seared with scars."

— Khalil Gibran

People say aging contributes to memory loss. But with a brain injury, it is more pronounced. A word or idea dissipates into nothingness. Since my mTBI, remembering recent events and day-to-day occurrences has been challenging. Short-term problems include forgetting details in conversation, where I left things, losing track, forgetting what I read or heard. I cannot remember appointments, arrive at incorrect times, disrupt schedules, forget what I intended to do. I write everything down, remember little unless cued. I struggle to retrieve correct information when needed, such as a name or word when talking, my past, almost entirely erased. Do not ask me to remember. I cannot multi-task. Is it memory or inability to pay attention? The latter is Jeniffer's suspicion.

After getting coffee in my Thermos, I wonder why it tastes different. Halfway finished, I realize it is water. I do not know which is worse; the fact I did not put the coffee in or that I did not realize until I was half-finished. Typical of me, but I am learning to laugh, otherwise I go under. When we are recovering from any injury, no matter how slow the progress, choosing to focus on centimetres or inches done each day is healthier than wallowing in self-pity attached to yards, miles, or kilometres not met.

I work on memory by repeating words, phrases, names, dates, but they refuse to stick. Recall is a deepening problem. Mid-air, I lose my train of thought and the lump in my belly grows. Please let it not become a worry. I search for a good show to watch, find the title, seconds later it disappears out the kitchen window, lost in the crab apple tree. Every time! Even if you tell me, I lose it. Grrr! I pray it gets better. If I watch or listen to an interesting show, I share with my husband. Retelling is an excellent tool. I play matching cards online. Developing strategies, such as jotting things down, is crucial. I watched my thirteen-year-old daughter do the same after her concussion. She and I always make lists, cross off as we complete each task. The experience carries with it a feeling of control, pivotal for those with head injury, as we constantly strive to regulate our brain and body. After she experienced a fall on that winter day, she started suffering migraines. She learned when they were about to hit by recognizing preceding auras.

Compensation Strategies to Help Memory

1. Get rid of distractions.
2. Ask others to speak slower.
3. Speak up.
4. Clarify.
5. Practise, repeat, rehearse.
6. Use organizers, schedules, calendars, to-do lists.

7. Write down and keep copies of phone numbers, pass-
    words, pins.
8. Keep important items in a specific spot. Tell someone.
9. Use a pill organizer or blister pack for medicine.
10. Use checklists.

Too often when we say, "I can't remember," folks add, "Happens
to me too." They want us to feel better, but it makes us feel worse.
It diminishes what we are going through. Please stop saying,
"Remember?" Or "Don't you remember? I told you that!" Those
words grate, nails on a chalkboard.

> If I forget, which I do within seconds, please do not remind
> me that I forgot. It makes me incredibly sad and reminds
> me of my difficulties. Instead, cue me, and the thought will
> come back. The best form of communication is direct, to
> the point, no extras. This allows the brain to work at its own
> pace instead of continuously trying to catch up and piggy-
> back thoughts which are more difficult when not our own.
> Talk slower. And please remember—body language speaks
> volumes, often reflecting a negative reaction. Let's be wary
> of the messages we send.

March 28, 2018

After a referral from Dr. Cudmore, I see Dr. Slater, a psychiatrist,
to be sure my injury did not generate further problems. Not going
to lie, leading up to the appointment, I was a bundle of nerves,
terrified he would conclude I had the same level of insanity as

Lewis Carroll's Mad Hatter or Cheshire Cat in *Alice's Adventures in Wonderland*. I too tumbled into a hole; my current life surreal. My husband showed kindness by coming with me. Visiting mental health professionals should not be scary. Trained to work with clients, they know what they are doing. Mental health is as crucial as physical.

Dr. Slater notices my stutter and gait. In his report, he states I am cheerful and display a sense of humour, which makes me happy. He remarks that my thinking processes are rational, my cognitive abilities unaffected. He notes that I clearly exhibit signs of post-concussion syndrome or what he previously termed post-traumatic brain syndrome, including the atypical emotional volatility and sensitivity with prominent irritability. Depression, he remarks, seems less severe than his usual encounters with PCS, resulting from the treatments, therapies, and exceptional care I receive. He finds no psychiatric conditions, advises me to keep with psychotherapy and to be sure to pace myself, noting the frustrations and difficulties of PCS, especially with my stuttering.

Around the same time, I have an assessment in speech therapy. Marlee writes, "My experience of working with Francene has been challenging and rewarding. She came to see me six months post-concussion. Speech-language pathology itself is a young field, and our understanding of neurogenic stuttering limited. We work through and adapt to traditional stuttering treatments. Although I have guided Francene in her recovery, she has taken it upon herself to adapt strategies, find new ones to best help her in her recovery. She has helped me better understand the value of client-centred care and the strength of working together. She continues to show her spirit and determination. I am lucky to call her a client and friend."

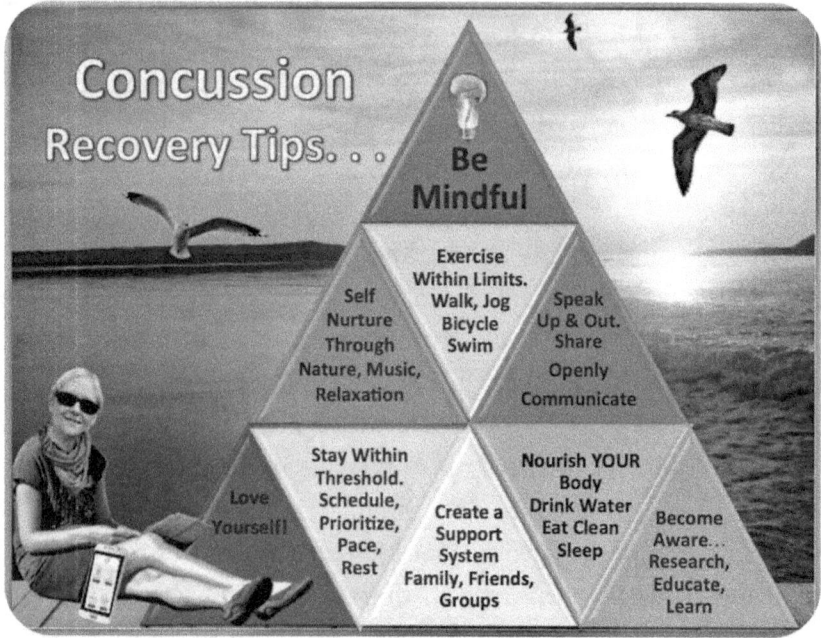

Concussion Recovery Tips...

Be Mindful

Self Nurture Through Nature, Music, Relaxation

Exercise Within Limits. Walk, Jog Bicycle Swim

Speak Up & Out. Share Openly Communicate

Love Yourself!

Stay Within Threshold. Schedule, Prioritize, Pace, Rest

Create a Support System Family, Friends, Groups

Nourish YOUR Body Drink Water Eat Clean Sleep

Become Aware... Research, Educate, Learn

For 2018, I continue going to Cathrine, Tanya, Marlee, Jeniffer, Liz, Dr. Mandelman, and Dr. Cudmore. Their friendliness and professionalism give me hope. Speaking of hope, my youngest daughter is expecting her second child in April, and we are beyond excited. I get approval from my doctor to fly with my husband to Edmonton. Nervous about flying I collect everything I need over months, pack in stages over weeks to cut down on becoming overwhelmed. I am best when I concentrate on one thing only. Hopeful, I think of how great it will be to fly; instead of focusing on what might go wrong, I envision what will go right. Feeling the push of the airplane taking off provides a sense of freedom as I escape two lost years, away from the world I once knew. In my glory I look down at giant, cotton balls below, a change in scenery what the doctor ordered.

Huge hugs all around, we anxiously await our second grandchild. April 30, 2018, Jack Robert Furlong joins our family. We are ecstatic. My daughter is a physiotherapist trained to help with any symptoms I experience. Although it is difficult to deal with the increase in stimuli, excitement of a newborn baby on my lap to cuddle and hug is the best therapy I could receive. The fresh scent of a bathed infant, cocooned in a blanket is the most wondrous feeling. Skin, the softness of petals, nothing like it. Papa and I fight over holding him. Aden loves his baby brother and us.

My body pays, some costs more than worth it. My grandbabies mean the world to me, as do my two daughters and sons-in-law. We are moving on up! My husband and I stay for a few weeks then fly back to our slower-paced Nova Scotia world and my therapies, eager for more progress. I feel like this might be a breakout year, as the practice and effects of strategies and techniques begin to show.

Scheduling

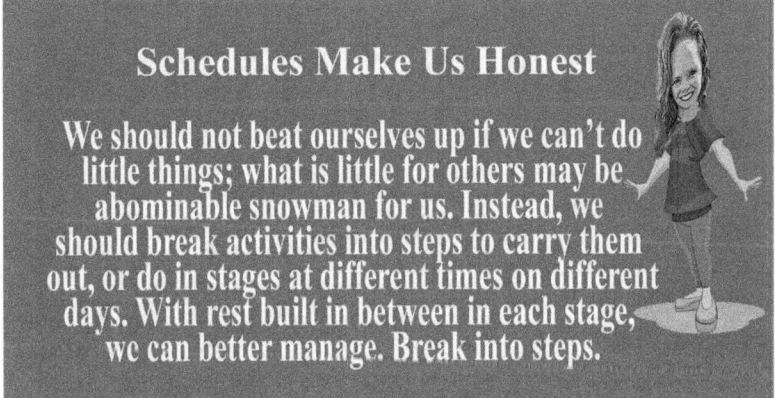

Schedules Make Us Honest

We should not beat ourselves up if we can't do little things; what is little for others may be abominable snowman for us. Instead, we should break activities into steps to carry them out, or do in stages at different times on different days. With rest built in between in each stage, we can better manage. Break into steps.

It is imperative to work within one's threshold—the level of activity endured before symptoms occur. Go overboard, pay the price. Figuring out one's threshold, my occupational therapist said, requires daily scheduling—tracking activities, breaking them into steps. The progress rapidly diminishes the sensation of inadequacy because I can conquer gradual steps. The learning process empowers me as I understand the level of involvement in the activity. Maybe I can throw self-chastisement away, as understanding crystallizes into improvements. Cooking dinner is not one activity, but a collection. Most activities are. When healthy, we take them for granted. When injured, the steps are no longer automatic but taxing. Breaking procedures into manageable units is crucial as is watching for the boomerang effect of doing too much at once. Scheduling provides insight, helps me avoid the boom-and-bust trap. It helps with cognition and setting goals but is exhausting and demands a pull-up-the-socks, no quitter attitude. I fight scheduling for a time, think it is too much work, discover how necessary it is.

May 2018

That time of year again. I receive my teaching assignment for September. Reading stirs upset; my duties without my input have me teaching new courses, a too-heavy schedule. I must let them know I will not be back, but hope to return sometime through the year, then I cry for a week.

June 2018

Not my fault! I dwell on substitutes filling my position. I want it back. I rarely missed a day. Storm days I worked catching up on lessons or correcting . . . loved/love teaching. I am deadwood. Brain fog, behemoth claw, and extreme fatigue pull me down as I attempt to balance, practise therapies, stall on the side of the mountain, enormous tree across the road. I need a break from everything.

July 2018—Boom & Bust

I stay within my threshold through summer but stop recording. Too tedious! I figure I can keep on top of activities without writing things down. Crash! Without a daily written reminder, I add too much. Symptoms escalate. The BOOM & BUST behemoth knocks me down. I cancel appointments, too sore, too fatigued, too anxious, too, too . . .

Later, I admit the benefits of a schedule, daily at first, then weekly, depending on symptoms and activities. They help keep us honest and aware. Therapists use them to gauge our next steps. Without a schedule, we Type A personalities bust. Every time. Yup . . . Type A. Lesson learned . . . maybe.

September 2018—Big Little Thing

Dr. Mandelman lowers my prisms, shifts the angles. My lens prescription changes. The reading glasses enlarge print, reduce strain. The distance glasses pull me to the right, compensate for the midline shift. Important I feel my heels and toes, so I do not flounder front or back. She expresses satisfaction with my improvement. Glimpses of the old me, heartening under the care of concussion experts, I smile. There is hope.

"Find magic in the little things, and the big things you always expected will start to show up."

— Isa Zapata

Thank you, dear therapists for making me smile during trying times. Kind acts are heartwarming to someone with a head injury. First small delight, after demanding work—the pleasant sensation of moist warmth on the back of my neck. Add acupuncture and that part of the body sings for fifteen to twenty minutes. A TENS machine helps aching muscles. I am ready for a bigger challenge.

It is September, a new school year starting without me. I want to be back seeing fresh faces. Lost without my kids. Can I curse? A roller coaster explains my feelings, attempts to return to life. Some days, I consider myself better until I get up. How fast I fall! My head throbs, full of thousands of ideas swimming and buzzing, I wake at 5:30 a.m. after a reoccurring nightmare of being fired under terrible conditions!

October 2018—Group Program, Antigonish Concussion Clinic

After months of therapy, my rehab team places me in a group program with other PCS patients. I am hopeful but concerned, familiar with activity stations, but not that they will be timed. In ten-minute intervals we are to finish one station then move to the next. So worked up I cannot concentrate or remember if it was blocks, puzzles, or step-ups. Senses on overload, sounds ricochet. The pace, rapid; I hold everyone back, time intervals too much pressure. I cannot finish the task in allotted time while others watch, wait, wonder. Inept. Do they stare at me? I cannot tell. A brick wall shuts me down. I struggle when asked to do activities involving crossovers—opposites, left and right. A fish out of water, I gasp, choke. How to do this? An inflated balloon with a tiny pinhole equates to a fatigued psyche . . . gradually losing air until deflated. I attempt the public program. I find it too challenging. I run away. Two hours takes a toll on mental energy; my insides squeeze water and tears as I race away from overstimulation, an intentionally noisy, distracting environment. I detest being last. Reaction rampant, trauma, rejection resurface, activate my nervous system, spins me down the rabbit hole. Jeniffer sees my upset, and we instead work in her office.

Next appointment, each group member rotates through the stations; therapists provide individualized activities. If I cannot keep pace with the group program, I must voice my concern. Best not keep things bottled inside. The rehabilitation team works with me, but I flounder, stomach in knots, heat burning my face. Too difficult; second attempt, I complete four of the adapted eight stations, feel lousy, last again, while others wait.

Determined to advance through stations designed for my areas of shortfalls, week two explodes. The noise level too high, even with earplugs. Lights too bright. I cannot perform the stages with time constraints, my energy level depleted from travelling and waking too early. A tempestuous storm brews, failure of the program constant on my mind from the week before. Inside the clinic, right at that moment, I have an emotional meltdown, filled with renewed ridicule, unable to speak my truth. Humbling. Awful! Jeniffer assures, it is not my fault, but PCS. I cannot handle the chaos, leave the clinic, walk outside to gain control. No one comes to check on me, assuming I left. With deep breaths and fresh air, I calm myself enough to go back in and apologize.

At home, I watch Dr. Phil challenge a young man to not let pain, hurt, destruction be his personal truth, to do what he can to turn his difficulties around. It makes sense. I must not let my personal truth be my injury. Waking next morning I am emotionally bankrupt, cannot stop ruminating. Tears stream. I want the floor to swallow me whole. Fibro flares, body pain draining energy as I try to deal with it and PCS symptoms. Too much pressure. A heavy, tall timber falls on top of me. I must speak up, hate confrontation. Stuck, I am closing in on a ridiculous three years. Will I make it?

January 2019—Snow Angel

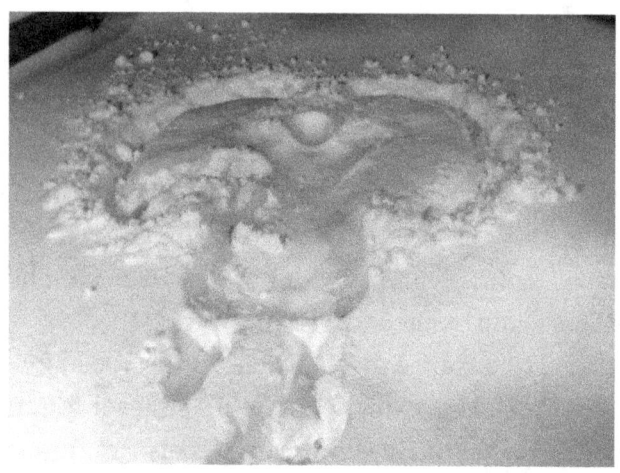

"No matter how bleak or menacing a situation may appear, it does not entirely own us. It can't take away our freedom to respond, our power to take action."

— Ryder Carroll, therapist,
"Resilience—bouncing back when facing adversity."

New Year's Day, a bizarre idea pops into my head. In a short-sleeved dress, bare feet, I step onto my snowy deck; the temperature, minus ten degrees Celsius. I manoeuvre into the drift, lay down, flap my arms up and down in two half-circles. Exhilarating. Liberating. I struggle to sit, attempt to stand. No go. Shivering like a chihuahua, I yell to my husband. At the patio glass doors, clown grin pasted—he points, mimes "locked." When good and cold, Bozo helps me up and into the house, laughing all the way.

I continue with my physiotherapy team in Inverness. They are excellent. Tanya works the knots in my neck, provides heat and acupuncture, gives me exercises to work my core muscles. An inchworm, I start again. Guess that means the only way I can go is UP! I rotate PT in Inverness and OT in Antigonish, PT in New Glasgow with counselling in Antigonish, visits to Dr. Cudmore with ones to Dr. Mandelman in Halifax. At the end of a busy week, I need rest. I beg doctors to let me return to work. No go! The brain needs to heal. Might carve that into my kitchen cupboard. Trevor Poirier replaces Liam as the Inverness physio assistant. I appreciate the gentle encouragement from my practitioners, their ability to put me at ease, even with my speech impediment.

To aim high, I must look after myself. I do basic activities and chores, vacuum, write, tidy, make sandwiches. Pace, pace, pace. I listen—fewer appointments more rest—much appreciated. Advice echoes, don't do everything at once, slowly work toward walks, household activities. I reduce flushes with a breeze blowing in my window or use a fan, take naps to rejuvenate. We control our reactions and our behaviour, but I struggle getting the concept to sink in. Regardless of the challenge, unfairness, illness, or injury—we control how we react. We have options: Wilt and resort to less desirable methods of coping or learn and transform lemons into lemonade. Words make the situation sound easier; we must respect that we do not all hit the same points at the same time.

None of us can be sure of the road we will travel, change unexpected, but we can choose, when able, how we crawl, walk, cycle, drive, or fly. I find reading or watching true stories helps me gain courage, fortitude, motivation. Success involves an open mindset. If we fall a thousand times, we rise a thousand and one. Rachelle Chapman's incredible documentary on TLC cable network is one of the first stories to wake me up. I observe captivated, immense admiration growing as I listen to this determined woman. What spunk and tenacity! In heartache growing up, I turned to inspirational books to pull me through. My rock! May her story, which I share later, provide motivation for anyone experiencing a long recovery from injury, illness, loss, and/or hopelessness.

With support (key to victory), we can rise above life's treacherous storms, however destructive. The body may suffer, but no one can rob us of our spirit. If we stay strong, use suggested tools, triumph is likely. We cannot change others, but we can change ourselves, influenced by our words and actions. If we do not try, we will never know our capabilities. I read my story when overwhelmed, a reminder to have a never-give-up attitude, to be grateful, recognize good people. I learn mountain loads, encourage healthy thoughts, recognize slips, try not to beat myself up, follow my own learnings.

February 2019—Wiggle Your Toes

I am eager to start fresh after my setback in the group. Once back in Antigonish, we alter my program, not yet ready to return to group activities. Even after I return from my oasis buried inside a mountain, pressure wraps my forehead; the cool breeze fluttering my hair in my face, sound of robins twittering outside my window, glorious heat of the sun my solace. I will arrive at my destination wherever that may be.

Jeniffer shows me a PowerPoint related to thought processes after head injury. Were they peeking in my window? Every slide causes pause. Amused, she reads the quotations, both of us knowing my doppelgänger rests plastered on the poster displaying damaging self-talk. No denying I had fallen into the blistering, feedback trap. Being aware is the first step. Isolation feeds harm, as does insecurity. Blame, shame, regret serve no purpose. It takes work to pull ourselves out of dark holes; we owe it to our loved ones and ourselves to navigate our world with sunshine eyes. Jeniffer—with her mighty duck, dynamo demeanour—gives me her raised eyebrow. I smile, body language speaking volumes. I must rephrase my words, stop inner voices. Jeniffer gives me a resource called TIC (Thinking Impeding Cognition) and TOC (Thinking Optimizing Cognition) created by the Canadian Back Institute (CBI). I observe how reasoning influences behaviour, I need to pay attention to my self-talk and interactions. "Tap into your creativity," Jeniffer says, "Wiggle your toes."

March 2019—Fancy Glasses

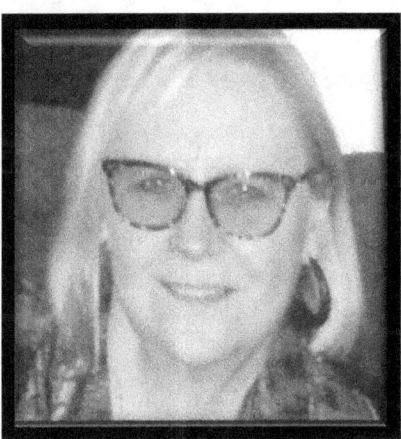

I see better with my fancy glasses; they cut the sun's glare. Before I had little depth perception. Wearing them, gives me a clearer sense of where I am in space; prescription sunglasses allow me to go out on bright days. I am pumped. We hope that by doing exercises, I will continue to restore visual function. I am ready for a new set of prisms. The estimated time for most people to identify improvement is three to six months. I enjoy my glasses. Three years out, I find differences with reading, text bigger, not as flat, or blurry. I cross my fingers. Dr. Mandelman has enough excitement for us both. We will see. An intentional pun? Not at all. Soon, I will drive; I can feel it in my bones.

Drum roll, please. I can read paragraphs, understand uncomplicated information, and research a little at a time! Complex text and complicated ideas, I syphon in baby steps as extra effort tires me within minutes, and the beastly pressure appears on my forehead, always appears when exuding extra effort. On my computer screen, the letters play with me. Sometimes sections of text are larger or smaller and shadows distract. Luckily, I can change font size so that is a good tip when vision is affected. I use the black background on my screen. If the font keeps playing tricks with my eyes, I stop, use visuals or a ruler to keep my spot, change font colour, or soften the background.

Spring/Summer 2019—Overload

Four appointments with my occupational therapist, four sessions with my ocular therapist, two trips to my physiotherapist, one for my speech, one to my psychologist, one to my concussion doctor, in two weeks! I cannot let my enthusiasm to be well sabotage my efforts. Peering back at the therapies and recommended exercises, the reason for my total fatigue becomes clear! Finally, I understand. Appointments are mentally draining, and putting me on overload. Faced with the dilemma of doing too much, I must weigh benefits against cost to my well-being. I speak to Dr. Cudmore. Finding a balance best for my circumstance is tricky. He suggests by paying close attention and listening to my body and symptoms, I will discover the answer.

Fall 2019—Through the Eyes of Others

Injuries take a toll on families. Be sure to find someone to confide in, share how you feel. I am too scared to share my true feelings with family or friends for fear of judgment; instead, I remain lonely and sad, tell my counsellor, but it is not the same. The perpetual idea of people judging is a dark shadow looking over my shoulder, an unwanted companion that causes immense shame, compounds feelings of low self-worth. I should be better, back in my classroom—should! Did the hit dislodge childhood trauma? The vivid green, red, brown leaf, once so exquisite and fascinating, blows perilously, at risk of blowing away. My goal is to be better, resume teaching, engage in life. I yearn for freedom, to sit and drive without constraints, like a bird in flight. Independent—no therapy, appointments, thresholds, schedules. Freedom! But I need medical help. If I push, juggle multiple activities, I hit a wall. Predictable, everything floods. Progress a slug's pace. I am ready to improve, but how?

My family is wary of changes in habits after my head injury. Shopping is no longer retail therapy, although I shop online. Not the best coping practice. I must get rid of physical, mental, emotional debris. Outside perspective helps me examine my situation in a new light. Those with concussions often perceive the world through the lens of physical pain, emotional hyper-reactivity, an obscured view. Through the eyes of others, we gain a wider lens, a beginning not an end. I reiterate, a crucial aspect to recovery— receiving prompt, proper treatment. Getting back to where we used to be takes time. I want to decrease the number of bruises from misjudging distance, a symptom I did not originally relate to concussion.

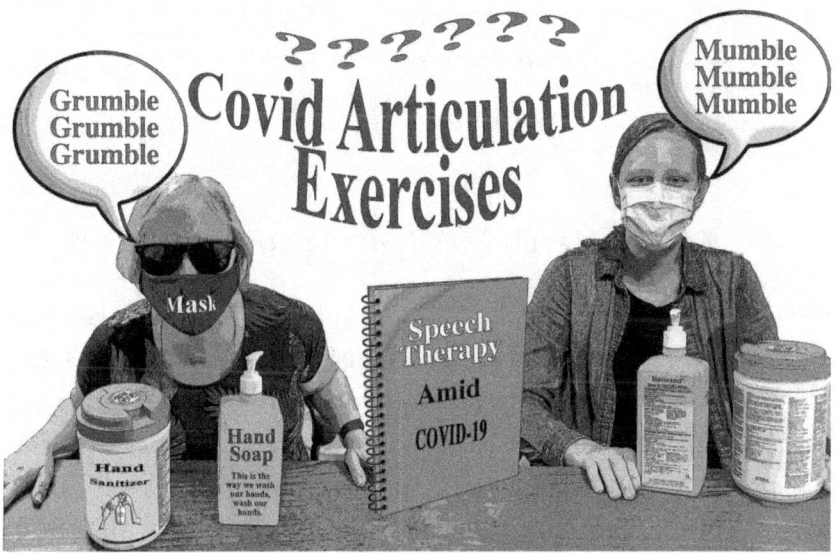

2020—Terror Strikes

With limitations comes fierce, tiger-striped inner dialogue, anger, frustration. A concussion startles and confounds, makes us believe we are inadequate. Getting help takes strength, but injury, sickness, and in 2020 a worldwide COVID-19 pandemic, complicates. Panic of the unknown strikes; hospitals fill, people die. Governments advise us to isolate at home, my injury minor in comparison. I hit a wall, stop. The root of my anger comes from outrageous expectations, which I do not reach, then frustration makes me irritable. Retrospective wisdom—my plan—look for the sunshine during distressful times. When I contemplate my snow angel, I take chances, expose myself to stimuli longer. I strive to coexist with myself, falter, but I am resolved that 2020 will witness faster growth, or am I setting myself up for a big fall?

"Isolation is aloneness that feels forced upon you, like a punishment. Solitude is aloneness you choose and embrace. I think great things can come out of solitude, out of going to a place where all is quiet except the beating of your heart."

— Jeanne Marie Laskas

March 2020—Isolation

It is disappointing to observe advances yet remain isolated during COVID-19 lockdown. My focus must be taking the strategies learned and putting them into action. Therapists stay in touch via phone; not the same. I miss the social aspect, affirming smiles, encouraging words. The habit of negative self-talk is hard to break. Stinking thinking—a term from AA (Alcoholics

Anonymous). My life closes in on me, shrinks because of the Beastie—as the stranded boys in William Golding's, *The Lord of The Flies,* refer to the invisible monster—that which they cannot see. Shrouded in ominous images, the lads are terrified. The visual representation of the thing remains unknown. Its name is fear or isolation, hours, days, weeks, months of post-concussion, PTSD, and COVID.

Increased isolation and discontinuation of office visits set me back. Hospitals no longer open to outpatients. My journeys to Inverness end as the hospital closes the PT unit. Tanya is such an exceptional physio, a home away from home. Liz V and her receptionist become cheerleaders; they take care of me. Liz continues multiple therapies. One of the best, we need more centres that offer multiple treatments like hers.

Exposure

I need more exposure, but COVID-19 and being isolated from loved ones does not help. I compare myself to before. How can I not? I begrudge the incident that shook my world, swaying, teetering in the wind.

> *"Anger is a wind which blows out*
> *the lamp of the mind."*
>
> — Robert Green Ingersoll.

I am well equipped after learning strategies to navigate frustration and fatigue. With adjustments, I handle sensory overload, revisit my own words when overwhelmed, practise my breathing to slow hyperactivity. Being aware of how we breathe allows us to calm ourselves, lower risk of reactions when at our threshold. Something so simple helps a nervous system gone awry.

April 2020—Humour & Breathing

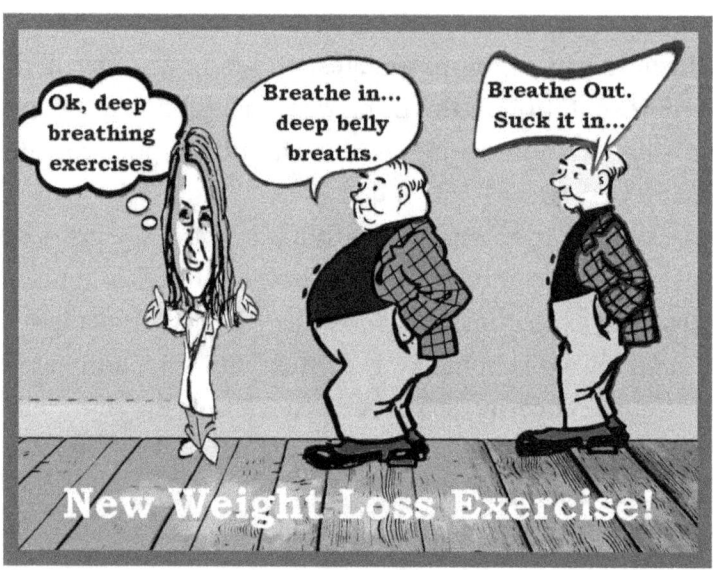

Humour sneaks in. I have a mischievous, lighthearted side few have seen. Might as well laugh at ourselves, better than crying. Please accept my humble attempts, but I realize the importance of it, even if it means watching reruns of *All in the Family*, *Everybody Loves Raymond*, or *Mr. Bean*. Humour is essential! Watching with friends or family provides even more laughter as the giggles of others are contagious. And playing board games can be a hoot! Life becomes easier when we learn to laugh at ourselves, not take our mistakes so seriously. I learn the hard way, am still learning. A dangerous battlefield, when bombarded with pain, we need to plant flowers and get out of our own way. And then, I find this gem posted on BrainLine from December 8, 2009. All BrainLine materials, including this, are a godsend. "Three-Minute Breathing Space: Use this quick meditation whenever you need to settle yourself into awareness of the present moment.

"Step 1: Becoming Aware. Try sitting up straight in a chair with feet resting on the ground if possible. Closing your eyes, bring your awareness to your inner experience. Ask yourself: What is my experience right now? What thoughts are going through the mind? What feelings are here? Are there any sensations of tightness or stiffness? Step 2: Gathering: As best you can, redirect your focus to your breathing. Feel the belly moving in and out, expanding as the breath flows in, and falling back when the breath flows out. Follow the breath all the way in, and all the way out, using the breath to anchor yourself in the present moment. Step 3: Expanding: Now breathe into the whole body so you are expanding your awareness. Sense your body. Breathe in and out, feeling the whole body rise and fall with each inhalation and exhalation. Feel the body. Take in your whole body and your facial expression. Just as it is."

Breathing helps to ground me, even if at first, I fight the weirdness. Fatigue cripples. Only when distracted or overloaded by sensory messages do I stagger, or if I move too fast. If I control my environment, I can function, but add people, sounds, bright lights, and overstimulation, like a candle I melt to the floor.

June 2020

Even as I write this, I am not sure if I shared this story—brain farts, lingering leftovers. At least I am aware. Difficult to pay attention and focus when someone talks to me. My mind blanks out at the worst times. I buy an item and go to pay but cannot remember my PIN, cruel when I cannot recall in front of strangers. Several times in a store, wrong PIN, my credit, or debit card declined, eyes burn into me as the cashier wonders about my financial situation. Flustered, I cannot remember the password or how to tap. She points it out. I cover my embarrassment. My brain, unable to multi-task, performs best in glorious silence. Some store clerks handle consumer confusion well, others not so much. After three tries of my PIN, I am locked out.

Silly things annoy—right or left, how to check voice mail, put car windows down, remember cold or hot tap, or replay a phone message. I hate saying the wrong word, uncanny, always with the correct first letter. Ask me a name I will say Bob for Billy or Mike for Mathew. Constantly I say mushroom for marshmallow. Even simple questions draw a blank. Am I a sorry, sad, country song, typical, atypical, or a few screws loose? I gain understanding. I would not have survived if my fall snatched my ability to write. With practice, practice, practice, I improve. Good to rant on paper. Keeping a journal helps self-awareness, a sense of purpose, as does designing visuals. Thousands suffer with PCS and mTBI (my official diagnosis), so why am I alone in my battles?

July 2020—Worth

With each unpleasant social experience, we cringe, consider not going out at all, play and replay our experience. I yell at my toothbrush, scream at my clothes, curse Alexa for not understanding me as she makes fun of my words with her crazy interpretation.

Then I go on a hour-long rampage of belittling myself for not being able to . . . I fall in a ball and sob myself to sleep. Storm clouds and torrential rains over the mountain, nightmare of someone chasing me, big black belt. Next morning, dragged through a rat hole, I try to hold my head up, turn 360 degrees in the kitchen, see if I can shake it off. Sometimes it works and sometimes I need someone to help. Do people exist to help disabled individuals regain independence? There are no practitioners or volunteers to come to my house. Phooey! Through these trials, I learn to find the light amidst pain. My family supports, cheers, reminds me it will get better, although I am not so sure. I choose how I respond if not taken off-guard, but it is damn hard. Another insight. I can slow my reaction by counting one to five if activated, lower the risk of saying or doing something not true to my nature. It works, unless over my threshold, or under 30 per cent energy level. More explanation on that later.

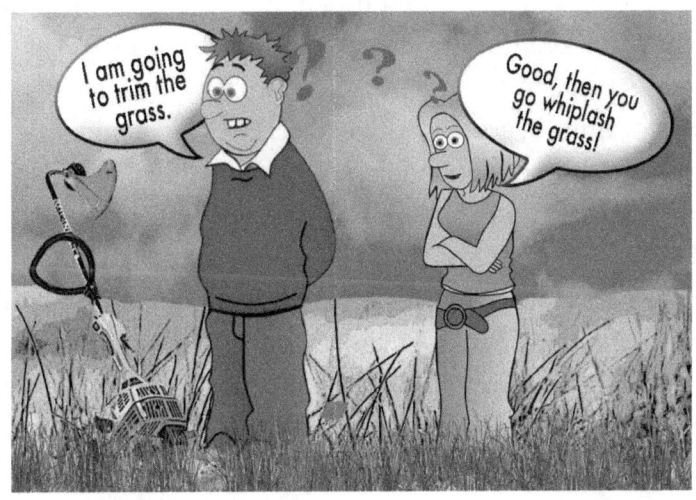

Am I the only one who ties my worth to what I can do? What a lethal word—Worth! What if I cannot do anything? Where would that leave me? Like Velcro, I attach it to everything. Is that why I struggle? Society places intense pressure and value on people's actions. What happens to those of us who cannot perform the way we used to? When we no longer contribute to our families, friends, work, community, or society, and flounder because we cannot keep up? What about relationships? How do we keep them when symptoms prevent visiting and reaching out because of unpredictability? How do we help others when we face challenges helping ourselves? Many families find it overwhelming. For the brain-injured left with residual symptoms, divorce rate is high. Another BrainLine resource called "Mindfulness, Meditation, and Prayer After Brain Injury," McDonough, Victoria Tilney Senior Editor, helps me see I am not a basket case.

McDonough shares the story of Melissa Felteau. All I can do is shake my head and cry.

"For almost six years after her car crash in 1993, Melissa Felteau spent much of her energy wanting things to differ from what they were . . . She would dream about her 'old' self, only to wake up a new, confused version of that self. Prior to her crash, when she sustained a traumatic brain injury (TBI), she had been a master swimmer, skier, and kayaker. She had held a top job as director of public relations for Lakehead Psychiatric Hospital in Ontario, Canada, and she had a robust social life. Little seemed out of reach. But after her crash—at age 31—she could not read or write. She had a tough time following conversations, and she could not get organized or remember anything. 'It was a long, slow, painful, depressing recovery,' she said. Worst of all, the mental chatter in her head would not quit. It was relentless—all the talking, criticizing, judging. 'The injury was devastating to my self-image. I told myself over and over that I was no longer loveable, that I was no longer good enough,' says Melissa."

I cannot control my sobs; someone besides me felt the cut of that "not good enough" derogatory phrase. Through watery eyes, I read. "'More than anything else, the brain injury left me with a residue of unworthiness—a deep soul wound. I was desperate to get back to myself, to find some kind of inspiration.' When a friend invited her to a yoga class to help with her persistent physical pain, she discovered meditation, felt a change immediately." (McDonough).

A light switch turns on as my tears saturate my pillow. I am not an anomaly. Who would have thought? In the article, McDonough discusses non-traditional treatments, and Melissa shares the incredible difference yoga made in her recovery. Bravo for her and much appreciation to her for sharing her story as we work to provide education and awareness. I am not alone. Others have felt it too, that deep slice of unworthiness. My new goal . . . lose weight, join a class, increase my steps, target that elusive recommended ten thousand steps a day. Oh my! I will start with one thousand, increase as I am ready, but I blow the entire outdoor walking season. Two rounds with COVID-19 set me back. I strive to reach an incredible five thousand, to get in shape for my grandchildren. Not where I want to be. God, give me the fortitude and physical strength.

August 2020—Surprise

Several mysterious packages filled with homemade soaps, candles, and sweet-smelling moisturizers appear on my front step. No name. No sign of the givers. I hear footsteps, start to cry at someone's thoughtfulness. Someone understands. Thank you. Small acts have massive effects. Another day I receive a pot of bright yellow mums; I had been suffering the boom-and-bust scenario. There can never be too much kindness.

Every night before sleep and morning upon waking I pray and express gratitude to the Supreme Being for life. I am on the delicate path of releasing pain and resentment. It is necessary to have peace about my fall, crucial to move forward. If I slip, slide, slump into a blanket of blahs, I perform a kind act, make sure to spread kindness, compliment, offer a smile, pat on the back. Is that selfish? It makes my spirit sing. We need more kindness in the world. If we each did one daily good deed, imagine the synergy we would generate. The ripple effect exploding, if we bring a smile, erase tears, lighten a load. We can afford encouragement. Everyone appreciates a goodwill gesture. It need not be big, but it is.

I fell today, bummed I did not have my glasses on, leaned left, down I went. Angry at myself. Grrr! I strain muscles, am sore, no broken bones. That is a break! No pun intended. I am on muscle relaxants heat or ice, which helps. I must be more careful. The symptoms hide within the functioning of the brain, fooling others and medical staff.

September 2020—Syntonic Phototherapy

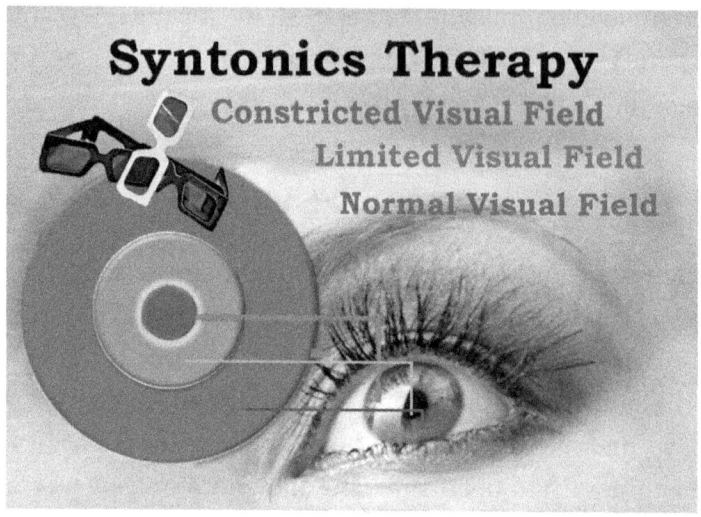

Word comes from Dr. Mandelman, I am ready for further therapy. "Syntonic phototherapy uses specific light colours, frequencies, and wavelengths to improve the body's regulatory centers in the brain. When light enters the eye, it travels through the brain to the pineal gland and hypothalamus—areas of the brain responsible for chemical and hormone balance. According to studies, applying light to these areas can stimulate the brain and help to restore the balance within the body's nervous system, thereby improving vision problems." (Lazarus, Dr. Russel, Dec 20, 2020).

I have an appointment in Bedford for my first round on September 12, running for eight weeks, trips every two weeks. A big commitment driving three-and-a-half hours one way, an overnight stay in a hotel, less than ideal for someone with fibro and PCS. Dr. Mandelman measures my peripheral vision; then I gaze into a coloured cone for twenty minutes, come home equipped with a halogen light bulb and plastic, coloured lens in a cardboard frame. For two weeks straight, every night through tinted glasses, I sit in darkness and gaze at the light. The violet colour soothes. Dr. Mandelman guides the colours throughout. If the therapy works, it will improve peripheral vision. Desperate to get back to school, I'll try anything. Will it be the difference?

November 2020

My rehab team root for me, but I feel discouraged when my best is not sufficient. I believe we do not know our best until pushed. Difficult to balance too little and too much. What works for one person may not work for another. I am on overload, another fall taking a toll. That feeling of dread just happens, rolls in like fog over the ocean.

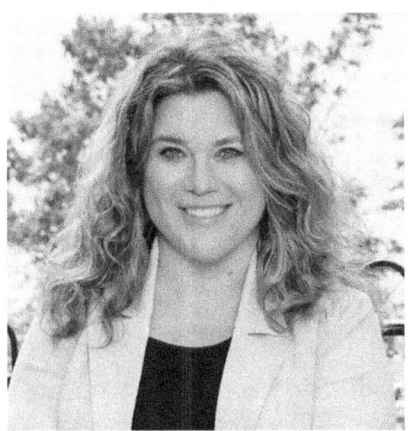

Dr. Erin Sheppard

Dr. Sheppard takes over Mandelman's practice working with TBI patients in 2020. I will meet her in 2021. In December, travel restrictions interfere with seeing my grandchildren for Christmas. Isolation leads to more struggle in dealing with the world's woes threatening to pull us down during challenging times.

January 2021—Moments

I only travel for appointments. Reliant on my husband to drive, is not fair to him. He never complains. I am the proverbial burden. He cooks, cleans because of me, although I now chip in making meals, vacuuming, changing bed linens. A start! But him having to do so much, rips me to shreds. Sorry for the pity party; it happens. Many things he cannot do because of me. Why can't I motivate myself? My goal to start each year anew, but I am reactive. A left-over plant, I wilt. No obvious reasons. Then I remember all I did; my fatigue makes perfect sense. I try to roll with the punches, do my best—without guilt, but it's a battle. So, I eat well, drink water, cross off lists, exercise, practise neuroplasticity, walk, and talk to someone. I am a one-second movie. Time for rest . . . Although the engine breaks down, radiator overheats, car has a flat, the scenery intrigues. Through my fascinating journey, I learn a tremendous amount about head injuries, whiplash, services available. I did not know. Most do not. In that, is purpose.

March 2021

In 2021, Dr. Cudmore closes his concussion clinic, remains a knowledgeable resource and consultant. A powerful advocate for the concussed and for concussion clinics, he worked with experts across Canada and the United States. A champion for the concussed, in his area of sports medicine, he advocated for the medically supervised team management model. His finger on the pulse of concussion, he referred patients to specialists focusing on specific areas of difficulty. Through his clinic other doctors received training. He stipulates the sooner treated, the better the outcome. We miss him. I would not have recovered without his guidance and expertise. I am lucky to have worked with him and Tara Sutherland, who along with her many credentials was an athletic therapist for thirty-one plus years, working at St. Francis Xavier University.

July 2021—Social Anxiety Disorder

Dr. Cudmore keeps seeing me until July, then officially releases me. I feel like I am losing my anchor; it is bittersweet. I will make him proud!

> *"Slow breathing is like an anchor in the midst of an emotional storm: the anchor won't make the storm go away, but it will hold you steady until it passes."*
>
> — Dr. Russ Harris

Social anxiety disorder is huge with stereotypes surrounding mental conditions and fears associated with a global pandemic. Fear and ignorance put people on edge, as do face masks and vaccines. It is a new beast. With invisible injuries, folks are judgmental, critical, with no knowledge of the impact of their ill-chosen words or actions. Most keep challenges unspoken, close to the heart, fearful of reprisals. We need to care enough to at least say, "Hi," or "How you doing?" People are more distant with COVID, a dangerous society shuts itself off, reason for the cautionary adage, "No person is an island."

Prior to my accident, I did not experience anxiety, but I had a healthy nervousness when doing a presentation or working in an unfamiliar environment with different people. That edginess kept me alert and on top of my game. With diligence, I aimed to articulate my thoughts and foster comprehension and connection. But after the fall, social anxiety is a new beast. Trying to handle multiple tasks, frays. Stressors added, I crumble. Need to calm down and be okay. I find reassurance in the stories of others, like Melissa's.

"Melissa Felteau's world, ten years later is still returning bit by bit . . . There were awkward moments when she cried at the slightest provocation or snapped at her assistant. 'I was overwhelmed,' Melissa confesses. 'I was having major problems and didn't want people to think I was stupid, so I stopped hanging around people from work.' Social engagements became opportunities for embarrassment and ridicule, causing Melissa terrible personal conflicts. She wanted to be out among the crowds, but simultaneously felt vulnerable and frightened by them. Melissa sank into long sulks and quiet withdrawals. The invitations stopped coming and the phone rarely rang. Of the sixty-five well-wishers, only one person remained a friend. On a visit to one doctor's office for her pain issues, she happened across literature on brain injury listing the wide-ranging side effects of brain injury: mood lability, agitation, poor attention, memory problems, coordination difficulties, and disorientation. 'I saw it and realized, 'Oh my god, this is what I have,' she says." (Mason, Michael Paul, 2009).

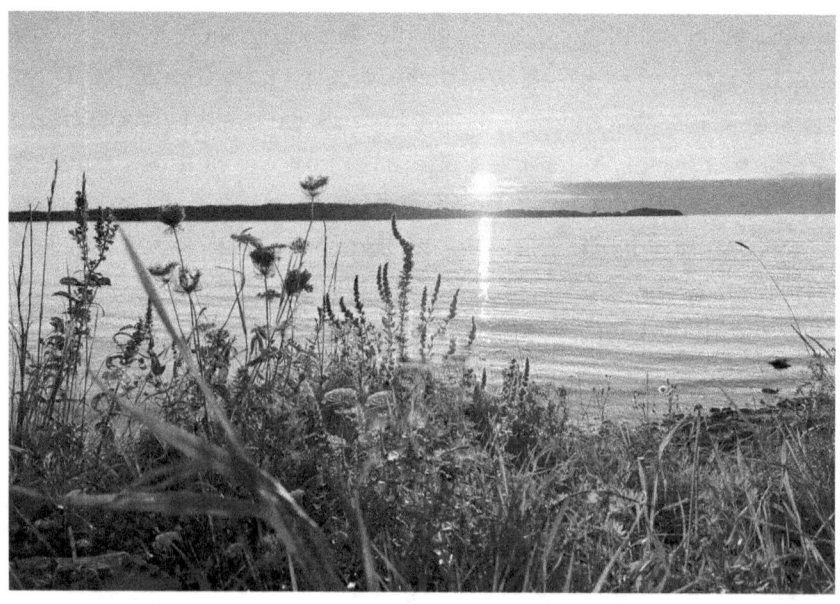

August 2021—Alexa to the Rescue

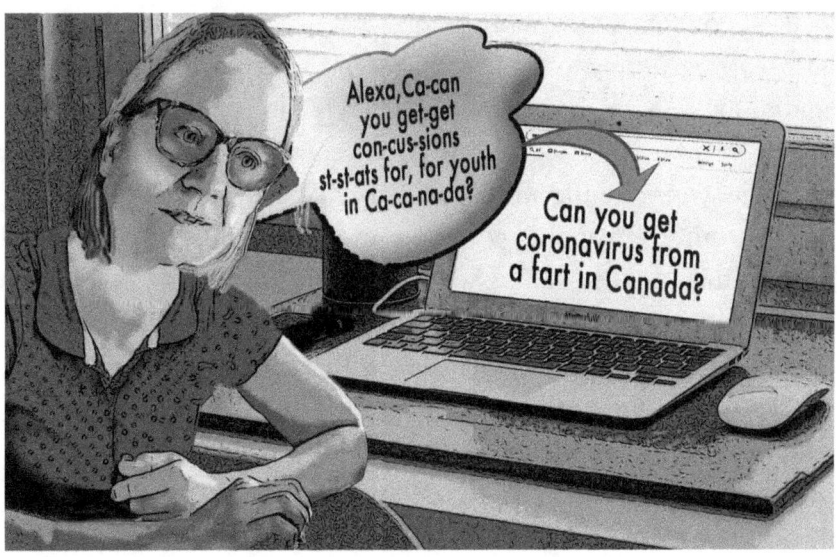

My speech pathologist and I discover Alexa and Siri can be useful in speech therapy. I practise, practise, practise; neither will respond to garble. It proves valuable and I begin to find it funny, instead of upsetting, as both misinterpret stumbling speech. I become more fluent starting in September 2021. I practise around the clock, no longer sounding syllables like a toddler, excited to stick with a new strategy. One identity stolen; another gets ready to emerge. Now, to carry out the steps, and head for the summit.

As the years edge farther away from my fall, so do my students. Although I think of them, those I taught are graduates of trade school and university; difficult to wrap my head around that. I miss them and my classroom, have not given up. If I had someone close to home to be a mentor, I would recover faster. My husband does more than his share. I would pay for a part-time companion to guide me into a healthier lifestyle, help me start my day, walk with me, show me healthy, easy recipes, urge me to do more, help me during fibro flare-ups, and hold me accountable. That heavy wall keeps me stuck. The result must be worth the mental effort of getting ready. To escape reality or what is too difficult, I create visuals, condense information for those of us challenged by text and reading. A suggestion from my optometrist to improve my spatial awareness, it makes me happy! The laptop rings at the fifteen-minute mark. I stop, refuel in silence, walk the house, move on. Relief comes in the word "will"—I *will* get better.

My family is my catalyst to do more. I want to chase after my grandbabies as they look back in gleeful playfulness. Exploring nature with them, seeing the world through their eyes, allows me to appreciate never-ending wonder, embrace the gift of others.

The Betty Clooney Foundation for Persons with Brain Injury created an excellent behavioural chart for people with mental difficulties and/or head injuries, used with permission. I feel a sense of comfort knowing why my brain is so reactive (https://www. facebook.com/BettyClooneyCenter).

Behavioural problems of people with traumatic brain injury, TBI complicate recovery. The list of behavioural dysfunction ranges from mood swings, depression, and hyperactivity to aggression, sexual inappropriateness, and elopement (running away). Even lack of activity or lack of initiation, can be a behavioural problem. In addition, psychological reactions to trauma, traumatic brain injury as well as predisposition to psychiatric abnormalities can be factors in behaviour complications. The locus of the traumatic brain injury is a key predictor of behaviour problems as shown in the diagram. Adapted by Francene Gillis with permission from the Betty Clooney Foundation for Persons with Brain Injury.

Frontal Lobe

(Behind Forehead)

Injury can cause changes in emotional control, initiation, motivation, inhibition, frustration, aggressive behaviour. Promiscuity or lethargy. Injury may lead to inability to plan a sequence of complex movements to complete multi-stepped tasks.

Cerebral Cortex
(Gray Matter)

Layer of cells on the outer surface of the cerebral lobes. A diffuse impact injury, such as a vehicular accident where the head is subjected to rapid, forceful movement, can impact the brain's ability to process emotions and behaviour.

Cerebellum

(Base of Skull)

Loss of ability to coordinate fine movement, ability to walk, reach out and grab objects

Temporal Lobe

(Side of head above ears)

Aggression is typically unprovoked and very abrupt. Damage causes long-term and short-term memory loss, difficulty in learning. Right lobe can cause persistent talking

Parietal Lobe

(Near Back/Top of Head)

Processes body information. Damage impairs ability to identify objects by touch, Causes clumsiness, inability to draw/follow maps, give directions

Limbic System

(Deep Inside The Brain)

Damage here distorts emotions, physical desires, difficulty with organization, perception of environment, problems with balance and movement. Can cause breathing difficulty

Occipital Lobe

(Located Posteral End of cortex)

Vision. Damage can cause blindness, difficulty locating objects, colours, recognize words, difficulties reading and writing, produce hallucinations

Behavioural Problems Of TBI

Adapted from the Betty Clooney Foundation for People with Brain Injuries

Success

I did it, figured out a problem on my husband's laptop! My brain works. It took hours of thinking and pacing, but I did it. First woman on the moon, baby! First time in years I did something productive. A turning point. If I take things slow, pay attention to body signals, pace properly, I might beat, no surpass, this beast. High-fives to everyone who accomplishes a challenging task! Power to you, and to me. I would inject an emoji if I knew how. Not yet! That too a good mantra. I need to accept the new me, rede-fine myself. I have big plans to get more support. The summit is within view.

I am over the moon. Ready to drive. Eureka. Pumped. My husband sits in the passenger seat, neither of us knowing what to expect. It is a welcome, cloudy day. After familiarizing myself with the car features, I turn and drive for fifteen minutes in a parking lot, feels great, no issues. To be cautious, I only get behind the wheel when within my threshold. I may have slowed, taken a different road, but I learn, grow. Head hitting pavement from a standing position can do that to a person. Hard way to knock sense into me! Not sure it did. I drive modest distances, for short periods of time.

Dwelling on an injury or what one cannot do puts emotions in a state of disorder. I am fortunate in Nova Scotia to have experts available to me, albeit far in distance. Missed initially, many people deal with a concussion on their own, confused when days or weeks later symptoms appear. As the clock ticks, I fear permanent deficit, feel sick reading of people years out with issues. When I fell, I was fifty-seven years old, had pre-existing conditions, exasperated by injury. Fatigue and pain remain a formidable brick wall.

Enough said. Let me see the ocean, its gentle fluidity, an ongo-ing process. Do not go there! I learned oodles along the twists, hills, valleys, treacherous hairpin turns edging out of ragged cliffs, falling to the Atlantic below. I must accept the new me and move forward, embark on the next stage of my recovery and life. Grateful, I am, for my lessons, although acceptance a thorn in my side.

Candid Camera

Wow! I cannot believe it, yet I can. During the heat wave of August, my younger sister packs me up and takes me to the beach at Murphy's Pond. To my absolute delight, stairs poke out of the path. My sister provides a chair, and any necessities, so I am content, disguised in my big, rimmed sun hat and dark glasses, sitting Hollywood style.

After about fifteen minutes, she says she is going to swim. I have a choice. Stay in or out? I follow, do not bring my walking poles with me to manoeuvre the sand. Do not realize I need them. We wade in, knee-deep, then out to hip level. I focus on the sky. I am in heaven after longing to swim for five years. Incredibly relaxing. She dips. No, sorry, she does not. Cannot remember the sequence, preoccupied with a slight current. Something nibbles my foot, a lobster or crab, and forgetting myself, I jump, lose my balance. I fly through the air like a flying trapeze, collapse backwards floundering in hip-high water trying to keep my face above the surface, hands and arms swirling helicopter blades. A not-so-graceful acrobatic dance, with my extended arm I search for the bottom to steady myself, provide a solid hold as I try to breathe as water spills over my face. I furiously bicycle my legs backwards underwater, trying to get my balance, the current moving me in chaotic circles—It is worth the price of admission. No risk of drowning, my sister laughs and laughs; I do not blame her one bit. Head over heels, ass over teakettle in water, quite the jolly scene. What a re-introduction to swimming! A classic blooper moment. Candid Camera! I am glad she does not film and share on Facebook. Once I get my bearings, we spend twenty minutes swimming in the water under cloudy skies. It is divine,

awakening a childhood memory of grabbing a bathing suit, rushing off to the ocean, diving in. I am pleased I not only get to the
beach, but I duck in the salt water that has been screaming invitations since the summer I fell.

That excursion ignites a flame snuffed out. Getting ready is the
hardest. Easier to prepare one day, grab and go the next, my sister's wise suggestion. She has a lot of them. Less than five minutes
away, the next day I drive, make my way solo to the Port Hood
Breakwater Beach, love of my childhood. First time in five years,
after those, lonely, envious long, hot days, weeks, months, years
of looking out my back door, wishing. And I make the best of it
floating, eyes closed, on top of the water, on top of the world.

The weather holds a smile, and the next day, my spirit flying
high I swim again. It feels fantastic, improvements showing themselves. I am uncomfortable in my straw sun hat, dark glasses, and
walking sticks. People, I am sure, wonder about the quirky woman,
but the hug of the ocean outweighs any judgment of extra weight,
COVID-19 rolls, or brain injury leftovers . . .

I figure out strategies to minimize the risk of headache and
forehead pressure from the glare, back-and-forth movement of the
water. I shuffle backwards using my poles to better manage and
navigate while trying to keep my balance. Too long a walk at low
tide, I watch for high, keep my eyes on land, and the sun worship-
pers nestled in warmth. So how do I do? I struggle to get in and
out. The process of collecting my belongings tires. By the time I hit
the path, I am depleted, need to stop and rest.

I cherish where I live, I love my beach. Even when despised
after Frankie's drowning, it pulled me back. I am content knowing
when I pass, I will be in Saint Peters' Parish Cemetery overlooking
the island and ocean I stared at most every day of my life. It is in
my veins. Armed with walking poles, a brick constitution, I try to
swim more often. Practise. Practise. Practise. Neuroplasticity! It
will get easier with a stiff upper lip, pacing, pacing, pacing, and

an outlook of possibility. I am in a good place. "Synapses among excitatory neurons begin to form new circuits within seconds of the events to be remembered . . . neurons that fire together, wire together." (Kennedy, Mary B. 2013)

Eating Properly—September/October 2021

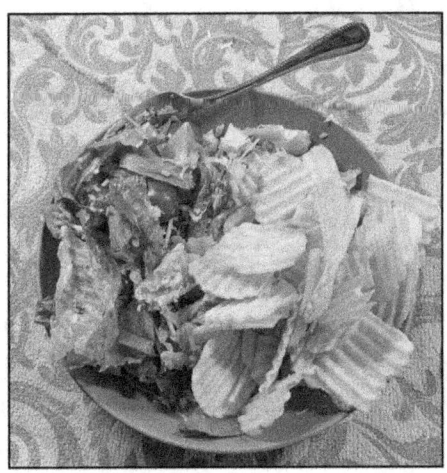

Yes! That photograph reflects my battle with food, convenience, and junk versus healthy eating. I love salads and vegetables, but preparation is a chore. Sad, I am being honest; please do not judge me. Going in public requires more energy than I have. For five years, I do not visit my local grocery. Brightness and dense shelves make searching for items too difficult. My husband grocery shops and is his mother's son with meals.

No sense in recreating the wheel. Excellent guidelines exist, like Canada's Food Guide (food-guide.canada.ca). Following them is difficult. Convenience reigns supreme. Bottom line—when you feel rotten, you care less. Handing over the role of chief bottle washer to my husband does not make me feel good. I beat myself up, even though he claims it is no problem. Wasn't I nice to give him the opportunity to learn to cook?

I help wherever I can. We try a meal delivery plan, enjoy the meals, a generous gift from our daughter—much appreciated. The Internet explodes with companies offering affordable meals. Junk food my nemesis, impossible to open chips, not eat the entire bag. I curl and hide, snacking, crunching. Experts say we are what we eat. Guilt oozes, as clothing sizes mock; rolls of flesh form spare tires. Hmm. Only solace is food. How can I lose weight if exercising puts me in a fibro flare? We become experts at excuse. You know what I am talking about. I would, if I could, but I can't. I try to watch what I eat, fruit and veggies every day, but that lasts a brief time, comes in cycles. I am a yo-yo.

November/December 2021

Mentally, I keep a food diary, track my eating habits, necessary for me to change and increase my energy. So why is it hard? Does seeing my reality on paper point to laziness? Am I? Inadequacy? I cannot even get my diet right. Why? Is it because of the underlying blame in the slogan, "We Are What We Eat"? Damn. After re-reading this section, I must stop making excuses, improve my diet, improve well-being. No more ifs, ands, or buts about it. Health comes first, directly connected to food and healthy choices. I pray I find the culprit that holds me back.

Studies show for many people five smaller meals are better than three bigger, skipping my response to the overwhelming preparation involved. I recall Jeniffer's reminders that cooking involves many steps, too many for me at once. I get everything ready the evening before. The secret to eating better—KEEP JUNK FOOD OUT OF THE HOUSE!

January 2022—Return to Possibilities

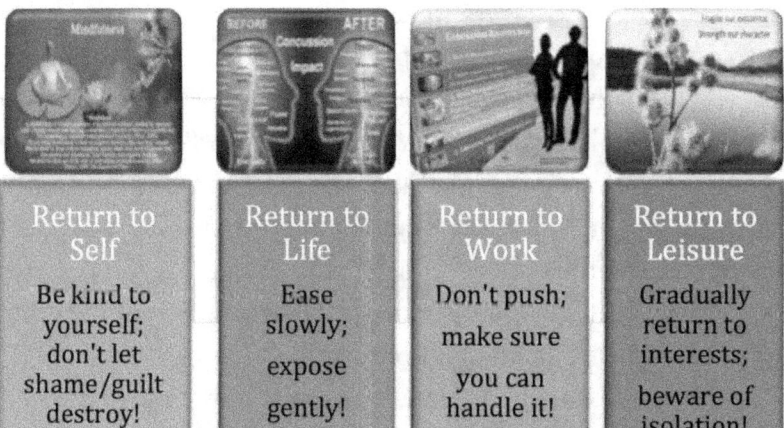

Return to Self	Return to Life	Return to Work	Return to Leisure
Be kind to yourself; don't let shame/guilt destroy!	Ease slowly; expose gently!	Don't push; make sure you can handle it!	Gradually return to interests; beware of isolation!

My speech therapy, continuous practice with Alexa, and dictation of my columns pays off—my speech becoming more fluent, only stuttering when tired or excited. With dictation I have to go back to correct countless mistakes, which adds time to the task but is good therapy for my brain. It helps my self-confidence even if a long way to go. My creative work comes more easily as my vision and brain function improve. I find comfort in being creative in quietness, work on self-nurturing as I climb through a dark, dreary, dense fog. A curious entity this beast, writing ingrained over years of practice. I have difficulty reading books, but I can read my work on the computer by adjusting the screen. Changing the background colour, and the font size helps. Black, blue, or purple the most soothing. I understand chunks of information in a silent environment. Filtering is a challenge. Isolation and loneliness engulf. I cry. Inch by inch, row by row like in Mallett's "Garden Song." I learn lonely is not a place you stay, but a place you walk through.

February 2022—Silly String

I will get where I need to go—a new mantra. Talking to others, consoles. They understand, experience similar grief, frustration. How can someone be absent from work for years because of a head injury and whiplash? Too many variables with PCS, PTSD, fibromyalgia, chronic pain, and fatigue. Disheartening. The silly string analogy comes back; I need release from a pressurized can. Colours fly everywhere, mismatched, faster and farther, represent nerve cells, fibres, electrical impulses needed for brain function. Difficult to gather, sort, stretch for communication and renewed function.

I still mute ads on television, look away, close my eyes because a gorilla squeezes my head. My OT recommended watching television as therapy. I do not feel productive until I assess my day and compare it to previous months. Therapies are helping. Creating lists of my day's intentions and checking them off prevents overload. I plaster quotations on my computer and around the house, read short, inspirational stories, find websites, self-help books, take responsibility for my wellness. When questions surface, I educate those around me. If screens or text bring on headaches, I ask someone else do the digging, read, provide a summary. My husband is excellent at finding information.

On bad days, I find quotations and strategies to help with residual symptoms, remind myself how far I have come. There is hope and sometimes transformation when hope seems lost. The gas tank analogy works—a full tank of fuel for the day. Other analogies include a $100 bill, coins, spoons. Once gone, time for rest and refuelling. Pacing requires keeping track. Even when we assume we are not using energy, we are.

March 2022—My Hickory Wagon Wheel

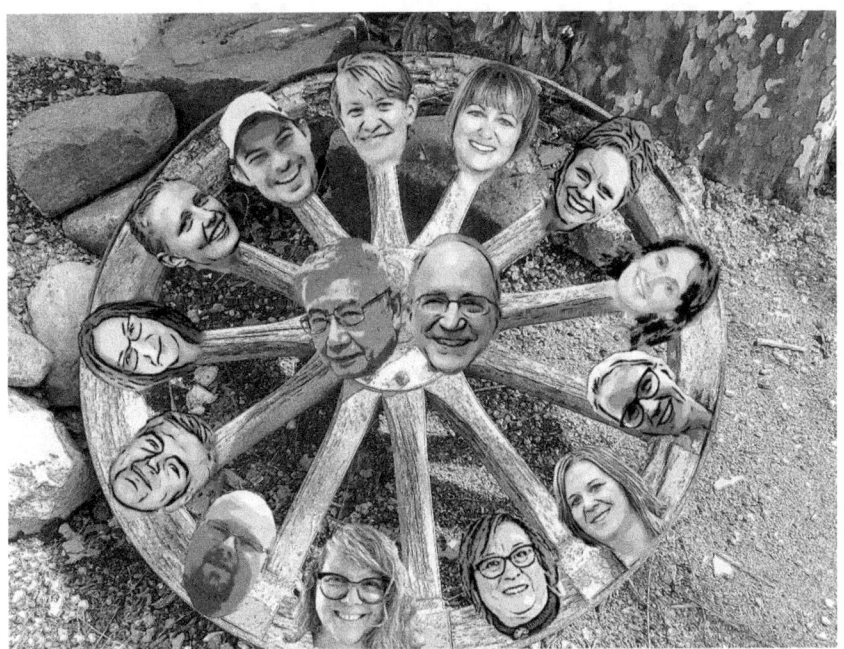

**Clockwise: Dr. Mandelman, Jeniffer, Shannon, Liz MD, Liz vZ,
Linda, Cathrine, Trevor, Sandy, Wendy, Marlee, Liam, Tanya
Center fulcrums & captains: Dr. Raymond Lok, Dr. David Cudmore**

Indulge me! I was isolated. My capable rehabilitation team grows from my desperation to get back to teaching and to move onward and upward. Spokes include doctors, physiotherapists, a psychologist, occupational therapist, speech pathologist, optometrist specializing in head injuries and post-traumatic eye injury, and my husband as he carried me through those tumultuous years and journeyed with me.

On days without appointments, I wake mindful, take time to ground myself, get my bearings. I make coffee or tea, sometimes a combination, wash up, exertion depleting the gas tank. Laying items out the night before removes morning pressure; times I am

too tired to do even that, and I cry. Am I slipping, symptoms inten-
sifying? Mornings have me overwhelmed before a mountain, melting into a puddle. A typical day has me checking messages, going
online to browse, walking around the inside of the house. I rework
old writings to keep sane, writing new material not yet possible.
Must let it go . . . I know what I must do, cannot get there. Why?
I cry in silence, begging the echoes to reach the Great Oz. In constant war with myself about returning to work, not able to handle a
classroom cuts—a serrated blade slicing flesh, drawing blood.

April 2022—Return to Self

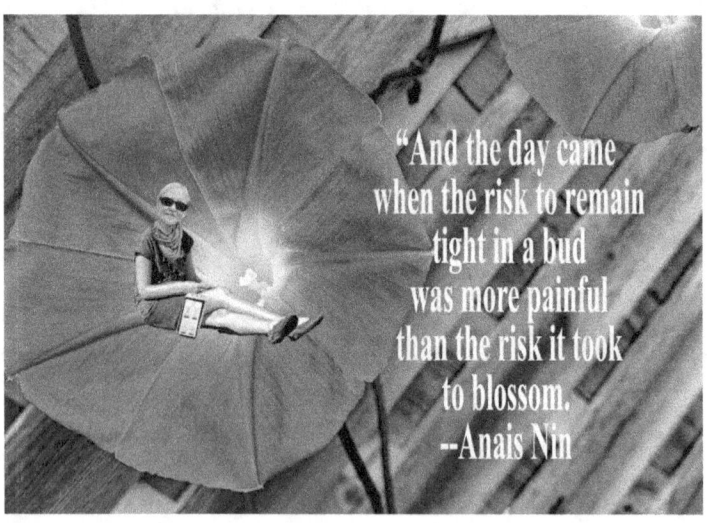

"And the day came
when the risk to remain
tight in a bud
was more painful
than the risk it took
to blossom.
--Anais Nin

"If you are always trying to be normal
you will never know how amazing you can be."

— Maya Angelou.

Return to self . . . requires implementing relaxation techniques. A
hardcore workalcoholic and perfectionist, I fall overboard, know it
is detrimental. The exposure involves risk, stepping out of comfort
zone—going beyond to match activities with capacities, staying

within safe thresholds. To proceed, I must be wary of four aspects: starting point, when symptoms arise, duration of rest, level of exertion. Self-care, life, leisure, mimic the skills and strategies we need. Thanks, Jeniffer, my encyclopedia!

May 2022—Return to Life

Since I fell, isolation is my reality; COVID-19 exacerbating it. Today, it is all about pacing and caution. I cringe at the thought of falling, refuse to let that hold me back. Whether skinned, bleeding, or burned, I must persevere, run errands, go grocery shopping, hang out laundry, visit friends, believe in the possibility of *normality*. A little at a time, I expose myself to noise, lights, crowds, stores, multiple conversations. Soon I will be ready to try activities requiring steps and stages, more complex thinking and exertion.

Return to work? The thought has me petrified; I know what is involved in teaching high school English Language Arts, times five days a week, one hundred students, administrative responsibilities, obligations, lesson planning, massive correcting, constant interruptions, questions, student and parental issues. The sentence alone, overwhelms. Potential images and fears bring on the claw and headache. I am not where I need to be.

My daughter tells me I am only 40 per cent of where I was before my head injury. I get emotional when I think of the job I can no longer do. My passion was robbed. To have that taken away slices me open. Tears flood. So effing unfair. I soon have to go off disability, return, or retire. Thank God I have my column, which I write weekly for *The Inverness Oran*. Sometimes I recreate old ones written over the past thirty years, use them as a stepping stone to a current view of the topic. I can space writing my column over a week, which I used to do in a morning. I am grateful such a fine newspaper kept me on.

Silence and darkness are my best friends. When I undertake any demanding task, I work in silence and break it down into stages. I write more with each sitting, which shows recovery. That excites me. I hope to regain my abilities soon, but now, I must concentrate on getting fit. For those with no choice in returning to work before ready, ask your boss and colleagues for adaptations, control your environment, take brief breaks away from busyness, and speak up for what you need to be productive.

June 2022—Return to Leisure

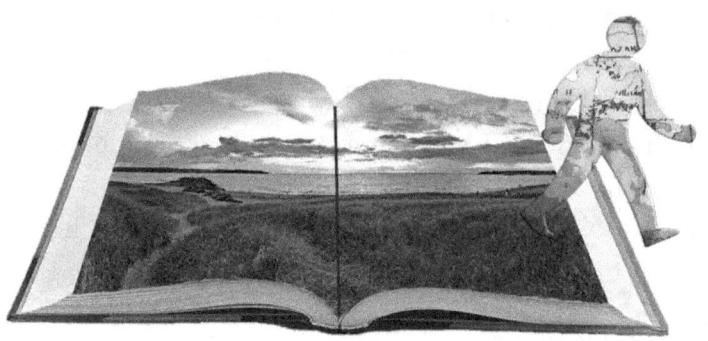

I am more physically active, exercising, stretching, walking. I try to keep within my boundaries with a goal to increase intensity, determined by my ability to tolerate levels set. Other goals in leisure activities include listening to instrumental, soothing music, watching television, movies, walking, and, please, God—more driving. I yearn for that freedom. I want to attend a concert, watch a movie in a theatre, take in festivals. Dreams on the back burner. Goals involve re-entering life, but planning is hard because of unpredictability. Whenever I plan something, the headache, pain, or fatigue might ruin it. If I follow the advice of experts, I have a fighting chance, if I do not give up on myself. One of the worst battles in this post-concussion war—losing passion, livelihood, ability to do what once came so easily. Even if in increments, I must look for the sunshine. I am losing touch with students and school. My world is snail-small, although my speech is improving, my eyes happy, I manage tinnitus and PCS symptoms. Another school year winds down. I struggle with frustration, sadness, anger. They no longer send teacher assignments. Retaining information remains a challenge. I say and do dumb things. Nightmares flood like the Atlantic Ocean during a storm. Night after night I deal with chaos around my inability to teach, monsters chase me. No one understands my words. Dark lessons morph into horrific situations. I fall into a deep chasm, struggling to hang on. Dozens of nightmares spiral in vivid detail and animation. I wake soaked in sweat.

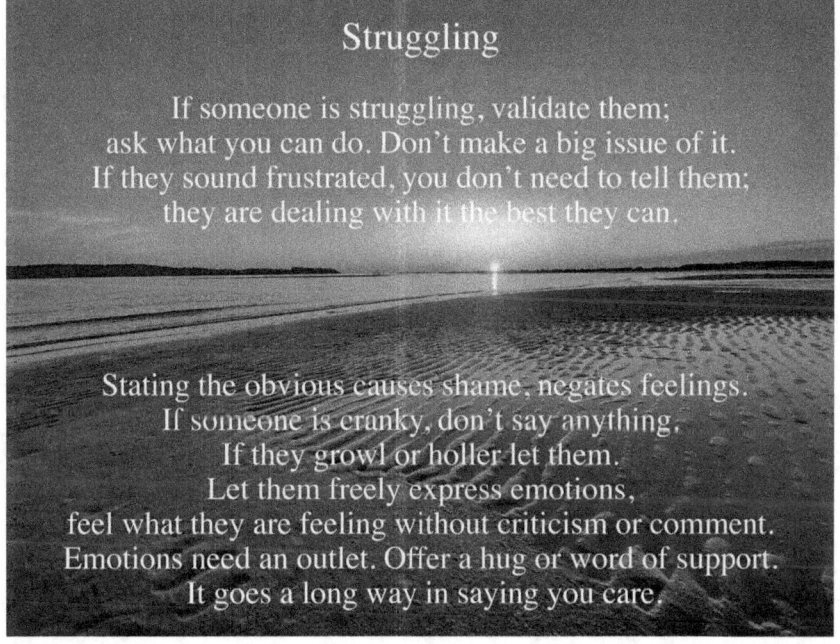

Struggling

If someone is struggling, validate them;
ask what you can do. Don't make a big issue of it.
If they sound frustrated, you don't need to tell them;
they are dealing with it the best they can.

Stating the obvious causes shame, negates feelings.
If someone is cranky, don't say anything.
If they growl or holler let them.
Let them freely express emotions,
feel what they are feeling without criticism or comment.
Emotions need an outlet. Offer a hug or word of support.
It goes a long way in saying you care.

July 2022—Reinjured

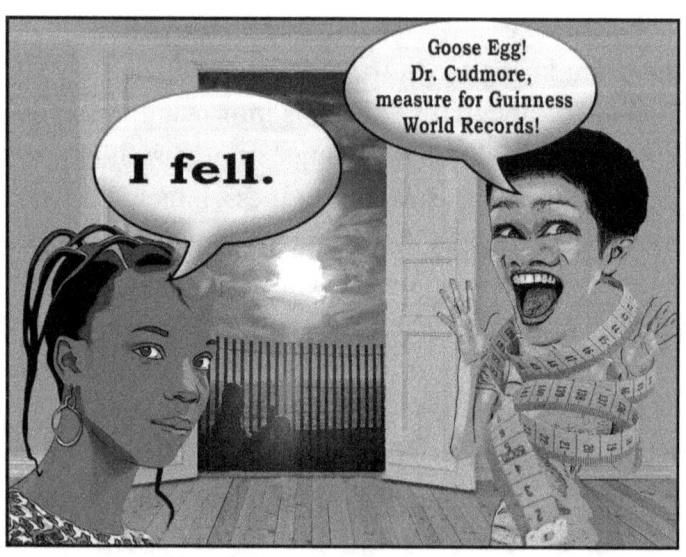

Walking and talking at the same time causes balance issues. If I get excited and forget, I stumble. On a hot, summer day, I smoke my head on pavement on the way into a local restaurant, fall headfirst, onto my knee and then my forehead smacks the pavement, stuns me for a minute or two. Damn, not again. Thankfully, I do not lose consciousness. I cannot drive home, so I sit on a bench outside as an immediate goose egg grows. The owners urge me to go to hospital. Instead, my husband picks me up. I consider going to outpatients but feel I know what to do; doctors would only prescribe the same care. I rest, thrown off a bit, take it easy for a few days, and pace, slowly start doing more as headache and symptoms allow. Caution, Francene, you are at risk. My third fall since my mTBI. I also fell walking on the Port Hood Boardwalk; my foot stuck, I went ass over teakettle, wrenched my muscles, was sore for days. The first time I was bending in the flower garden, lost my balance. Ouch! I suspect I will always have balance issues.

August 2022—Acceptance

"Our greatest weakness lies in giving up.
The most certain way to succeed is always
to try just one more time."

— Thomas A. Edison

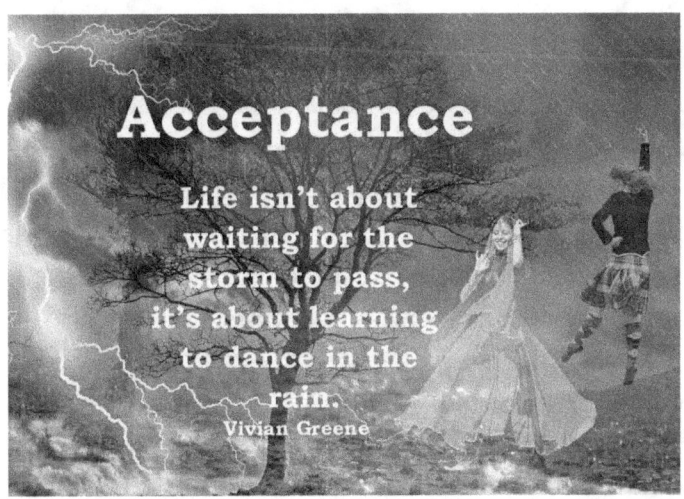

Acceptance is a process. I do not realize how angry I am, that deep down I refuse to accept what happened. Why is it so difficult? My gut tells me, I am not there yet. I long for someone to visit, suggest a walk, lunch, or drive. I am vagabond lonely. Writing is therapeutic, keeps me in touch with my feelings, helps me celebrate daily successes. I have taken a positive turn, climb the mountain path hugging rocky heights. Am I nearing the top? My younger, fellow-PCS friend Cara Palmer inspires me with her never-give-up attitude, refusal to stay down. During recovery, I contact her. It helps me not feel so alone. Inspired by her improvements, I share her story. In fact, I connect with Joanne Schmidt as well, she too has PCS and fibromyalgia; her story, "Naysayers," is included. The artist's brush creates a different masterpiece each day. I learn from others on a similar journey; they understand, help me see myself. I need to soak it in, rekindle my spirit.

September 2022—Favourite Spot

I find myself sitting in my favourite spot on my deck, overlooking the magnificent Atlantic Ocean and Port Hood Island. Bright light still hard on my eyes so I sit in my corner under the shaded enclosure. The whispering breeze kisses my face while sparrows and goldfinch play games in the holly bush; the ocean flows, waves reflecting and echoing my temperament or mood for the day. The water is a calm blue grey, a ripple coming to shore, a few dark patches, faster-moving white caps hitting the end of the island. It is my quintessential paradise. On the horizon, I hear the longing echoes of the millions drowned on a voyage to a new world, my view once a bustling shipping port. Closer to shore I hear the sighs of my baby brother in the lapping waves. Comfort comes in the mysticism of the vast canvasses of the evening sky, no two the same.

> *Red-orange wispy wings,*
> *hints of pink innocence, eminent magenta,*
> *transient transcendence,*
> *the sun as if God, draws the eyes, beats*
> *captures the wow of the heart in stillness.*

I drink in the tapestry, breathe in nature's beauty with her many brush strokes. The salt water reminds me of life—how we must be ready to flow with storms, undertows, currents, cross-currents, tempestuous seas. Calm, awe-inspiring, serenity spreads when we do our best, show appreciation, remember to thank everyone who crosses our paths. Affairs of the heart make life brighter. Being grateful for challenges and lessons helps us grow.

October 2022—Today is the Beginning of Your Tomorrow

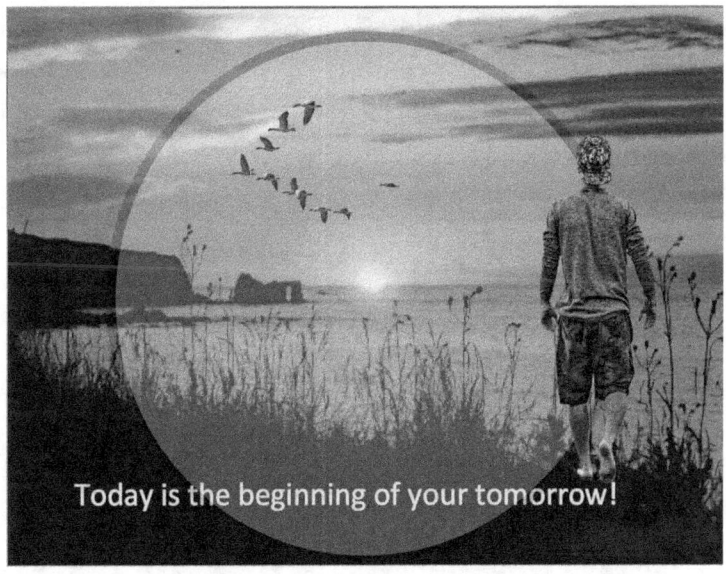

Today is the beginning of your tomorrow!

Follow your dreams
and believe in yourself.
When you start to doubt,
remember each page is blank
until written upon.

Some pages say more than others,
what yours will say is up to you,
for it is Your Tomorrow!

Francene Gillis

For years I posted that verse on my refrigerator. I need to focus on it. The fridge shares wise sayings, speaks beside photographs of family. For them, I must do what I can. Ditching guilt associated with lengthy recovery is a major battle, but necessary. Being in the present is my goal, not dwelling on the past. I set SMART Goals: Specific, Measurable, Attainable, Realistic, Timely. Without them, I become complacent. Or am I lazy? That detestable word. Does my age affect my difficulties? A loss of friends? Depression? I do not think so. Like the commercial on television of an older woman who falls and hollers, "Help me I've fallen. I can't get up!" Something holds me down . . .

November 2022—Exercise

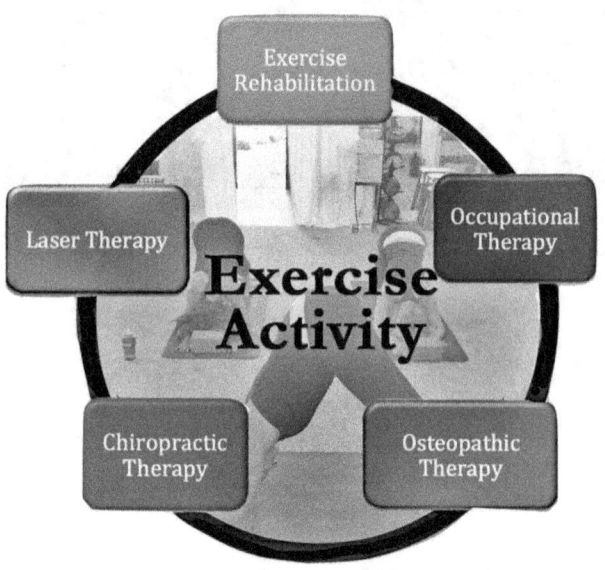

I enjoy exercising my brain. The control centre needs it, crucial to keeping us young. And it can be fun. I like playing solitaire, cards, checkers, or chess. Putting jigsaw puzzles together, the old-fashioned way with cut-outs, takes prowess. I manage sixty pieces, anything more overwhelms. My writing exercises my noggin. Mixing routines forces us to think rather than do activities automatically. Read, study, learn, teach. Another mantra—We can do more when rested. Exercise helps the body stay healthy; the mind sharp. So why can't I practise what I preach? Franny, Banny, pudding, and pie, pulled out her thumb, "What a hypocrite, am I?" I certainly hope not.

Exercise does not like me or I, it, even though I know its value. My jeans, skirts, tops, pants detest it. Shame, I gain sixty pounds, had always been a skinny miny miller. A common guilt trip for women, I feel like I must explain my weight gain. I am *inferior* if wrapped in extra layers of padding. Societal norms have me brainwashed. No place for body shaming. We do not know history or story; everyone has one. Slow and steady says my turtle friend, but what is my excuse after that? I love walking. The problem is in starting, the effort it takes. So, combine exercise with fun. My husband and I work in our yard; I supervise, he labours. We plant flowers, add decor to match our personalities. An innovative approach to exercise . . . stretch and bend until, as I tug branches, my back goes out. My body goes in spurts. I do well some days, crash on others, so unpredictable.

December 2022—Senior Citizen

A tumultuous time, I turn 65 on December 29; I must come off long-term disability or retire. My contract states, I can substitute. Is that worth holding onto, or time to call it a night? The pandemic, school system changes, leave me with mixed feelings. I know I cannot make it through one sixty-minute period, certainly not busy hallways, new protocols, rules. When teaching, I developed high school resources; maybe I can focus on them. A pressure valve released, catching up to do with my writing.

After several years, I compile my thoughts and experiences into a guide for those with mTBI, PTSD, and fibromyalgia, along with inspiring stories from wise individuals. Yup! One door closes, another opens. I have been crawling too long, treading water. It is time to run, dive, swim, and float, spend quality time with my best friend out my back door, my cantankerous ocean, or drive up the mountain instead of poking along.

> **Do the following to help create a positive mindset:**
>
> 1. Every morning or evening make a list of people in your life for whom you are thankful;
>
> 2. Make a list of the situations, events, and happenings for which you are most thankful.
>
> 3. Say thank you or something to that effect after each and every day.
>
> 4. Feel the good sensations that come with positive thoughts; nurture them with a smile.
>
> 5. When you close your eyes to sleep, think of the opportunities and people who have come into your life to allow you to grow, and learn, and develop into a better person.
>
> 6. Strive to be happy and live each day giving the gift of self.
>
> *If we can rise above our circumstance to be there for others, chances are our own heartaches will dissolve into that sweet magnanimous breeze with which Mother Nature so enjoys tickling us. She can blow our cares away with the same invisible energy that churns the waves, blows the sand, nuzzles the leaves, and urges flowers to dance. Nature, respected never lets us down. We may still struggle with symptoms, but a positive mindset helps.*

For those suffering months and years out, multidisciplinary treatment clinics capable of managing PCS are the answer, if you have insurance. They can be expensive. When first injured, I needed a concussion map. Now I know where to look.

January 2023—Moving On Up

Typing this, I am completely different from the person in those first post-injury years. I learned an encyclopedia full of valuable information, two more therapies added this year help with leftover symptoms. Of the utmost importance, I do not allow myself to go under a 30 per cent energy level; it has made a world of difference in handling fatigue and emotional reactions. You know you are at that mark when symptoms explode. This I need to explain. In summer, I sought a naturopath for extreme fatigue, pain, and limited activity. We discovered I misunderstood the professionals who worked with me prior. I thought my threshold was when I dropped to zero. I was wrong.

Dr. Glenna Calder suspects my fall depleted me because I was in a cycle of boom and bust. She makes sense. I reflect on the moments my emotions became fragile; frustration overwhelmed—when drained. I have learned to never go below 30 per cent energy; the body needs some to build on. I never thought fatigue could cause a person to slump on the bathroom floor and cry, doubt I saw above 20 per cent in those first years with the mayhem of medical appointments three days a week.

Now, I am super aware, do not let myself fall below if I can help it. When close, I retreat, rest, replenish. What a highly enlightening moment. Dr. Calder assesses and recommends select supplements to help with issues pertinent to me. A high dose of adrenals helps with lingering mental and physical fatigue. The naturopathic approach revolutionizes the way I go about my day. I gain strength, start doing things I love. I begin my one-hundredth health regimen. Perseverance with a capital "P." I find another type of massage therapist closer to home. My motto—keep trying.

With head injury, it is vital to figure out what works best; the brain affects every system and requires therapy to address deficiencies. Each year, new treatments, therapies appear. The ultimate way to help ourselves and those we love is to stay current, read about real people, actual cases, although we are more than "cases." If my trek up the mountain helps, I will wear armour to deflect criticism. I recognize the shock of what happened to me, my journey, struggles, hardships. This is my story, the stories of kind souls who share with the same intent. Sift, and please be kind. Now, I absolutely love showering! Instead of an exacerbating chore, it relaxes, feels good as the water, like rain, falls on the top of my head, pulsates over my body. I rest after.

March 2023—Mindfulness

Mindfulness helps when frustrated or overwrought. I have been in a boxing match with self-compassion my entire life. With each attempt to stand tall, I feel the punch of childhood accusations.

Stained worth spills chastisement. I try to redesign a belief seared into my mind during my most vulnerable years, cannot look in a mirror and say pleasant things. If I try, I tear up and run. I am not alone in facing demons from the past that ricochet into the present. Head injuries can cause past trauma to resurface, complicate recovery, cause a George Foreman knockout. Despite dealing with them, they reappear. Therapy helps me reclaim my voice, bury the demons, even the insidious ones.

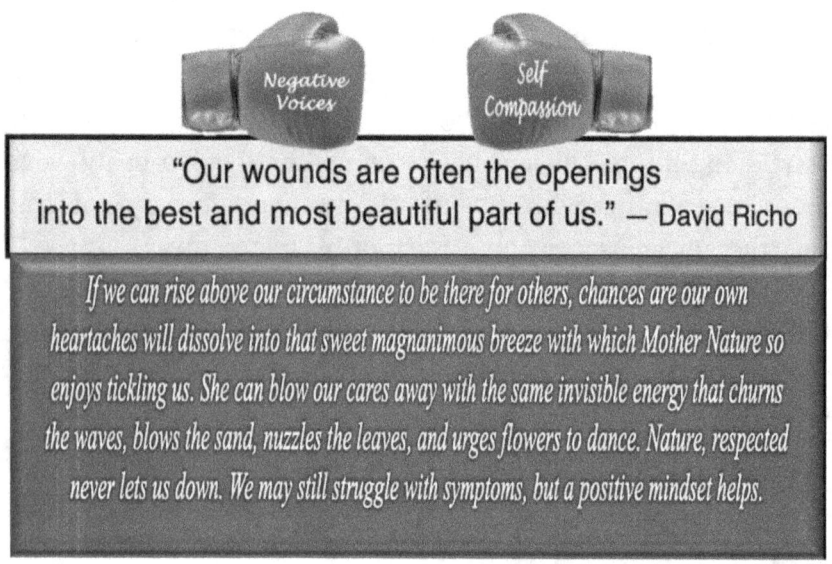

"Our wounds are often the openings into the best and most beautiful part of us." — David Richo

If we can rise above our circumstance to be there for others, chances are our own heartaches will dissolve into that sweet magnanimous breeze with which Mother Nature so enjoys tickling us. She can blow our cares away with the same invisible energy that churns the waves, blows the sand, nuzzles the leaves, and urges flowers to dance. Nature, respected never lets us down. We may still struggle with symptoms, but a positive mindset helps.

May 2023—Myofascial Massage Therapy

We are never too old to learn. The knee bone connects to the hip, thigh to the shoulder . . . wrong. Some of us live with chronic pain, in bed on a sunny day when we would rather hike the coast, feel spring's first breath. This therapy has to do with fascia—the thin sheath of fibrous connective tissue wrapping every single nerve ending, muscle, organ, bone in our body, a coating around a wire . . . a massive cobweb of them.

Jolene MacDougall owns Issues in Your Tissues, Myofascial

Release, which considers the whole body-and-mind connection, the way we view pain, and intricate relationship between thoughts, energy, and tissue function. Jolene says the key to pain is the fascia. Gentle massage has me sinking into the hurt to clear tension and feel better. Myofascial therapy uses gentle, constant movement. Jolene finds trigger points, knots, tenseness in the fascia tissues, applies butter-soft pressure until it releases. She also recommends barefoot shoes, wider for our toes to spread naturally, allow our feet to feel the earth. They help with balance, posture, and keeping the feet and ankles strong.

Joy! Joy! I pull off a baby shower for my oldest daughter in May, with several guests coming to the house. Huge for my daughter and me. Months of preparation, my husband and one of her friends helped. I feel *empowered*, an important word on the road to recovery. Sure, it takes a week to rest up, but the glow on her face was worth it.

May 26, 2023—A Toast

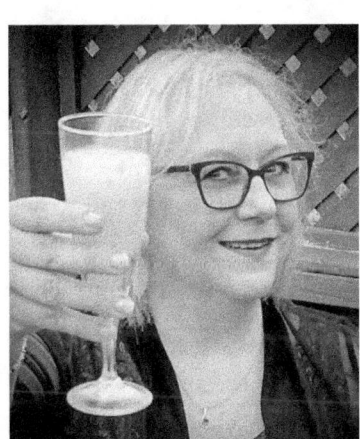

A tumultuous time arises, puts emotions in a tailspin. A retirement dinner. Weeks and days prior, I cycle through battles of not being good enough to attend. Blistering unworthiness attacks. I wrestle—go or not go? I chastise myself. Students and parents over the years showered me with accolades, student success speaks for itself, but challenges occurred as in all professions. The good and bad we take with us. I was more attached to the students than the system; if I do not go to the dinner, I will regret it.

Encouraged by family, I go, excited but scared, far too conscious about appearance.

Easy to understand benefits at an intellectual level, not so easy to deep-down change. That is where precocious Fran comes in. A scrapper, until forced to retreat inside herself for safety. Had I realized prior it was a district-wide event for all retirees, I would not have gone. We find a neighbour, sit together. I fear being called to the front to stand before strangers, a few acquaintances to receive a token plaque while listening to a few general words delivered by someone who does not know me. I should hold my head high, but stare at my feet. Need to reframe my thinking, revisit—I am worth something beyond what I can do. Sad how judgment affects even into our senior years, harsh voices haunt, thoughts linger, therapy silences, but not always.

May 27, 2023

Next night, a second retirement dinner for teachers in our local region. I go to find closure. When my fall forced me to stop teaching, I lost my identity. Not how I planned to end my career, passion, and purpose, working with vibrant young people with the world before them. I wanted to give them the best chance possible. Where do I belong? I fall into a tailspin, domino of emotions cascading, bursting a Yellowstone geyser, triggered by inadequacy. That phrase, forever rings in my head. Will it ever shut up?

The teachers and executive from our local region welcome me with smiles, greetings, and open arms. A smaller group, I feel at ease. My vice-principal, whom I ask as a guest and friend to say a few words, makes me smile, laugh, and cry, anecdotes of our time together on the green, (or red wing?), notating sections of the school. I absorb her words because they are genuine, from the heart, no platitudes. They allow me to realize the work I did throughout my career helped students and the educational system. It is the affirmation I craved. Having our school secretary as a guest at my table, comforts. I am back in school, chatting before heading upstairs. I celebrate with other retirees, wholeheartedly feel valued among my colleagues. The atmosphere, warm and inviting, is a most enjoyable send-off. A toast to all who reach such a milestone!

June 2023

In June I begin psychological psychosynthesis therapy with Susan Walsh, counsellor, MEd, RCT, CCC after feelings explode during my myofascial massage sessions. Because emotions connect to our fascia, sometimes it evokes feelings we hold too tight. Unable to deal with them, I search Susan out, see her every two weeks, and reinforce the benefits of her therapy with an online program. I have accepted where I am, but forever strive for more. Is that a contradiction?

I follow a five-day MindWell-U course through Wellness Together Canada available to anyone to help with inner dialogue, importance of taking five minutes a day, or five times a day to ground self in the present moment, a cue to help change unhealthy thinking patterns. We need to change thinking patterns and behaviours, an entirely different beast to wrestle and believe. Some cuts bleed deeper than others.

At sixty-five years of age, self-esteem issues still rise. Can you imagine? Do I have something wrong with me? Appearance so engrained? I must stop focusing on it. Not all intend to embarrass or belittle. Most folks are friendly, care. I must fill my plate with a heaping of goodness; more conscious of the doom and gloom cloud, a leftover of growing up, it does not need to be my present. In time, I hope to trust, hope people see my compassionate heart. Catharsis common, Susan, a remarkable practitioner.

A cautionary tale—no matter how an individual might seem on the outside, we seldom know what inner pain they carry. I have been writing—my source of sanity—this book, so readers might better understand the trauma from invisible injuries. Driven by what I needed after my fall in 2016, I dug for answers, learned oodles.

July 2023

Second joy, July 13, 2023, our first and likely only granddaughter, Maeve Mary Anna Burgess, comes into the world, another wee one to brighten our days. Luckily, she lives ten minutes away. I get to see budding wonder. My energy tank fills more easily.

September/October 2023—Bravo

Pat on my back! I fulfill two monumental goals I set in 2016 involving a passion and crowds, and I carried out every step by my lonesome, although my husband drove. I went to an overnight writing retreat on two separate occasions, and the flickering embers inside burn again. Reading this, I am excited, no longer questioning worth, although when down I still do. When first injured, I did not know whether my thoughts were garbage or insightful; that was anxiety—not knowing, fearing judgment, accepting a changed physical body, dealing with life's aging process, and the realities of PPCS. But that does not mean I shrivel like an armadillo. It means I rediscover my essence and truth.

January 2024—Finding Myself

Bell Canada, Let Us Talk Mental Health Day—January 24, 2024, reminds us of the importance of destroying taboos of mental illness and getting help, a thought that goes hand in hand with invisible injury and illness. Not everyone has tools and coping mechanisms. This worthy campaign brings awareness at a time of escalating crisis.

I have respect for the beast that is concussion—its companions: post-concussion syndrome, whiplash, post-traumatic vision syndrome, vestibular issues, inner ear nerve damage, VMS, depression, PTSD, mental difficulties. All require treatment. Nitty-gritty time. Can I accept where I am? Which begs a bigger question: Who am I? What happened? A yo-yo—up and down. My father would say faster than a whore's drawers. Is that okay to say? I try to be *normal* . . . do I have to be normal? What is normal?

A mild winter, I return to my deck, place of solace and contemplation, my turtle smiles. I should have given it a name. Bobblehead. I get angry at myself when I find an activity hard. Grrr! I trip on a circuitous route, weaving around stumps. Fallen trees block the road. My husband wants to fix everything. I wish he could. He tells me my eyes look like two piss holes in a snowbank (a colloquialism used in Cape Breton) because they are half-closed, tired. Thank you, dear. I am now able to laugh.

April 2024—Lessons Learned Over the Years

Lesson 1: Practise acceptance

Life is full of mysteries, and the reason bad things happen is often unanswered; the sooner we accept our circumstance, the faster we can work on the changes needed. It sounds easy, but many of us pound against the anvil of unexpected change—what we never asked for or intended. Moving forward is letting go of haunting reasons and what-ifs. Acceptance, attitude, and forgive-ness keys to recovery and progress. Creating lessons from which to learn, signifies growth along the way, the greater the chance of success. Do I need to forgive myself for falling? Maybe.

Lesson 2: Be aware of the gift of time

Life is short; make the best of it, live in the moment, share with others. Slow down. Leave the past where it belongs, or if crud keeps resurfacing, get counselling. Growth comes from the advice of others. If desires burn, develop them. All we have is today, this hour, minute, second. Why waste it? We should be aware in social and family inter-actions of our words, actions, so we have no regrets.

Lesson 3: Practise gratitude

How many of us offer thanks for the air we breathe? Do we avoid comparison and appreciate what we have? Max Ehrmann states in "Desiderata," "If you compare yourself with others, you may become vain and bitter; for always there will be greater and lesser persons than yourself." Being grateful switches the mindset when challenges rush in, allowing a focus on what we have rather than what we have lost. When practised, it lightens difficulties, changes perspective.

Lesson 4: Develop patience

We need to be patient, especially when waiting for something important. A powerful struggle, when frustrated, irritated, or emotional. We may want to reach a goal before it is realistically feasible. Patience makes it less frustrating. A bobble-head turtle on my deck symbolizes my forced slowdown, requiring tremendous patience, which I did not have. Patience calms the emotions and counters reaction.

Lesson 5: Find a purpose

Every one of us needs a reason for being, or a place to belong. Purpose is born in passion and crisis. Without it, we feel lost and restless. We need to ask ourselves deep questions to arrive at answers. Mindfulness helps. Through introspection and meditation, our inner voice speaks, gets down to our core and what means most to us; with opinions of loved ones, we can discover our why in life.

Lesson 6: Be compassionate

Life sings when our heart is in the right place. Love given and love received make the world a better place. When we care, we feel our emotions rather than shutting them off. We become vulnerable. The media depicts humanity's shortfalls and witnessing it in the world is difficult. Easy to become cynical. We choose how we react. Compassion opens the heart rather than closing it. The quality of caring for others, allows us to care for ourselves, to understand, empathize, and treat others with common decency, dignity, and respect. We all need to love and feel loved.

Lesson 7: Be vulnerable

Post-pandemic we have become emotionally distant, block emotions as if wrong to display them. When emotionally touched, we experience life's greatest gift. We need freedom to express ourselves; it makes us human. Scared, we wear masks. Deep wounds caused by unresolved pain and emotion blister, scar, make us miserable until dealt with. Joyful emotions carry us through trying times. Where would we be if we could not experience laughter, love, happiness?

Lesson 8: Look for the humour

We need to look at the lighter side of life, to laugh at ourselves and not be so serious. Too many of us have our nose to the grindstone and miss the fun. Telling jokes, sharing stories, feeling connected through humour excites the spirit, exudes gladness. It helps us let our guard down, unwind, relax, be childlike. Looking at the lighter side reduces pressure and stress. It can help us heal.

Lesson 9: Avoid wishing

The danger here is the onus falls on the outside, rather than the inside. Wishing for things implies what we have is not good enough, which may well be, but abstractions get us nowhere without action. Instead of wishing, creating workable goals or pursuits along with determination gets us further. The fulcrums of the engine behind fulfillment are belief, tenacity, preparedness, and faith. When at my lowest, I prayed and asked for understanding, acceptance, courage, and guidance. Unlike a wish, faith helps ground us, gives us something to hang onto when flood waters rise.

Lesson 10: Seek support

We need support—emotionally, mentally, physically—which comes through love, love, love, or at least care. No one should suffer alone. It increases pain. Any of us can ask the questions: Can I help you? What would you like? What can I do? We need others to feel alive, part of something bigger. Making connections with family and friends, having good working relationships allows us to thrive, not just survive. Through the support of others, we learn honesty, humility, and what matters. We need a special someone we can rely on when times get tough, to share when time sings. In dark, dire times, we may need an entire hallelujah chorus of angels to teach us dignity and respect for ourselves, and to remind us of the good in ourselves and in the world.

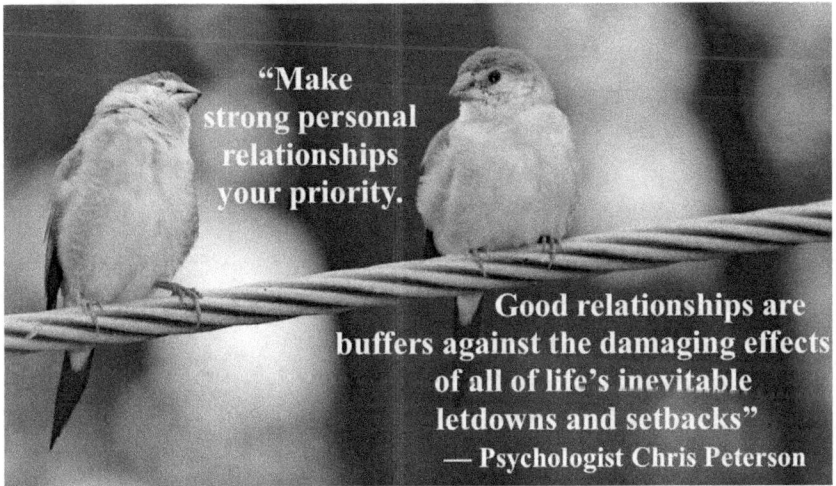

"Make strong personal relationships your priority.

Good relationships are buffers against the damaging effects of all of life's inevitable letdowns and setbacks"
— Psychologist Chris Peterson

The Almost New Me

I must accept my present self, let go of the past. Not changed, but different. My anniversary date no longer holds power. I still get emotional late August, early September, old song and dance—I want to teach, miss the energy of the young. Teaching, consulting—summer used to be my educational playtime as I worked, learned, trained others to take provincial exams, reviewed, wrote curriculum for advanced courses, and more. It felt good doing something valuable. What happens when you can do little? Does that mean you are no longer worthwhile? Our value is not in what we can do, but in who we are, our character, personality, beliefs, spirit, and contribution to a life well lived. Convince me!

A typical day used to involve that internal struggle. I can still teach in a different capacity. I still ask people to lower their voice, soften their tone, slow down. My brain, focusing on more than one task at a time, becomes a sloth. And that is okay; I work around it, manage leftovers. My lifestyle involves pacing and balancing. I read my work and write, am diligent, know when symptoms escalate I need reprieve. I control my environment. We are puppets on a string, our brain the master puppeteer.

I learn to laugh at myself, thus the silly comics infused throughout this book. April Fools' Day is one of my favourites! The fun of tricking someone and sharing belly laughs is wonderful for the psyche, as is watching comedy reruns on television. A laugh a day, essential to well-being. Board games, jigsaw puzzles, colouring books, word games help with anxiousness. I love playing chess with my six-year-old grandson in person when we visit, and online. It is a hoot because he honestly beats me.

Physical exercise challenges, even walking. I am motivated, but then I make excuses. Contradictory? Are they excuses? Hard to know anymore. I need to figure a way through, imagine nature's exposure as I climb higher on the mountain. Around every turn, magnificent scenery as I meander through meadows revealing amazing creatures—fox and fawn, rabbits, blue jays. A stroll to the edge of a cliff exposes the ocean—her vastness, wild or tranquil temperament dependent on the wind.

May 2024

Interviews I did for feature articles in the early 1990s and again in 2022 and 2023 create powerful moments in my adult life, help me realize we all feel happiness, pride, love, light; on the underside—we struggle, suffer. The difference in building character, is what we do with the situations given to us. The importance is not what happens on a particular day, but what we do with it. What a mystical challenge. Even as I work on the last draft of *Where Did i Go?* my editor pushes me to do more. I sit in the driver's seat, a few bumps, and ruts later, in 2024, I am up to the task.

Thoreau says, "Keep your worries on your thumbnails."

What a challenge! My body has fallen behind my brain, which fermented for over seven years. It needs exercise. I hope to share my soul with those who will take it cupped delicately in their hands, protect my most sincere intent. I look at my daughters, wives, mothers, professional women. My chest fills with overwhelming pride. Watching familiar traits come out in my grandchildren, life does not get any better. It does not need to be complicated. I hope to bring what were once dreams into reality. May we transform our journey of suffering into one of recovery, acceptance, growth, and triumph? Research is evolving, scientists and governments giving more attention to the world of brain injuries and concussion. In that, there is hope.

"Unlike a broken bone or a torn ligament, a moderate to severe TBI is not a one-time injury with a linear recovery; rather, it is a chronic neurological condition leading to significant life-long disability." (Muradov, Jamil, July 5, 2024).

My injury does not define me, is only one part. I cannot forget that. I do not want to be known for sickness or an mTBI. I am more. Like puzzles and mosaics, I pick up the pieces, make innovative designs, ones that sleep deepest in my spirit and heart. It happened *to* me, is *not* me. Time to pick up the fragments, decide what self-mosaic to build. Mine will include the ocean, open arms, and an open heart.

The Willow

There is a being
like many
standing undefined,
searching in others
for purpose.
A tree bending,
in the winds of other's tongues.
Unresisting to their definition
too scared to reveal the willow,
in striving to be an oak.

One?
What can he/she/it/they do?
Yet, a tiny light, flickers
in the eyes,
others catch a glimpse, do nothing.
Like the saint of yore, Christopher,
someone does.
He bends the branches,
Teaches
Waters, nurtures, accepts
the uniqueness
of this being.

Watches in wonder
each bough and branch blooming,
as in spring—
November's frost,
shimmering, shining glass ice,
musically crackling, in a silver thaw.

The sleeping root,
November dormant,
is touched, awakened,
with the inner wellspring of self—
Each branch newly encased
iridescent, singing
BURSTS into bloom.

The willow stands
as others look in awe.
Joy leaping into their hearts
at the wonder
of what had been hidden …
or perhaps had been there all along
before they took time to look.

He/She/They/It stands self-defined
Tall, yet still bending,
Applauding, accepting, affirming
A strong, powerful root
for other willow saplings.

Francene Gillis

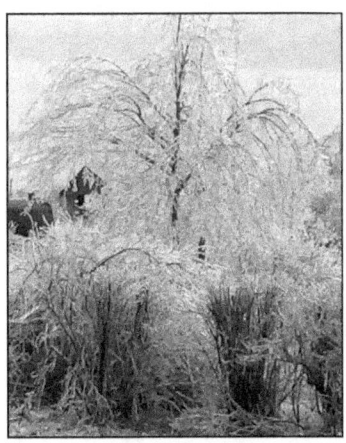

Education and Awareness

"Knowledge is power, and it can help you overcome any fear of the unexpected. When you learn, you gain more awareness through the process, and you know what pitfalls to look for as you get ready to transition to the next level."

— Shetty, Jay 2024, British podcaster, author, and life coach, best known for his podcast *On Purpose*

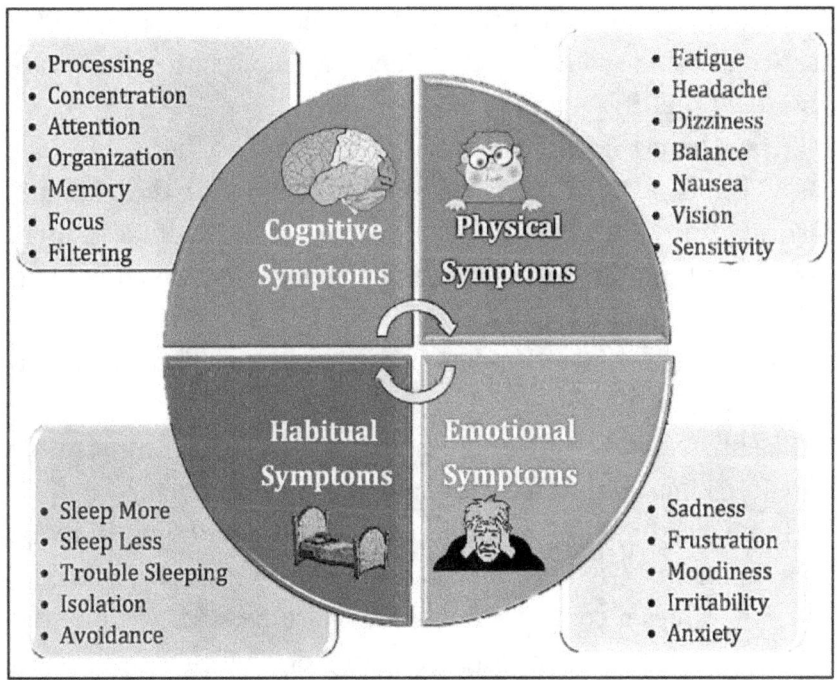

- Processing
- Concentration
- Attention
- Organization
- Memory
- Focus
- Filtering

Cognitive Symptoms

Physical Symptoms

- Fatigue
- Headache
- Dizziness
- Balance
- Nausea
- Vision
- Sensitivity

Habitual Symptoms

Emotional Symptoms

- Sleep More
- Sleep Less
- Trouble Sleeping
- Isolation
- Avoidance

- Sadness
- Frustration
- Moodiness
- Irritability
- Anxiety

*T*errified with strange symptoms I did not understand, I felt lost and alone, did not know where to turn. Four dreadful months I wondered if I was normal or would ever be. What follows are take-aways from my experience, treatments, and advice from health professionals, plus research into my condition(s). I needed to learn how to recover. As a teacher, it makes sense to share so the journey might be shorter for others who sustain a head injury. This does not replace professional or medical advice. Please see your doctor. Its intent is to share stories that provide insight into injuries from patients, therapists, and health practitioners dealing with head injuries on a regular basis. I share what helped me.

I hope this section allows people to become more literate about brain injuries while providing needed tools. Even with help from local, regional, and national brain organizations and groups, we all benefit from further education on concussion, whiplash, mTBI, TBI, acquired brain Injury (ABI), sports-related concussion (SRC), post-concussion syndrome (PCS), and persistent post- concussion syndrome (PPCS).

Please know practitioners and therapists use the words concussion and mTBI interchangeably. According to the National Institutes of Health (NIH), U.S. Department of Health & Human Services, "Personal health literacy is the degree to which individuals have the ability to find, understand, and use information and services to inform health-related decisions and actions for themselves and others."

Scientists need to do more as brain injuries continue to go unseen. Thousands suffer with ambiguous symptoms, go to their doctors who sometimes misdiagnose, send them home thinking their problems are "in their head," a multi-layered implication which devalues a concussed patient. Those injured become part of a bigger statistic of people returning for medical care to treat symptoms, without getting to the root cause. Read Peg's story, how doctors missed or downplayed the possibility of a TBI. She had other major injuries, but she knew something was awry, much more going on.

The Concussed Brain
Information Processing
Integrating All Systems for Functional Gains

Sensory Input
Breath, Mindfulness
Pacing, Symptoms
Adding More Senses

Environment
Management
Distractions
Obstacles

Attention
Sustaining
Alternating
Dividing

Execution
Incorporating
Saying, Doing
Concentration, Focus

Memory
Short Term Storage
Long term Storage
Retention

Hilling, J., OT, December, 2016
Gillis, F., January 2017

Goal: Matching Capacity With Demands

"Traumatic brain injury (TBI) needs to be viewed and managed as a condition, not a onetime event, and it needs to be seen through a framework that considers multiple factors which affect a person's access to care and increased likelihood of negative outcomes after TBI . . . The health care system needs to function as a lens to direct or redirect the trajectory of a person's care and recovery after TBI toward an optimal path." (National Academies of Sciences, Engineering, and Medicine, 2022).

1. Literature suggests seeing a doctor as soon as possible after head injury, within one day of ongoing symptoms: confusion, dizziness, nausea, headaches, sensitivity to sounds, inability to process information, or concentrate. It is necessary to be diagnosed and to be treated promptly and efficiently.

2. The brain and how ABI's and whiplash affect us is very individual. Injury can be overwhelming. Organizing symptoms into categories can help us become better aware of how our injury is affecting us.

3. Tracking symptoms which appear in any of the four categories provides awareness. Cognitive and physical symptoms show up first.

4. Making connections to what is occurring in the body allows for awareness and recovery. Knowing main issues can help in choosing the best treatment.

5. Tracking symptoms is imperative. Memory is unreliable. We forget when distracted, tired, or overloaded by a flood of messages and demands.

6. Staying isolated increases challenges. It is important to expose ourselves to more, but to not overdo. Having to stay home, decreases social time and exposure but to recover we need to get out—talk to friends and family and provide self-care.

"There are more than 5.3 million individuals in the United States who are living with a permanent brain injury-related disability. That is one in every 60 people. At least 2.8 million Americans sustain traumatic brain injuries in the United States every year." (Brain Injury Association of America, "Brain Injury Awareness in the News and Media Inquiries," 2024).

Table of TBI severity ratings **U.S. Department of Veteran Affairs, 2022**

Severity Level	Confused / Disoriented State Lasts	Loss of Consciousness Lasts	PTA Lasts	GCS	Structural Brain Image Results
Mild	Less than 24 hours	Less than 30 minutes	Less than 24 hours	13-15	Not usually indicated; if taken will be normal.
Moderate	More than 24 hours	More than 30 minutes but less than 24 hours	More than 24 hours but less than 7 days	9-12	Can be normal or abnormal. A TBI can be classified as moderate if all other criteria are mild, but a CT scan is abnormal.
Severe	More than 24 hours	More than 24 hours	More than 7 days	3-8	May be normal but is typically abnormal.

Other classification systems exist: Mayo Classification System for TBI Severity, National Academies of Sciences, Engineering, and Medicine, 2019, + Others.

"Every year Canadians sustain about 200,000 concussions. With 15% resulting in post-concussion syndrome, that is 30,000 new cases each year. 'It's a gigantic number,' says Dr. Charles Tator, a world-renowned neurosurgeon and concussion researcher at Toronto Western Hospital. 'We used to think that everybody got better from a concussion, but we now know that is not the case. Only 75% get better from a concussion and the other 25% have what we call post-concussion syndrome, and we regard that as serious now because of how disabling it is. We find patients with eight or 10 symptoms of post-concussion syndrome and if these persist, you can be disabled. Sometimes they never get better." Grech, Ron; *The Daily Press*, Dec. 2, 2018).

Helpful Advice in the Initial Stages

They Know It

If someone is struggling in their relationships, school,
with self-esteem, depression, financial issues, addiction,
weight, they know it. It eats their thoughts each day.
Provide empathy, kind eyes, a smile of assurance.
Give them unconditional love where they are.
Be an attentive and respectful listener.
Create a safe place for others to open up and talk.
Be willing to listen, and not interrupt. If they are sick,
they know it. If overweight, they know it.
If reactive, they know it. Be there for them.
Show you care without judgment.
Share appreciation for who they are.
Help them see the shining sun on dark, wet days.

Recovery Chart or Tips

- Start each new day with gratitude and renewed determination and spirit.
- If you need help, or a pick-me-up, reach out to someone.
- Go for a walk or exercise.
- Believe good can come. Make it come.
- Be true to your best self.
- If you say/do something not true to your character, apologize.
- Listen to uplifting audio books, and music.

- Be your own friend. Pamper yourself. Stop worrying; it serves no purpose.
- Write essential information on paper; it is easy to forget.
- Keep track of healthy meals and daily activities.
- Find a driver. Staring out a window can cause headache and fatigue.
- Acknowledge symptoms, share frustrations to get proper help.
- Throw guilt of not being able to do anything out with the garbage.
- Set aside one day a week for quality time with a special someone.
- Nurture self and loved ones with words, actions, and validation.
- Buy or have someone pick up or make ready-made meals.
- Eat healthy foods, lots of vegetables, fruit, fewer processed items.
- Arrange for someone to clean the house and help with chores.
- Keep records, receipts, reports together.
- Ask someone to help with taxing paperwork.
- Get trusted help to apply for insurance, disability, pensions, claims.
- At night, share with your maker your prayers, concerns, rantings.

Canadian Government Steps Up

"With comprehensive national concussion guidelines and protocols, children and their parents, athletes, coaches, and healthcare professionals will have the information they need to help prevent concussions and manage them when they occur." (The Honourable Philpott, Jane; P.C., MP Minister of Health, 2016).

It is rewarding to see government interest, various provincial and national groups and organizations working to understand, educate, and make people aware of the impact of a head and/ or neck injury but there is a gap—most of the attention goes to athletes and children in sports. Disconcertingly, injuries in sports are high, but an increased number of seniors, adults, and children receive concussions outside of sports through vehicular accidents, falls, bangs to the head. They show up in emergency departments, debilitated, forced off school or work. The missing link—the need for education and awareness among medical personnel and general practitioners around steps, procedures, medical options, what is available, and follow-up treatments. Hopefully, coaches, teachers, and educational staff will receive more training.

Recovery varies among individuals. The older we are when injured, the longer it takes to heal, many variables in tow. "The Canadian federal budget 2024 announced renewed funding to the Brain Canada Foundation including a commitment of $80 million over four years. This investment will be matched by the Brain Canada Foundation. In total, $160 million will be funded through the Canadian Brain Research Fund." (Government of Canada, September 5, 2024).

What a wonderful opportunity for the concussed to get the services they need. Priority should be services for rural Canadians. Urban areas have programs and clinics readily available, but rural residents struggle to find professional help because of distance, transportation, or lack of guidance, creating an immediate need for online, interactive support groups, run by concussion experts, at least one per province. A proven link between head injury, depression, and mental health challenges makes the need for rural services more acute. Suggestions lead to questions, possibilities, and action.

Brain Injury Association of Nova Scotia offers several in-person drop-in programs in Bedford and survivor programs once a week online, a concussion café once a month, and people can sign up for Zoom meetings once a week, 11:00 a.m. Friday (as of writing), and a new virtual checkpoint with community educator and navigator on the first and third Wednesday of each month from 2:00–3:00 p.m. via Zoom.

This is a good start and example, but the concussed living outside urban areas need more. We need ready support, a place to ask questions, share symptoms, as no two days are the same. We need to make sense of a conflagration of oddities, and know we are not alone. From those who have walked the walk, we learn the most. A support group run five days a week with occasional special speakers would encourage and reach a broader audience, with specific times set aside for confidential video or audio sharing.

A platform just for people with PCS would be ideal. I appreciate what is available, but concussion website pages must be less ambiguous, easy to navigate with PCS symptoms, information clear, programs easily understood prior to signing up. Valuable brain injury resources need to be accessible if we are to find and use them when we need them most. The more steps involved, the less likely we will have access. Computer screens, daunting, we need more printed material, as many do not have their own printers, thus this book.

Whiplash

"Whiplash is more likely to cause serious or lasting injuries in two groups: older adults and women, people assigned female at birth (AFAB). It is more serious in older adults (over age 65) because they are typically more prone to muscle and bone injuries because of age-related muscle and bone deterioration and weakening . . . Sharp, sudden movements can cause your brain to smack

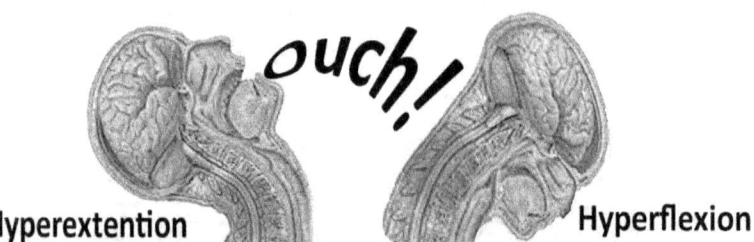

Hyperextention   **Hyperflexion**

What is WAD (Whiplash Associated Disorder)?

WAD is a term used to describe a range of symptoms resulting from whiplash. These can vary from no symptoms to severe.

WAD injuries are usually graded on a severity scale between 0-4.

Grade 0   No pain or discomfort. No physical signs of injury.
Grade 1   Neck pain, stiffness or tenderness. No physical signs of injury.
Grade 2   Neck pain, stiffness or tenderness and some physical signs of injury
           such as point tenderness or trouble turning the head.
Grade 3   Pain, stiffness or tenderness and neurological signs of injury, such
           as changes to reflexes or weakness in the arms.
Grade 4   Pain and fracture or dislocation of the neck.

(Quebec Task Force Classification of Grades of WAD, 2017)

against the inside of your skull, causing damage to your brain . . . Whiplash happens when inertia causes your head, neck, and body to move at different speeds. That forces your neck to compress or extend too quickly or in ways that push the muscles, ligaments, and bones of your spine beyond what they can tolerate." (Complete Concussions, Cleveland Clinic, 2024.)

"Whiplash can lead to long-term symptoms: problems with concentration and memory, ringing in the ears, inability to sleep well, irritability, chronic pain in the neck, shoulders, head. Some people experience chronic pain or headaches for years following their accident." (Johnson, Shannon, Healthline, 2023).

Pain

Pain can be
localized, or extend
down shoulders and back.

Headaches

Whiplash headaches usually occur
at the top or the back of the head.
Whiplash headaches can be
intermittent or constant.

Decreased Mobility

Neck movements are often restricted
following a whiplash as muscles contract
when the neck is painful.

Tender Points

Elongation, bruising or tearing of the neck's soft tissue
can lead to inflammation and edema. Inflamed and
swollen tissues are more sensitive to touch.

Memory/Concentration Problems

Individuals who have sustained whiplash injuries often report
problems with memory and/or concentration.

Whiplash Injury Issues

Reference: Recover Injury
Research Centre, 2017

The paper "The role of the cervical spine in post-concussion syndrome," reviews the existing literature surrounding the numerous proposed theories of PCS and introduces another potential and treatable cause of this chronic condition; cervical spine dysfunction due to concomitant whiplash-type injury. It discusses a short case-series of five patients with diagnosed PCS having favourable outcomes following various treatment and rehabilitative techniques aimed at restoring cervical spine function (Cameron M. Marshall, et al. 2015).

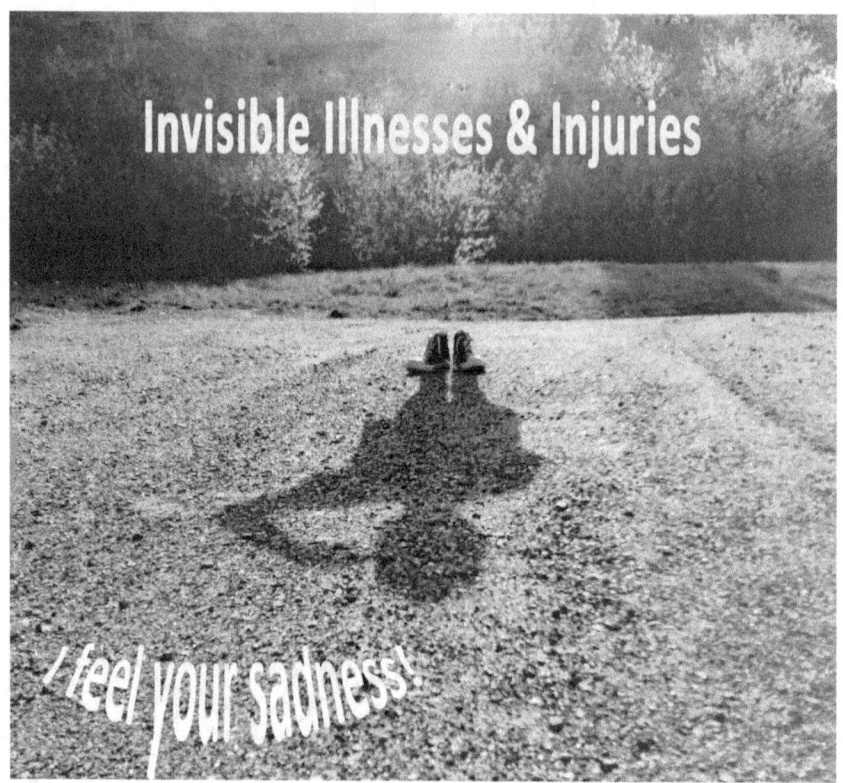

Invisible Illnesses & Injuries

I feel your sadness!

Invisible Injuries: Who Has Seen the Wind?

"Concussions are not like broken bones. We on the outside cannot see how the concussed individual is suffering, so, we must learn to listen and try to understand patients and their difficulties." (Sutherland, Tara, PT, Antigonish Concussion Clinic).

Many onlookers have minimal knowledge of concussion and whiplash, and inadvertently can be insensitive or obtrusive. "But you look great," a common statement, when trying to explain an invisible injury, can impose guilt. "You should," or "I don't think you should" are unhelpful statements.

Trauma On Trauma (Insurance)

Far too often invisible illness and injury can lead to trauma on top of trauma, when lawyers belittle the client who's submitting a claim. Insurance companies are cautious—rightfully so—but hardworking people devastated by injuries should not be subjected to the additional trauma of a battle, an unjustly denied claim, or put through the purgatory of a long court case. Unless people speak up and demand change, nothing will happen to improve this state of affairs. Perhaps government should consider legislating head injuries differently from injuries that are apparent through physical testing.

As it stands now, the people who treat invisible injuries are overwhelmed: they cannot keep up with the demand to access this kind of treatment and the injured are suffering. It may need court intervention to make the process of obtaining specialized treatment easier for victims.

Plaintiffs should not have to fight with insurance companies to collect what is rightfully theirs. The doctors and staff alike at TBI and concussion clinics are burnt-out with legal obstacles imposed on their patients and many close, permanently.

Even when a plaintiff documents and tracks their own symptoms, insurance adjusters and their lawyers demand that head injury patients show proof. Unless such injuries are so severe and overtly obvious, how can they prove there is injury without an opinion from a specialist in TBI and concussions?

Extremely long and expensive lawsuits can ensue, the onus placed on the victims. Independent medical examiners (IMEs), often hired by insurance companies, frequently endeavour to dismiss very real symptoms; it's the underbelly of personal injury litigation. As a result, patients are forced to fight, some, for years, which magnifies many issues caused by their injuries. Their elevated stress, the anxiety—patients navigating the system often feel they're drowning in stormy seas, bringing unnecessary regression of recovery. This is a hard truth.

A CBC News article by Marchitelli, Rosa; Blair, Jenn, posted online, Nov. 18, 2024, could be an important reference for people locked in these battles. "Insurers fighting injury claims hire doctors slammed for shoddy work as key medical experts," (*Health, Go Public* series). How's that for a title? A cautionary tale it reiterates what several claimants have told me. The judges hearing these cases must be aware of the insidiousness of invisible head injury to make fair and impartial determinations, but they rely on expert medical testimony, which may not be how it sounds. New timely legislation would help those who deserve and need the help.

"Doctors called out for being biased, faulty or careless expert witnesses in court are being hired by insurance companies looking to deny injury claims for people hurt in car crashes." That is how the first line reads, echoing what I heard of a certain neurologist in Nova Scotia mentioned many times by interviewees not only for unprofessionalism, but odd, erratic, and offensive behaviour.

The CBC report speaks of Jonathan Graul, from Fergus, Ontario, who found himself under attack in court by two doctors hired by an insurance giant, after he'd suffered a traumatic brain injury from a December 2017 crash.

The article goes on to say, "Medical experts have a duty to help the court by offering independent, objective and unbiased evidence in cases where opposing sides often clash on what the facts are . . . 'Everything hinges on these medical reports,' said DesRoches, who heads the not-for-profit FAIR Association of Victims for Accident Insurance Reform, which is made up of motor vehicle accident victims struggling with the auto insurance system in Ontario . . . DesRoches says the blame lies with professional colleges that oversee these doctors, the Ontario government and the doctors themselves. 'I think it's important that the public knows,' she said. 'The quality of the medical evidence used in courts is a big concern . . . I mean, they make a lot of money doing this, and they really ought to be sure about what they're saying.'"

It is time the system changes in order to protect plaintiffs from ridicule and added trauma. Questionable medical experts need to be disallowed. Most doctors take their role seriously, and have credibility and integrity, but the system seems broken when people have suffered invisible injuries, adding trauma on trauma. Doubting the injured leads them to push themselves beyond their capabilities, triggering a lifelong cycle of symptoms and self-judgment. Countless honest, qualified professionals exist, but to find them, to persevere, is vital. When an injured person is not treated with dignity and basic kindness, judges need to push the medical societies and lawyers' associations to initiate reforms of the medico-legal system.

Physicians who simply want to concentrate on treating injured patients are being forced to use their limited time and resources to provide proof of invisible injury to insurance companies and adversarial attorneys. In consequence, doctors are being overwhelmed by this ever-increasing interference and demand on themselves and their staffs. Is it any wonder we are losing so many dedicated and caring doctors? It is shockingly sketchy.

Fatigue

"When you experience a concussion (or any TBI), your immune system causes inflammation near the site(s) of injury . . . When you try to do something that those cells govern—like encoding a new memory or paying attention to a conversation—they will not be able to accomplish the task. Other neural pathways will then attempt to complete the process, even though it is a less efficient

path for that information to take . . . This tires your brain out, leading to post-traumatic headaches, feeling overwhelmed, irritability,
and other symptoms. For post-concussion syndrome patients, the
brain keeps using less efficient pathways to complete tasks even
after the inflammation has resolved. That suboptimal signalling,
like getting stuck in traffic or taking a side road which requires
more gas, is what results in long-lasting concussion symptoms.
The more your brain has to use suboptimal pathways, the more
likely you are to experience symptoms." (Fong, Dr. Alina, PhD;
Cognitive fx, July 16, 2024).

No wonder we get fatigued. "Tired" is a nebulous word. Tired
from . . . anything. "Many subtypes of fatigue have been identi-
fied, including cognitive, physical, emotional, and stress fatigue.
Secondary fatigue is fatigue due to, for example, poor sleep quality
or chronic inflammation. In contrast, primary fatigue is due to
the brain injury itself." (Wylie, Glenn R; Flashman, Laura A, Oct.
27, 2017).

What Every Survivor Wants You to Know

"Every single thing we do, whether physical or mental, takes a toll
on our brain. The more we use it, more it needs to rest. If we go
out to a crowded restaurant with a lot of noise and stimulation, we
may get overloaded and need to go home and rest. Even reading
or watching TV causes our brains to fatigue." (Zellmer, Amy, Dec
6, 2017.)

Zellmer suffered an injury from a fall in 2014 and has become
a powerful advocate for people with head injuries. She has written books and has resources available online. Her quotation sings
familiarity to the brain injured. At the time of writing, she was
editor-in-chief of *The Brain Health Magazine*, an award-winning
author, speaker, TBI survivor.

Mental Health

And what do we discover? Psychologists do not judge.

They...

- Do not criticize, berate, belittle or condemn
- Attentively listen, professionally observe
- Ask questions, make suggestions, offer advice
- Offer respect and compassion
- Counsel, allow us to see circumstances with fresh eyes
- Offer outside perspective, needed with charged emotions
- Provide tips and offer resources
- Ensure the pace is appropriate and comfortable
- Build in time to take a break, rest, reflect, recharge
- Teach mindfulness, awareness and strategies for coping.

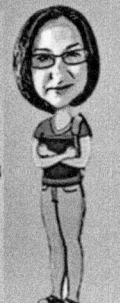

Life after an mTBI or concussion can be stressful as survivors cope with the loss of self-identity, a career or job, friends, social life, family, or community. Psychiatrists, psychologists, and brain associations can help by providing education and counselling to individuals and families in sectors focusing on various disorders that arise from life after injury. Some that are helpful include:

- The Centre for Addiction and Mental Health
- Canadian Mental Health Association
- The Post Traumatic Stress Disorder Association of Canada

Check out helplines and crisis centres. The United States also has plenty of evidence-based sites you can access. After a brain injury mental health is incredibly important, has an enormous impact on physical and emotional well-being, as well as recovery and rehabilitation.

"Consistent care and therapies over the long-term with mental health professionals and caregivers who are familiar with you and your needs are what help you continuously improve." (Brain Injury Canada, "Mental Health," 2022).

Emotional Irregularity

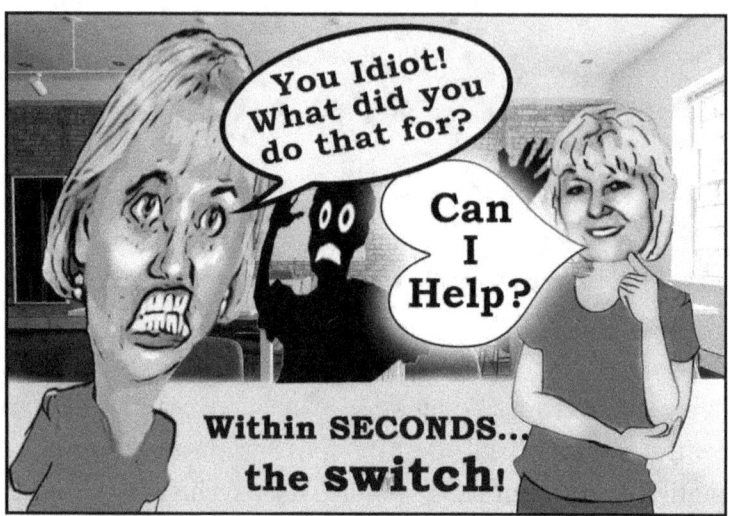

It is common to have issues with emotional irregularity after a head injury. If suffering, it helps to tell someone, reach out for professional input and resources if unable to regulate emotional outbursts. When injured we need to own the feeling and not attach shame, blame, or guilt; when we do, there is a risk of spiralling. It is helpful to practise strategies to calm the central nervous system, such as meditating, practising breathing exercises, or asking a loved one for what we need.

If in the company of someone who is emotional, ask caring questions: Are you okay? What can I do for you? Do you need help? Acknowledge the upset. Through gentle conversation, clarify needs, validate feelings without comment, judgment, or blame. Show empathy. Speak words of acknowledgement, affirmation, kindness. The concussed have difficulty with emotions as they try to gain control over what was once so easy, how their body reacts to stimuli and frustrations. Nagging inner voices and negative self-talk may lead to avoidance, non-participation, depression, or escapism as the fight-or-flight response kicks in. Afraid to approach the difficult, some never accept their injury or expose it, thus never master it. We must feel safe to open up. Took me a long time.

"There are many factors to consider when healing from a concussion—One is the body healing; the other is pivoting to a new definition of yourself which includes self-compassion while recovering. And subsequently, bringing values into your life with acceptance of the trauma and losses that you have experienced because of the concussion. The space of healing is what I coin as, 'aloeverish.' (The benefit of imagining the soothing impact of the aloe vera plant's gel.) It is important to have, aloeverish moments and aloeverish people in your life, to be aware of, what is not aloeverish for you at any given time. Listening to a negative friend providing unsolicited advice is not healing. Become aware of what and who is healing for you and proceed on a minute-by-minute basis, then proceed by making decisions aligned with your values. This is now a calm space that is helpful to your recovery. For example, go for a coffee with that aloeverish friend but not in a noisy, brightly lit, restaurant for two hours, but rather a cozy cafe, with soft lamps, and set a time limit of no more than an hour. Then plan an aloeverish nap or bath." (Murray, Sandra, BEd, MCP, RCT, October 28, 2024).

Anxiety

"Three types of anxiety can arise after a concussion: General anxiety, where you experience persistent, excessive fear and stress over health, school, work, or home life. It becomes difficult to control, and you can experience physical symptoms like restlessness, fatigue, muscle tension and sleep disturbance. Social anxiety

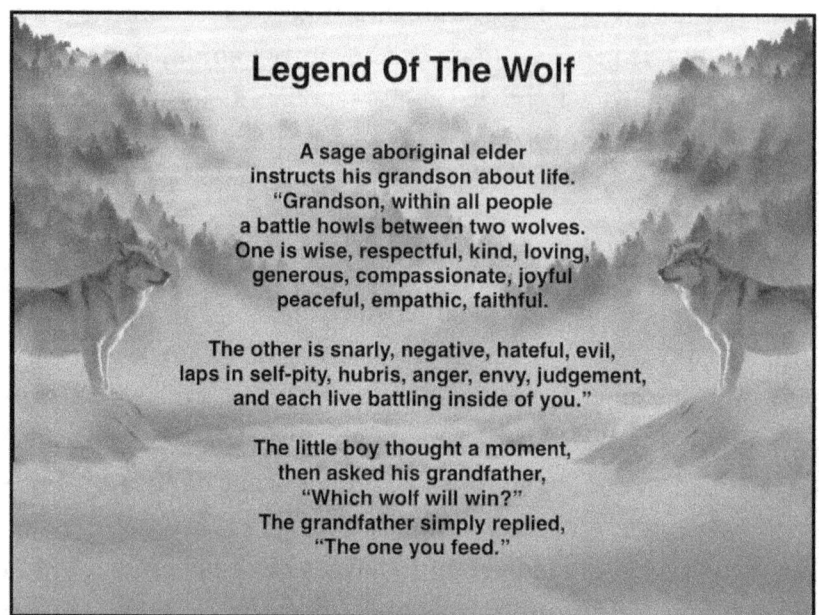

Legend Of The Wolf

A sage aboriginal elder
instructs his grandson about life.
"Grandson, within all people
a battle howls between two wolves.
One is wise, respectful, kind, loving,
generous, compassionate, joyful
peaceful, empathic, faithful.

The other is snarly, negative, hateful, evil,
laps in self-pity, hubris, anger, envy, judgement,
and each live battling inside of you."

The little boy thought a moment,
then asked his grandfather,
"Which wolf will win?"
The grandfather simply replied,
"The one you feed."

occurs when you are fearful about, or avoid, social interactions and situations; you worry about being judged, embarrassed, rejected. This often leads to isolation. Panic attacks are abrupt surges of intense discomfort that reach a high within minutes, accompanied by physical/cognitive symptoms." (Brain Injury Canada, "Anxiety," Government of Canada, 2022).

"The 333-anxiety rule involves observing three things you can see, three things you can hear, and three things you can move or touch. It is a grounding technique—a coping skill to manage intense emotions by steering the mind away from anxiety and toward the present moment." (Stella Centre, DC, 2024.)

Relaxation tips that worked for me: Visualization, learning to laugh, colouring. It helps to find a hobby, ponder gifts in your life, find role models or inspirational stories that resonate. Share emotions. Keeping things bottled leads to explosion. Listen to audio books, music, podcasts, TED Talks. Find credible resources. Declutter. Educate yourself. Validate your symptoms. Laugh at your husband's dry jokes.

Depression

"After a brain injury, abilities, and sense of self changes, and adjusting to a new self and situation is difficult, causing elevated stress, feelings of sadness, anger, loneliness, and depression. These emotions are normal and expected as the injured grieve an old way of life." (Brain Injury Canada, "Depression," Government of Canada, 2022).

"We think that depression and anxiety is a neurological condition. Fortunately, it can be treated effectively." (Tator, Dr. Charles; Middleton, Jackie, April 7, 2014.)

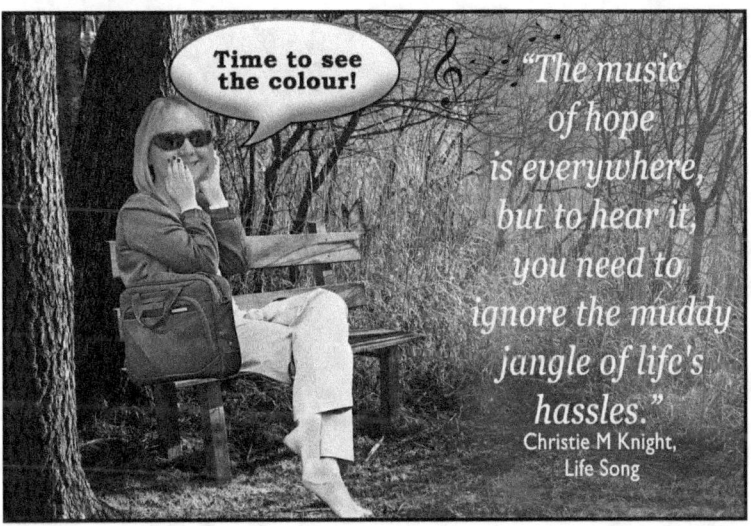

Suicide Risk

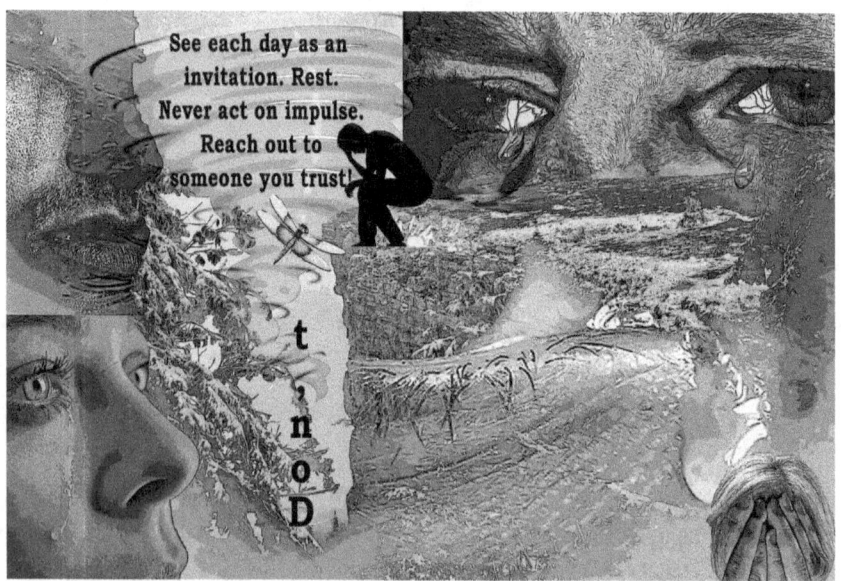

"Our prime purpose in this life is to help others.
And if you can't help them, at least don't hurt them."

— Dalai Lama

This is a painful topic. When a brain injury, illness, or overwhelming condition causes desperation, it is sadder than sad.

"Research shows an increased risk for suicidal thoughts, suicide attempts, and even death by suicide following brain injury." (Seale, Gary S., July 10, 2024).

"Depression is a medical problem, like high blood pressure or diabetes; you cannot get over it by simply wishing it away, using more willpower or toughening up. Best to get treatment early to help prevent needless suffering and worsening symptoms." (Fran, J., and Hart, T., Model Systems Knowledge Translation Center, (MSKTC) 2010.

"People with brain injury may feel anxious without knowing why. They may worry and become anxious about making too many mistakes, or failing at a task, or if they feel they are criticized. Many situations can be harder to handle. Being in crowds, being rushed, adjusting to changes in plans can cause anxiety... Difficulty reasoning and concentrating can make it hard for the person with TBI to solve problems. This can make the person feel overwhelmed. Anxiety happens with too many demands. Time pressure constraints heighten it. Situations requiring attention and Information processing make people with TBI anxious." (MSKTC, Model Systems Knowledge Translation Center, May 2019; msktc.org)

"Resilience theory refers to the ideas surrounding how people are affected by and adapt to challenging things like adversity, change, loss, and risk. Studies of resilience demonstrate it isn't a fixed trait. You can grow your capacity to practice resilience . . . Flexibility, adaptability, and perseverance can help you tap into your resilience by changing certain thoughts and behaviors." (Hurley, Katie, 2024.)

MSKTC publishes a guide on three types of resilience, and five principles that echo stories within. And what about people who do not have the skills they need to get through a dark time? I go digging and find the Canadian Association for Suicide Prevention (CASP), whose mantra on their website is: "Envisioning a Canada without suicide." Through their resources, I discover the new theme for World Suicide Prevention Day (2024) is "Changing the Narrative: How we can Reshape Public Discourse about Suicide to Save Lives." Long overdue, a universal problem, systemic of a society that breeds depression, trolling, bullying, cruelty, and addictions. Too many on social media hide behind a screen. We need to create empathy and give a sense of what it is like to be in the shoes of those who feel hopeless so more will care. Below are valuable guidelines from the CASP media, public service section:

- Encourage people to speak openly about suicide.
- Indicate that the life of a suicidal person is important.
- Acknowledge the suffering that is associated with suicidal thoughts and the conditions that give rise to them.
- Emphasize that suicide is preventable.
- Highlight the devastating impact of a suicide death on loved ones.
- Provide information about support for people thinking about suicide including how to approach/offer help to someone and crisis resources such as helplines.

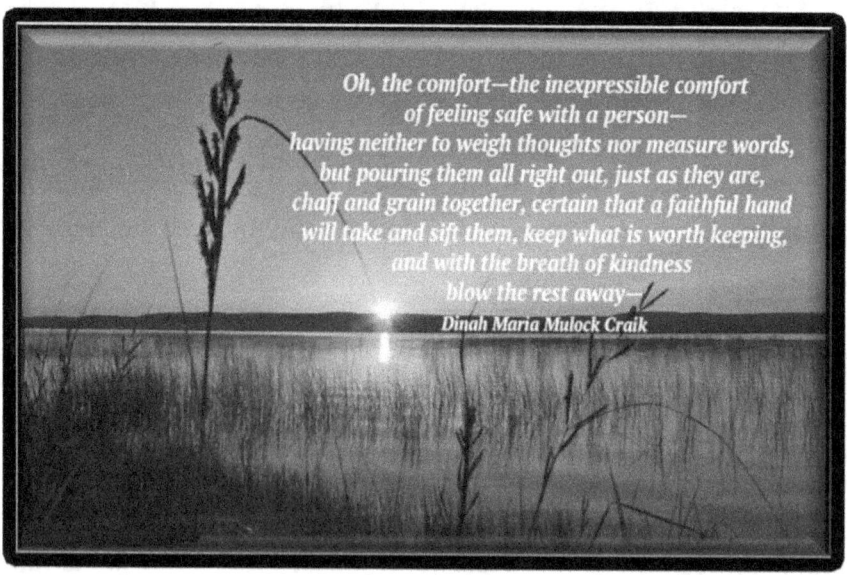

*Oh, the comfort—the inexpressible comfort
of feeling safe with a person—
having neither to weigh thoughts nor measure words,
but pouring them all right out, just as they are,
chaff and grain together, certain that a faithful hand
will take and sift them, keep what is worth keeping,
and with the breath of kindness
blow the rest away—*
Dinah Maria Mulock Craik

Visual by Marilyn Elison

Helpful Resources for Suicide Prevention

- Canadian Association for Suicide Prevention (CASP) https://suicideprevention.ca/resources/

- Roots of Hope, Share Hope Canadian Association for Suicide Prevention (CASP): Crisis Call: 1-833-456-4566, Kids—1-800-668-6868, Text CONNECT 686868.

- Vocabulary—"How to Talk about Suicide." "Suicide Bereavement & Postvention Alliance, Mission— resources, foster communities, support initiatives of suicide bereavement, postvention in Canada"

- Mental Health Commission of Canada: https://mental-healthcommission.ca/what-we-do/suicide-prevention/

- Talk Suicide Canada: 1-833-456-4566, or text: 45645, Quebec, https://suicide.ca/en

- Military Mental Health: You are not alone: 1-800-268-7708, https://www.canada.ca/en/department-national-defence/corporate/reports-publications/health/suicide-prevention-intervention-guide-caf-leadership.html

- Aboriginal Youth: A Manual of Promising Suicide Prevention Strategies downloadable; Centre for Suicide Prevention; Canadian Mental Health Association, Alberta Division

- Suicide Prevention in Indigenous Communities, Indigenous Services Canada, 1-855-242-3310 https://www.canada.ca/en/indigenous-services-canada.html

- Suicide Prevention, https://helpguide.org/

- NIMH—National Institute of Mental Health: United States https://www.nimh.nih.gov/suicideprevention, 1-800-273-TALK (8255)

- American Psychiatric Association, https://www.psychiatry.org/

- The Centre for Addiction and Mental Health (CAMH): "Let's make better mental health care for all a reality." https://www.camh.ca/

The onus is on people who care. We need to educate ourselves using resources from credible sites suggested and vetted. It starts by teaching our children to love instead of hate, stepping into the shoes of others and empathizing instead of judging. Important for us to stop comparing ourselves to others, falling for propaganda, trying to have the perfect child, or striving to be the perfect human being, all futile efforts. We and our children need to learn what mindfulness is, encourage mental health by allowing each family member to express and talk about emotions, struggles, best way to handle problems, or accept help. Schools should teach children mindfulness, self-awareness, resiliency skills and allow students to express themselves with teaching moments around responses. Preventing mental illness should top the government's priorities to effectively lower the number of people disabled because of mental conditions. Mental health needs to be in the forefront.

An Invisible Condition: PCS and Mental Illness go Hand in Hand

According to author Neff, Kristin (2023), "Self-compassion encompasses three interrelated components: 1/ self-kindness versus self-judgment, which involves being kind and understanding towards oneself during moments of inadequacy, suffering, or failure instead of being self-critical or neglecting one's suffering; 2/ common humanity versus isolation, which involves recognizing that mistakes and failures are part of the human condition and that we should not feel isolated; 3/ and mindfulness versus over-identification, which involves seeing oneself in a balanced and realistic way, without suppressing or exaggerating one's thoughts or emotions, rather than over-identifying with them . . . Self-compassion refers to being supportive toward oneself when experiencing suffering or pain—be it caused by personal mistakes and inadequacies or external life challenges. [Neff's] theoretical model of self-compassion [comprises] six elements: increased self-kindness, common humanity, mindfulness, reduced self-judgment, isolation, and overidentification. The first step towards changing how you treat yourself is to notice when you are being self-critical. Make an active effort to soften the self-critical voice but do so with compassion rather than self-judgment. Reframe the observations made by your inner critic in a friendly, constructive way . . . Imagine what a compassionate friend would say to you in this situation."

To our loved ones
- Please don't tell us we are lazy, or that you feel the same thing.
- Do not play comparison game, demeaning our situation, feelings.
- Do not disregard our struggles, efforts, constant adjustments, pleas.
- Please offer encouragement, praise, affirmation daily, hourly.
- Know our work, relationships, quality of life, have been affected.
- Validate, help us discover the new us, our gifts, talents, purpose.
- Spend quality time with us; we are lonely, extremely hard on ourselves; belittling our efforts causes us to fall, affirmation, to rise.

Trying new things, no matter how small; opens us up to opportunities to discover something new about ourselves.
(themighty.com, 52 Small Things, April 2019)

A most valuable resource I found to help me is a newsletter called *The Mighty*, an interactive, digital online community created to empower and connect people facing various health challenges and disabilities. You sign in, pick an illness, condition, or injury, and receive electronic newsletters on those topics. I signed up for post-concussion syndrome, whiplash, fibromyalgia, mighty morning, and pain. They fill their electronic newsletters with a wealth of material, tips, and personal stories, and on the main page, they offer affirmations and thoughts for the day. Their guides are updated, living documents combining expert and patient advice. They are phenomenal.

The Concussion Legacy Foundation

You can sign up for the CLF newsletter for insightful reading and updates. When I first investigated this website, I thought it was for football players. For a year I ignored them. Only recently did my brain click through the fog, and it dawned on me . . . it was the CLF (Concussion Legacy Foundation) not CFL (Canadian Football League). That is what brain fog looks like.

The Concussion Legacy Foundation (CLF) of Canada website contains excellent resources and invaluable stories. Their mission: To "advance the study, treatment, and prevention of the effects of brain trauma in Canadian athletes, youth, veterans, and other at-risk groups." Ignorant of concussions, we learn when affected, scour everything hoping to spearhead recovery. A story by someone who gets it is a life preserver.

Tricia Ruiz is a help line caretaker practitioner team officer (May 2024). The CLF helpline, launched in 2019, provides free personalized support and resources to those struggling with the outcomes of brain injury, as well as their families. They offer one-on-one partnerships and group support, including virtual support groups on Zoom, and excellent webinars. They also provide guidebooks for patients. It is a thorough resource for those suffering or battling brain injury. The more resources we get to help with head injuries, the more likely people will know where to go when they need help.

> *"The only person you are destined to become*
> *is the person you decide to be."*
> — Ralph Waldo Emerson

Looking for the sunshine and aloe vera go a long way to healing. An excellent resource is *Overcoming Mild Traumatic Brain Injury and Post-concussive Symptoms* by Nigel King, 2015. A self-help guide it uses evidence-based techniques rich with information, principles, and strategies. "Three critical principles outlined: reducing mental load, managing mood, accepting limitation and finding ways to get around difficulties," says King. Topics that resonate are acceptance, anxiety, dizziness, light/noise sensitivity, relaxation, brain training, pain management, achieving optimal functioning.

Family Affair

"The strength of a family, like the strength of an army,
lies in its loyalty to each other."

— Mario Puzo

Family is another intrinsic piece of the puzzle—the emotional effects on family and/or caregivers. We, as in those with head injuries, are not the same, and we can be difficult to live with. Smiles and nods of agreement. We get grouchy, lose our temper, feel violated—get frustrated, cannot do what we once could . . . insidious Tasmanian Devil shows up. Family should take advantage of resources developed by specialized professionals, talk to people who have experience with the head injured.

It is imperative to understand how injury affects each family member, support vital to well-being. If not present, important to find outside support. Recovery is easier when family know what to do or say when something or someone triggers an overreaction. Assumptions can be dangerous. The concussed feel guilty they cannot do what they used to. Spouses may be abrupt, confused as things halt in the household. Tensions build. Family members

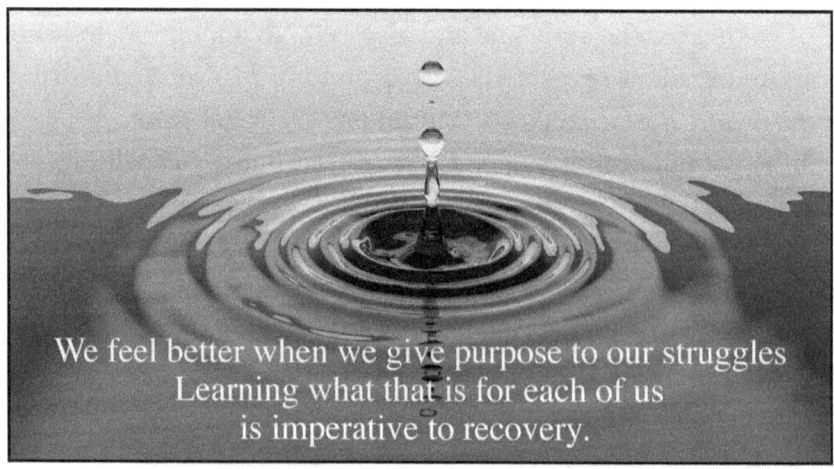

We feel better when we give purpose to our struggles
Learning what that is for each of us
is imperative to recovery.

might withdraw, become angry. The whole family suffers. It helps if loved ones make themselves aware so they can understand and do what they can to help, which means overlooking oddities, being patient, and forgiving. Including family members in the process leads to a better outcome. Be wary of slipping into patient-caregiver, a delicate role to balance. Family members may probe, try to understand. Ignorance slows recovery. Communication allows emotions to surface with less judgment, smoother sailing.

My husband and I faced rolling, challenging, crashing waves, tipping the boat, drowning us both, but our biggest cry—Do NOT take things said or done personally, even though they hurt. Sorry for that! My anger comes from a place of fear, pain, fatigue, frustration. Let go. Forgive. Forget. Move on. It is tough; it can be done.

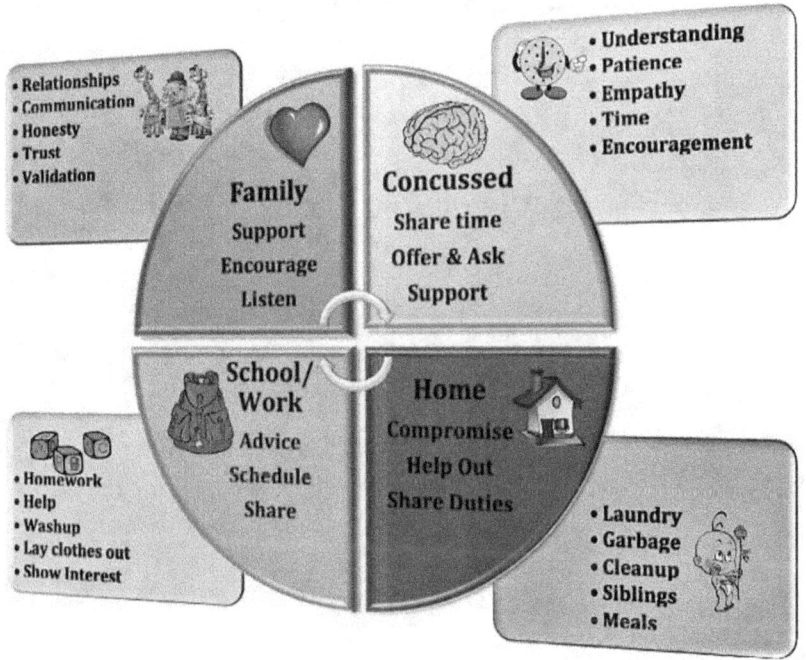

Although I cannot always avoid emotional intensity, I can navigate those moments without making myself or another feel worse. Head injuries wreak havoc on relationships; many do not make it through. Empathy and awareness need constant work. I try to be aware of who I fell in love with; pull from that, encourage the practice of acknowledging the skills of the other, show appreciation and gratitude, apologize when necessary. It takes patience, and an outside view to not get lost in a world distorted by chronic pain and PPCS leftovers. Injury erodes relationships. Thus, the importance of education. Priorities must be reassessed. A meeting once a week allows family members to raise concerns, deal with them before they build up. Everyone in a family must feel respected, heard, safe enough to share their perspective with no shame, blame, criticism, or analysis; vital the injured individual has a support system when the rain falls too many days, causing a mudslide of emotions.

Communication Tips

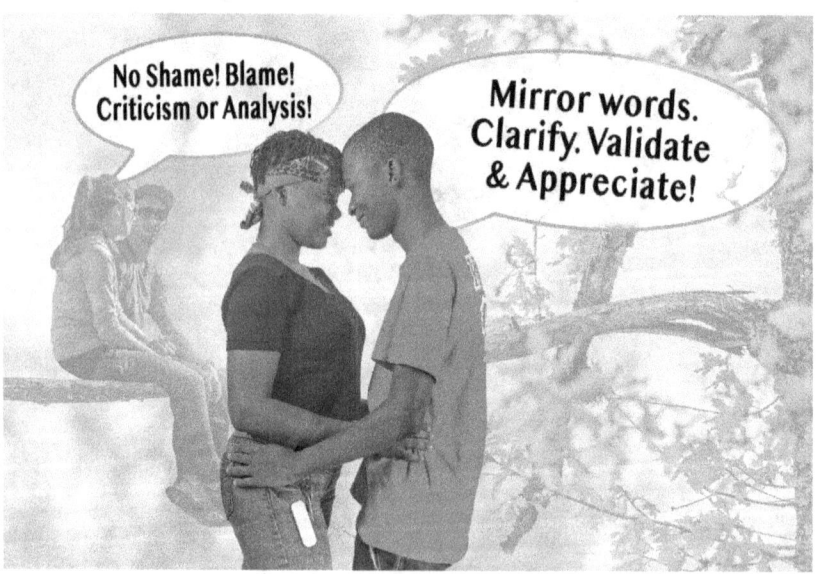

When talking to the concussed, simple, slow, to the point is best. Give extra time for processing and answering. Words pile one onto the other while sifting messages from other senses, background noise, clothes, expressions, gestures. Mirror words. An excellent strategy, not sure where I heard it, keeps communication open and respectful. Acknowledge, clarify, validate, appreciate throughout a conversation. It provides a good start when words are difficult, shared in a spirit of concern and respect.

Adjusting to change takes time, effort, and counsel from qualified medical practitioners, plus a willingness to be open, honest, and accepting of the injury. An outside perspective helps to see situations in a new light. Those with head injuries, often view the world through physical pain, hypersensitivity, and emotional hyper-reactivity. Through the eyes of others, we have a wider lens.

For anyone suffering with a brain injury, "before" is a wounded word, the only basis for comparison, and comparing we do . . . Navigating the unfamiliar landscape can crush the spirit. We need tools to break harmful habits, motivate, start and maintain healthy new behaviours, build healthy relationships.

Hurtful Questions and Comments

Hurtful	Helpful
1. What is wrong with you?	1. Is there anything I can do?
2. Just relax. You are too stressed.	2. I still love, (care) for you.
3. There's people worse than you.	3. That's tough. I am proud of you for hanging in. What do you need?
4. I wish you would...	
5. You should be...	4. I want to spend time with you.
6. I told you that. Don't you remember?	5. It's okay to not be okay.
	6. Compliment efforts, progress.
7. To be judged in any way.	7. Validate feelings and person.
8. Taking outbursts personally.	8. Provide a change in scenery.
9. Isolation, loneliness, made to feel less than, inadequate.	9. Acknowledging triggers, not casting blame.

Mindfulness

According to the Mind Space Clinic (2017): Growing empirical research shows that mindfulness meditation techniques can:

- Help cultivate compassion for self and others
- Reduce stress and anxiety
- Decrease emotional reactivity
- Improve concentration
- Strengthen confidence and resilience
- Promote peace of mind and well-being
- Help cope with pain and illness
- Enhance willpower and decision-making
- Help cultivate compassion for self and others

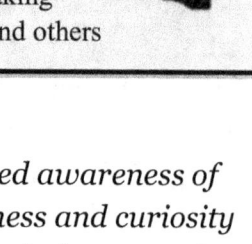

"Mindfulness, a mental state of relaxed awareness of the present moment, marked by openness and curiosity towards your feelings, rather than a judgement of them, is a powerful tool for experiencing happiness when practiced regularly."

— A.E. Wiltshire, 2023

Mindfulness is a great practice for anyone. It allows us to become more aware of how our body reacts to stimuli, how we sit or stand, observe our surroundings. Through introspection, we can consider why and what we are doing, practise deep breathing, noting what the body experiences. Because concussion causes overactivity and sensory flooding, paying attention to how we react slows our body's responses to a level where we can better manage the barrage of stimuli. Dealing with this hyperactivity in a healthy manner takes time, and it is beneficial to practise mindfulness throughout the day.

Some suggestions, and there are lots: wear an eye mask, focus on a water fountain or the rhythm of a clock, instrumental sounds, or music. The key—slowly breathe in and out, in and out . . . focus on a word or phrase. I inhale health, exhale stress. Inhale energy, exhale pain, then repeat with intent, concentrating on different body parts, smoothing out tension. Too often, we hold our breath, tense our body or hands into fists, and that can lead to soreness. With pain we have more difficulty being mindful. My mother shared a gem with me as she suffered with rheumatoid arthritis. Offer my physical pain as prayer or a plea to lessen the pain of someone going through a worse time, or as a catalyst for change. It helps me cope in major flare-ups. To see pain outside oneself also helps with understanding. Pain does not define, but influences. If chronic pain is a constant companion, ensure medicine and modalities are appropriate. Nurture self for tough days, and do not feel guilty. For too long my pain controlled my life. I am ready to control my pain. God grant me the serenity . . .

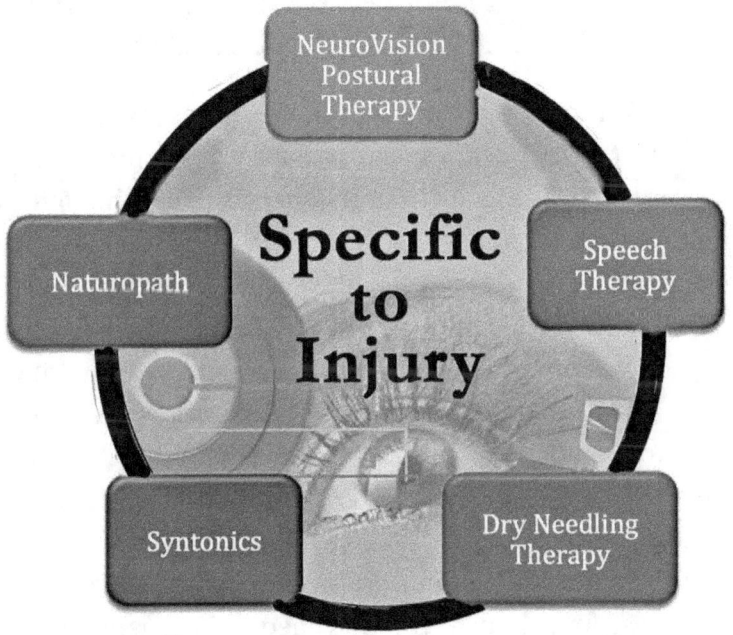

Gratitude

Oprah is right in reinforcing the value of gratitude journals. Creating a list of things we value, aids in cultivating a healthier mindset, provides strength and resiliency. Pausing at a lookout, absorbing the awe-inspiring panoramic view, we can invite Robert Frost to walk along a snowy wood in winter, or Emerson to converse over a glistening pond. Friends can come from anywhere— books, movies, documentaries, support groups, online.

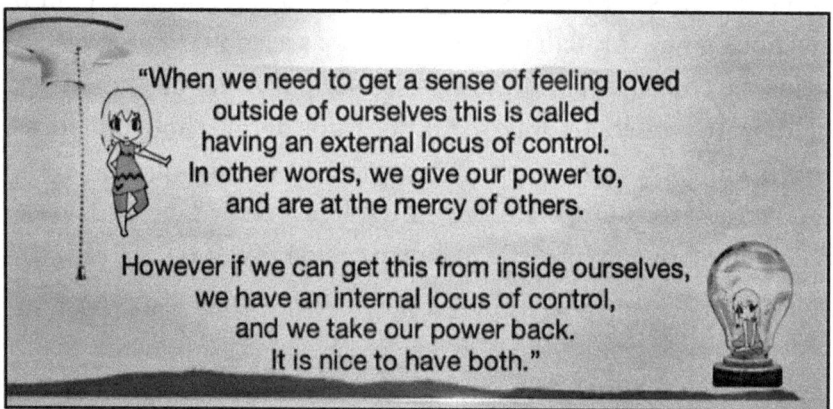

"When we need to get a sense of feeling loved outside of ourselves this is called having an external locus of control. In other words, we give our power to, and are at the mercy of others.

However if we can get this from inside ourselves, we have an internal locus of control, and we take our power back. It is nice to have both."

In her YouTube video, "Happiness Takes Work," Sonja Lyubomirsky (professor of psychology) suggests expressing gratitude toward someone in a letter or journal, visualizing our best potential future once a week, performing acts of kindness to lift the mood. She encourages us to imagine what or where we want to be. Visualize and it will come, like in the movie, *Field of Dreams*. She suggests we run through the mind several times a day what we have to be thankful for, especially when frustration bites because we cannot remember, sound like a buffoon, or fall below our 30 per cent energy level. Paying attention to that principle is an excellent strategy for anyone.

The Internet oozes mindfulness resources, especially on YouTube. Test first. You might find meditation or mindfulness weird, and fight it, but it has merit. Pinterest has a plethora of resources such as the 11 Mindfulness Worksheets and Templates to Live in the Present Moment. Making mindfulness a part of a routine helps our wellbeing, found at: www.developgoodhabits. com/mindfulness-worksheets/. These resources change, so please forgive dead links, and make sure the sources are credible.

Brain Foods - Wholesome Eating

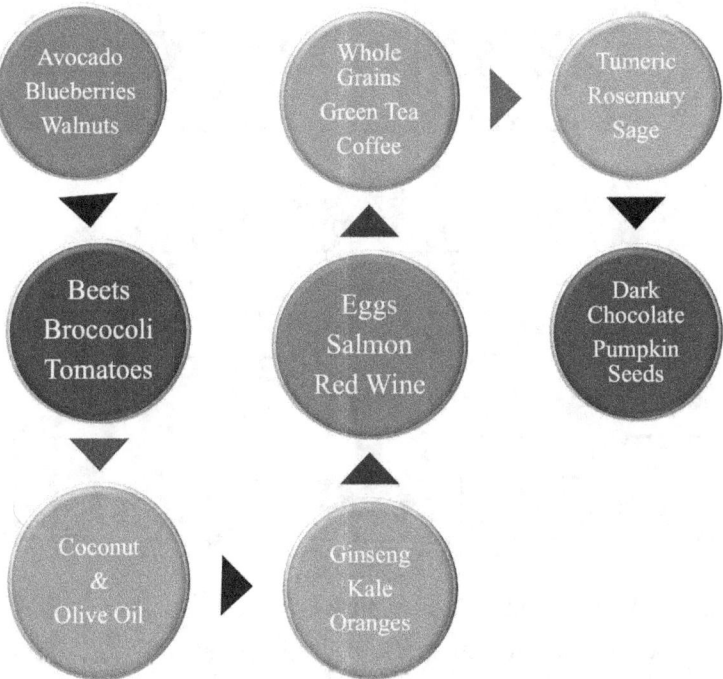

When tired and in a funk, it is too easy to eat fast food and junk. Once a week we can cheat, but to be as well as we can be, eating healthy foods is golden. Healthy also includes eating at the proper times and not skipping meals, which can lower blood sugar and affect mood and behaviour. Eating breakfast is crucial, as is checking and getting the right vitamins and minerals. Vitamin B1 (thiamin) from beans, whole grains, and pork; vitamin D, from fish, cheese, and eggs; omega-3 fatty acids, magnesium, Coenzyme Q10 from organ meats, Brussels sprouts, and cabbage.

I found lots of healthy recipes on the Internet. Find ones that work for you and your family. Add to your recipe collection. Accessing resources is easier today with the Internet and availability of ready-made, healthy meals. We owe it to ourselves to nourish the brain, flood it with the best. Picture the wilting plant receiving water, food, soil, sun. It is a catalyst for feeding that allows us to function and live.

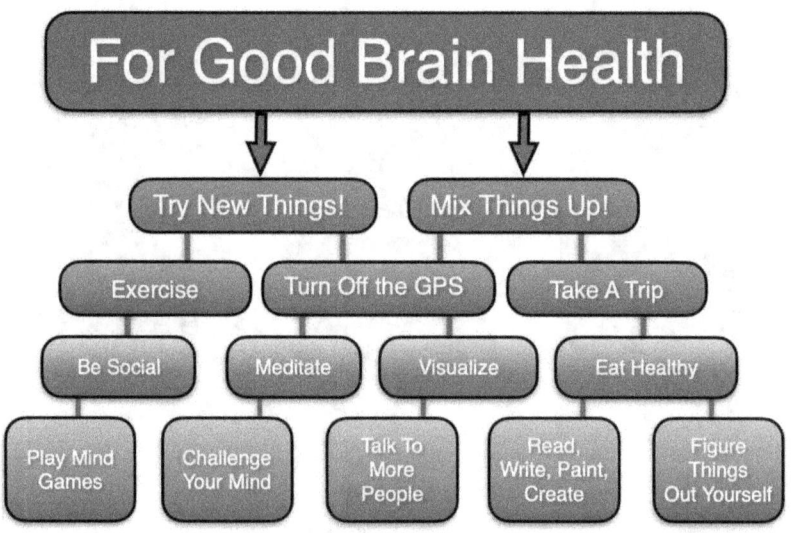

Eat fresh or frozen as opposed to canned. Be wary of salt and sugar, especially in hidden areas. If food brings enjoyment, indulge in moderation. Once every few weeks, make a double meal. Freeze leftovers or have the next day. Brain food can help with brain fog, cognition, nerve repair, brain health. Food that is rich in antioxidants, vitamins, minerals, and healthy fats, are important for us, boost energy levels. That right there is important, as chronic fatigue can be a killer. Brain foods increase alertness, attention span, ability to process information, and focus. Not a bad pitch for eating healthy.

Neuroplasticity

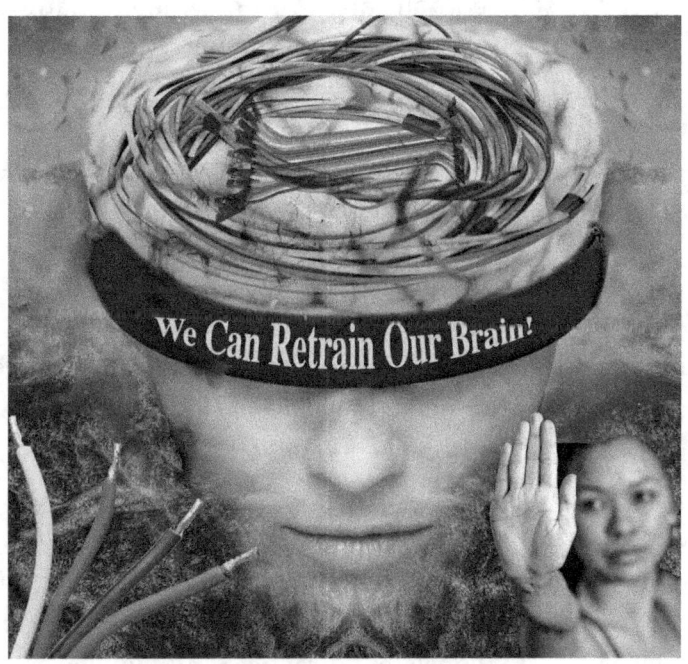

"By focusing on possibilities, you can see more than a potential light at the end of the tunnel. The light does not have to be at the end of the tunnel; it can illuminate an opportunity wherever you are."

— John B. Arden, *Rewire Your Brain: Think Your Way to a Better Life*

Neuroplasticity—a giant word—refers to the brain's ability to repair itself. It involves practice, practice, practice. Exciting news for anyone with a head injury or mental illness.

"Neuroplasticity suggests the human brain possesses the capacity for self-reorganization . . . new neural pathways are formed through renewed cellular activity facilitated by synaptic plasticity in adjacent regions." (Foojan, Zeine, June 2024.)

Proponents of neuroplasticity believe we train our brain with what we practise, that which excites us, motivates us, keeps us involved. Neuroplastic change occurs at the chemical, structural, and functional levels of the brain. These changes work together. Busy regions get more blood flow since they need more oxygen and glucose. Inactive neural connections wither away. Neurons that fire together, wire together.

The work of Donald O. Hebb (Canadian psychologist, neuropsychology) shows that synapses, the connections between neurons, get more sensitive, and new neurons grow, producing thicker neural layers. With consistent practice, individuals can have noticeable, lasting, positive effects. Practice shapes our brain, as exercise shapes our body. An intriguing resource on neuroplasticity and brain injuries is the book *The Ghost in My Brain*, a first-hand account written by Dr. Clark Elliott who suffered an mTBI and fought his way back. In his book, Elliott explains how his brain damage healed with a new set of eyeglasses and some brain puzzles. I skimmed pages but found the text too complex.

A 2017 review on Goodreads: "Doctors told him he would never fully recover. After eight years, the cognitive demands of his job, single parenting became more than he could manage. In one last effort, he crossed paths with two brilliant Chicago-area research-clinicians. One, a specialized optometrist, the other a cognitive psychologist—working on the leading edge of brain plasticity. Within weeks, the ghost of who he had been [re-emerged]."

Elliott found therapies and glasses dramatically improved his life. He worked with Deborah Zelinsky, OD; an optometrist noted worldwide for her work in neuro-optometric rehabilitation; functional neuro orthopaedic rehabilitation (FNOR); with a fellowship with the College of Optometrists in Vision Development. He also worked with Donalee Markus, PhD (a cognitive restructuring specialist).

"There are three ways that Zelinsky uses light to alter the way the brain operates: First she bends the light to various parts of the retina; this activates bundles of axons differently. Second, she changes the frequency of the light by allowing assorted colours through to the retina. Third, [she] selectively blocks signals from reaching the retina through occlusion filters that block out the light to certain parts of the eye." Working with Dr. Markus was crucial to Elliott's recovery. Her rehabilitation focuses on brain exercises, and puzzles of increasing complexity.

Some resources specific to neuroplasticity:

- Video: After Watching This, Your Brain Will Not Be the Same, Dr. Lara Boyd, Brain Researcher, University of British Columbia, TedX Vancouver at Rogers Arena on Nov 14, 2015.
- What is Neuroplasticity? Psychologist Courtney E. Ackerman, MSc, provides many excellent resources on her web page and blog covering neuroplasticity.
- Growing Evidence of Brain Plasticity with Michael Merzenich, TED Talk
- Video: The Sentis Brain Animation Series, neuroplasticity. YouTube, Recorded TedX Vancouver at Rogers Arena, Nov. 14, 2015.

Youth and Concussion

What Canadian youth know about concussions

Public opinion research with youth, ages 5-19, shows that:

- 9 in 10 understand that someone does not have to pass out to have a concussion
- 8 in 10 have little or no knowledge of concussion
- 7 in 10 identify that a concussion is a hit to the head that causes headache or blurry sight
- Canadian youth know very little about where to obtain concussion information or who is responsible for identifying a concussion and how to treat it.
- 7 in 10 incorrectly believe wearing a helmet will prevent a concussion
- 6 in 10 believe a harder blow results in a more severe concussion
- 4 in 10 think they should stop taking pain relief medication if they suffered a concussion

Information accessed June 20, 2020 Reference: Government of Canada

It's about self-improvement about being better than you were the day before!
- Steve Young

"The Impact of Concussions," an article by Jackie Middleton, *Canadian Living*, recounts stories of hockey moms. One mother, a Windsor, Ontario, schoolteacher, who did not expect the sport her eleven-year-old son loved would change his life, tells the story of how her son received a concussion while playing in an aggressive game in 2012, and her fight for better rules in hockey. "The concussion crisis has changed the face of sports as we know it and it has brought to surface the incredible importance of our brain health. The time is now for us to make our brain the number one priority so that education and awareness can take effect and begin to change the way we approach the health of our athletes from youth to professionals." Ben Utecht (former football player).

Concussion symptoms are multi-faceted; removing athletes from the game creates "an incredibly challenging time for them. They are under tremendous stress coming from all aspects of their lives. Their worries begin with not being able to play their sport, not practicing, losing their spot, letting their coach and team down, the social exclusion of not being around their team and taking away the athletes' biggest stress reliever—exercise." (Chen, J. K., et al. 2008: Harris, Katy, 2014).

Sports-related head injuries rank high among athletes in contact sports. Coaches, parents must teach young people how to take a hit or fall; they must wear proper headgear as designated by a particular sport. Education of long-term consequences of head injuries should begin long before the sport season.

Canadian Concussion Collaborative: "The mission of the Canadian Concussion Collaborative (CCC) is to create synergy between health organizations concerned with concussions to improve education about concussions, and the implication of best practises for the prevention and management of concussions. The CCC is composed of members from multiple relevant organizations. The CCC is chaired by the Canadian Academy of Sport and Exercise Medicine." (CCC)

The team, collaborative approach is exciting. I am proud of the incredible work being done by all members. Individuals like me will benefit, as well as our families, athletes, seniors, and youth.

Second Impact Syndrome

A great resource for youth is a podcast called, *Popping the Bubble Wrap*, on Apple, Spotify, or wherever you catch your favourite podcasts, produced by Story Studio Network, website in references. Young people think they are invincible, yet they need to be reminded to be careful, honest if injured, or suspicious of concussion. Please, so many sad stories of young athletes injured seriously and never the same. These stories are important to share. One, in particular, stays with me. I salute Rowan's parents.

"Rowan Stringer, known as Ro, was a 17-year-old, in grade twelve, and captain of her high school rugby team. During her last game, after suffering multiple concussions, she landed headfirst on the ground and fell instantly into a coma. It was May 8, 2013. She never did come out of it." (Hempstead, Doug 2015).

There are many articles written on Rowan, her tragedy a revelation for athletes, parents, coaches. The inquest into her death brought about positive change, as her parents fought, and pleaded for a change in the culture around concussions. A coroner's inquest held in May 2013, concluded she died from second impact syndrome, happening after two earlier concussions (not realized) in two games during the five days preceding the last match. She hinted to her friends she might have a concussion but did not tell her parents. An avid athlete and leader, she played ringette, soccer, flag football, lacrosse, and loved snowboarding. Rowan had been accepted into the RN program the University of Ottawa, her energetic desire to give back, as strong as her athletic commitment. Whenever I think of the dangers for youth, I see her smiling face, and the pain that must live in her parents. Determined to make her life count, they became staunch advocates and pushed for the formation and passing of Rowan's Law. They urge athletes to speak up and tell if they suspect concussions, further risk not worth it.

"Hearing the coroner's inquest . . . was difficult for her parents. It drove them to do all they could to make a change in concussion awareness, so no other young person suffers the same fate. A new mantra—when in doubt, out—can be heard in sports across the country; and to play smart, play safe." (CTV News, June 2016).

Gordon Stringer and his wife, Kathleen Stringer, suffered scenarios of what-ifs following their daughter's death, but it was not the end of their journey. They dedicated themselves to educating the public about the dangers of concussions. Kathleen Stringer,

Rowan's mom, reinforced the two would continue to do whatever they can to help.

Rowan's Law passed Ontario legislation in June 2016 and came into force on September 9. A committee worked on forty-nine recommendations made after the coroner's inquest, including education for athletes, parents, teachers, as well as guidelines to ensure a child's removal from play, and proper treatment if a concussion is suspected. Second impact syndrome is a rare, potentially fatal condition should you hit your head again before prior concussion symptoms have resolved. SPEAK UP! And parents –instill in your children the importance of speaking up.

"'She'd be very impressed,' Kathleen said Wednesday of the recommendations. 'And very happy and proud of us for all the hard work we've done for her.'" (Sherring, Susan, *Ottawa Sun*, June 3, 2015). And I would add for young and old people the world over. Thank you, for speaking out and up, taking a tragedy and using it to help others.

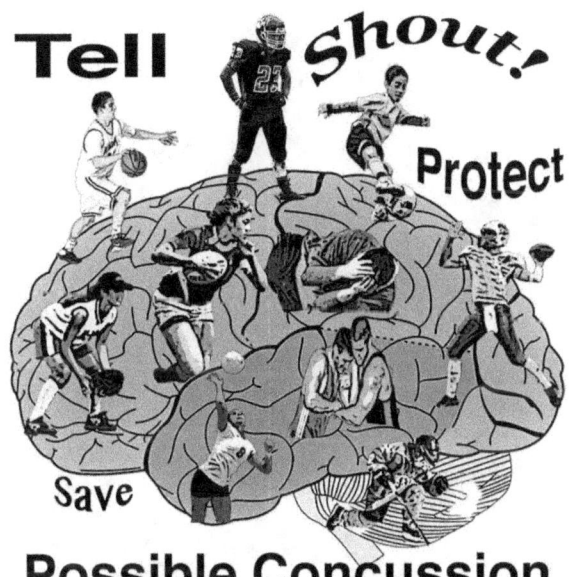

Tell Shout! Protect Save

Possible Concussion

Treatment

We are more than our injury or sickness, and we will no longer be defined as such. They are but fragments or shards left behind. With the proper treatment, we can take those fragile, delicate pieces and put them back together better than ever. May the following help.

— Francene Gillis

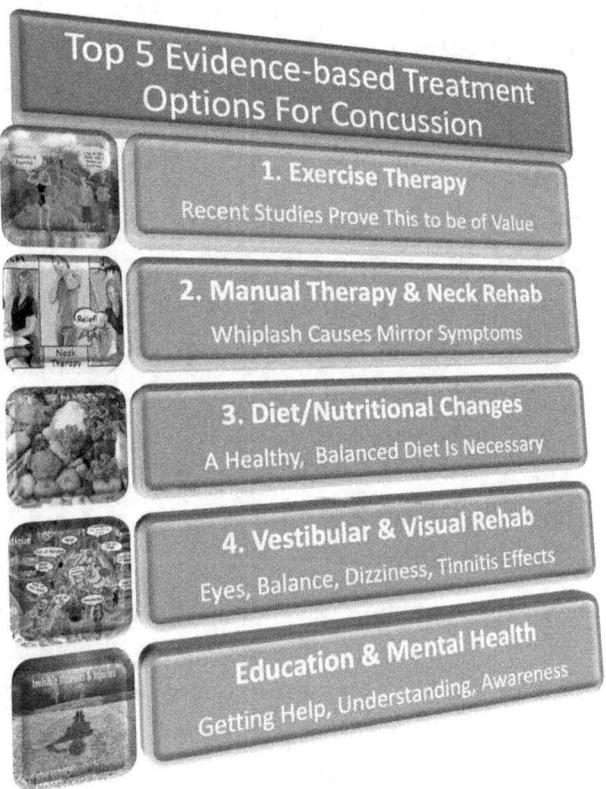

*W*hat is functional neurology? A new healthcare discipline, addressing the underlying causes of neurological
disorders, employing research-backed interventions to deliver
relief from post-concussion symptoms. Various techniques include
conventional treatment, visual and auditory therapies, physical
rehabilitation, progressive modalities to promote healing and
improve brain function. It addresses root cause of post-concussion
symptoms and promotes long-term recovery. Brain injury is unique
to individuals; multiple factors weighing in treatment, such as type
of injury, impact, gender, and age. For that reason, treatments deal
with the symptoms and issues that present themselves, or crop up
hours, days, or weeks later, leading to many therapies and specialists. What follows are treatments, some common, others on the
forefront of what helps in 2024, as well as self-help techniques.
Finding the best treatment takes time; what works for one may not
work for another. Recovery may be slow as the brain needs time to
heal, and exploring treatments is a process.

Research shows a team approach works best. Most with PCS
have several areas that would benefit from treatment. What follows are evidence-based treatments to enquire about, exercises
and activities to practise. Treatment should follow a thorough
assessment of symptoms by an experienced doctor or medical
professional. If you live close to a concussion clinic, or brain injury
centre, tap into their expertise. No matter where you start, find an
advocate to help. Prioritize what works for you.

Concussion treatments can be aggressive; some professionals
believe the sooner they expose the brain to what holds the patient
back, the sooner they will recover, thus forcing patients beyond comfort levels. Others take a steadier approach, as symptoms allow. No
one is better than another; it is more about which one fits the injuries
best. The balance between too much and too little is a conundrum.
Multi-faceted, multimodal clinical treatments are best with doctor
referrals based on individual shortfalls. Finding proper care should

not take months or years. When injured, we enter an ambiguous world, blind. Curveballs come at us. Answers need to be easier to find, oracles and their riddles too taxing on the brain.

Treatments & Therapies
MBI, MTBI, TBI, SRC, ABI, PCS, PPCS

It is important to note that many of these therapies have crossovers with one particular therapist qualified to offer more than one therapy.

1. Medical doctor specializing in head injury.
2. Naturopath to provide natural supplements and guidance.
3. Medical caseworker to help manage a road map.
4. Physiotherapist for physical injuries, soft tissue damage, pain.
5. Vestibular physical therapy for mobility, dizziness, coordination.
6. Cognitive rehabilitation to help with executive function, and memory.
7. Exercise rehabilitation to help with guided exercise, yoga, walking, hiking.
8. Occupational therapy to help with daily tasks, scheduling, pacing.
9. Osteopathic therapy to relieve pain through muscular system.
10. Laser therapy using focused light to help with pain and soreness.
11. Chiropractic therapy to help through manipulations of the skeletal system.
12. Massage using hands-on therapy to relax and activate muscles.
13. Myofascial massage, using light touch to make connections between body tissues.

14. Psychotherapy counselling to help with emotional regularities.
15. Psychologists to help clients with emotional problems.
16. Psychiatrists to help with mental health conditions and to prescribe medicines.
17. Psychosynthesis therapy to help with problems using creative expression.
18. Cognitive behavioural therapy, talk therapy to help with hyperactivity, PTSD.
19. Financial counsellors to provide strategies for financial well-being.
20. Legal advisers to help with lawsuits, insurance claims, unemployment.
21. Neuro- visual postural therapy to help with post-traumatic eye syndrome.
22. Speech therapy to help with speech, breathing, and swallowing issues.
23. Dry needling therapist to use acupuncture needles to activate muscles and help with pain.
24. Syntonic therapy using colour to promote brain cell activation.
25. Medication prescribed by a doctor based on individual issues.
26. Yoked prism glasses to help eyes focus and parameter issues, and improve balance and mobility.
27. Specialized earplugs to cut down on noise and too many signals coming at once—flooding.
28. Group therapy offered online or in person, sharing stories and hearing from others in a similar boat helps with courage, motivation, and recovery overall.
29. Concussion clinics offer a team approach to recovery with more than one therapy available.
30. Don't forget the positive influence friends, family, and caretakers can have on people with head injuries, as well as those who've walked the walk.

Cognitive Rehabilitation

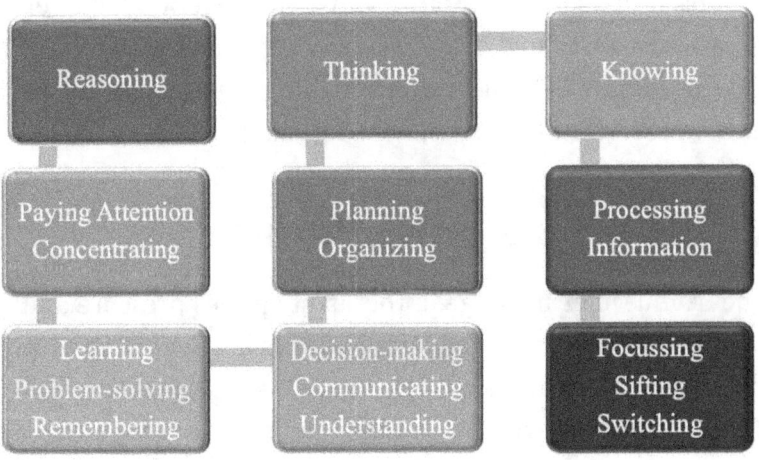

Practitioners weave cognitive therapy in with other therapies, encourage repetition, practice, cues, making notes. For therapy to be effective, it needs to be specific to individual needs and goals and focus on cognitive strengths and challenges. Card sorting and games, word, or math puzzles, playing board games with family or friends provide brain therapy as does reading, researching, and learning something new. Bonus, it is fun!

Physical Exercise

Before starting any exercise program, the concussed should have a thorough practitioner assessment done to determine the best form of exercise. Early suggestions can include gentle stretches, increasing mobility of the limbs, neck, and head as symptoms allow, and strengthening core muscles. Light exercise and walking provide a good start, gradually increasing intensity and duration. "It is important to know that symptoms can come later that day or even the next day, not necessarily during the activity." (Sunnybrook Health Science Centre, 2019.)

Exercise can speed up recovery by providing increased blood flow to the brain. Push through mild symptom increase, add more vigorous exercise when ready. Have your therapist "determine your exercise threshold; train just below that point. This is the best level to promote healing without making your symptoms significantly worse." (Smith, Jessie, Feb. 25, 2022)

Massage Therapy

In neuromuscular massage, a therapist applies pressure and friction using the fingers, knuckles, or elbows to release trigger points in the muscles. The Massage Therapists' Association of Nova Scotia (MTANS) sums up what is on many websites. Massage therapy is the manual manipulation of the soft tissues of the body, to achieve a therapeutic response. It enhances the function of muscles and joints, improves the circulation of the blood and lymph, relieves pain and stress, and can reduce blood pressure. It has a sedative effect, designed to rehabilitate, maintain, improve physical function through manipulation techniques. Massage therapy is not a substitute for medical examination or diagnosis; a doctor or nurse practitioner should make the referral.

Myofascial massage has to do with the fascia in the body and involves a soft touch approach to injured tissues. "Fascia is the organ of form. It has six to 10 times more sensory nerves than muscle. It does not show up in MRI's, CT scans, or x-rays. The fascia system connects the skeletal system to the muscular system. The fascia is the 3-D spider web of fibrous, gluey proteins that binds those cells all together in their proper placement. Facial restriction causes pain." (Sterling, Dana, 2024)

"Dehydrated fascia causes pain because we do not drink enough water. It shrinks, restricts, makes us achy. Myofascial release can improve pain, and reverse damage." (MacDougall, Jolene, 2023)

Yoga

Yoga, taught by a licensed instructor, is a mindfulness activity that allows a compassionate connection with the body, meant to relax, calm, and empower. Yoga focuses on breathing, mobility, balance, stretching, and slow repetitive pacing to condition and improve core strength, helping with problems such as sleeping, attention, concentration, memory, fatigue, and pain. Positive mantras used often help change negative patterns of thinking. High-functioning clients can do traditional or chair yoga, but for lower-functioning, one-on-one instruction is best.

The Internet and YouTube offer a wide range of yoga videos, meditation, and breathing exercise apps that make it easy to incorporate into daily life, but a health professional should supervise their usage in terms of adaptability and suitability. Slowing down, quieting the mind, and focusing on body awareness is good. With several types of yoga, it is advisable to get expert opinions on what might work best for you.

> "A study exploring existing research into the effects of meditation, yoga, and mindfulness-based interventions on minor traumatic brain injury and concussion symptoms finds these interventions can have beneficial outcomes." (Acabchuk, R.L., 2020)

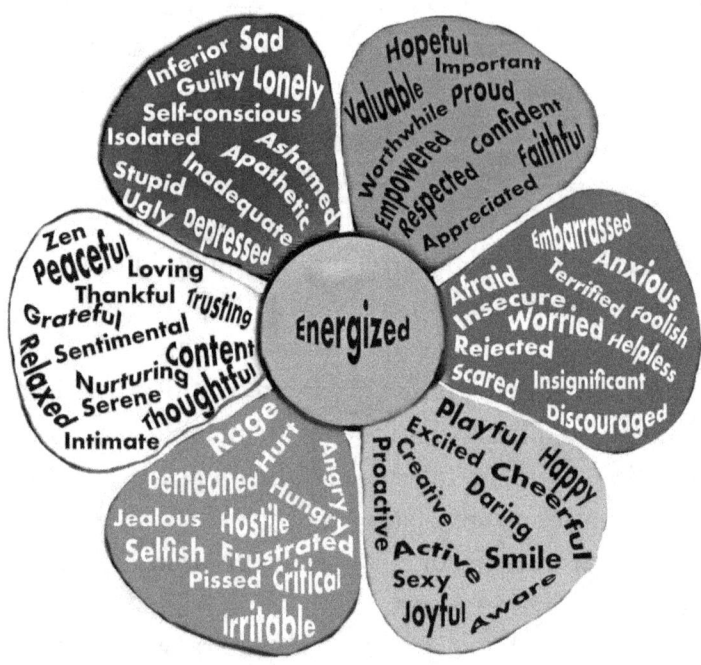

Psychiatrist, Psychologist, Psychotherapist, Counsellor?

With head injury, mental wellness is at risk. Who to go to for help? A psychiatrist, psychologist, counsellor? A smorgasbord of mental health professionals exist, so where to start? Your doctor may recommend a specific mental health professional. A psychiatrist has a Doctor of Medicine degree, specializes in diagnosing and treating mental health issues, is the only one licensed to prescribe medication. A psychologist holds a Doctor of Philosophy (PhD) in psychology, or Doctor of Psychology (PsyD). Registered psychologists can counsel and perform psychological testing and diagnosis, treat mental health and other health-related concerns.

Mental health counsellors hold a bachelor's or master's degree in psychology, counselling, social work, or related field. These counsellors can evaluate and treat mental health concerns by providing psychotherapy or counselling. Cognitive behavioural therapy (CBT) is used to treat the concussed to change harmful thought patterns. In persistent post-concussive symptoms, thought patterns often manifest as fear, guilt, frustration, or unworthiness. Much of the therapy centres on emotions and body awareness and restoring equilibrium and control of the mind and body through recommended techniques. Understanding this process is crucial to wellness. Thoughtful practice and behavioural repetition help with rehabilitation and recovery. It helps to get an outside, professional perspective.

Psychological psychosynthesis therapy—big words derived from psychoanalysis, a branch of psychology that identifies a deeper centre of identity. It considers each individual unique in terms of purpose and explores personal growth and human potential. Psychologists have clients examine what holds them back, such as trauma, unresolved pain, or inner conflicts, and work with them toward healing and discovery of self. The therapy connects the psychology with spirituality and offers gentle, creative methods toward self-realization and awareness, especially after a head injury.

Sometimes we need a family counsellor if injury causes upset within or for a family member. Ask your doctor for a referral to a psychologist or counsellor who does individual and/or family counselling and who is familiar with head injuries. We need to speak of the effects of concussion on a family openly, often away from the home.

Speech Rehabilitation

Help when Speaking/Listening

1. Gently get the person's attention before speaking.
2. Maintain eye contact.
3. Avoid body language, moving hands, gesturing.
4. Minimize background noise (TV, radio, and conversations).
5. Keep voice and tone in normal range, soften, unless asked to be louder or lower.
6. Keep communication simple. Do not ramble.
7. Allow time for response; silent air is not a reason to jump in.
8. Get to the point quickly.
9. Don't talk down, belittle, or demean effort.
10. Simplify sentence structure.
11. Emphasize keywords.
12. Reduce rate of speech to allow for processing.
13. Give individual time to speak, pause, process thoughts.
14. Resist the urge to jump in, interrupt, or finish sentences.
15. Ask if you, yourself are too fast, too loud, confusing.
16. Encourage drawing, notes, writing.
17. Use yes and no questions rather than long open-ended ones.
18. Praise attempts and downplay errors.
19. Allow the injured or sick participant to control the conversation.
20. Encourage independence and avoid being overprotective.

(Reference: Speech Language Hearing Associations)

"Neurogenic stuttering is a type of fluency disorder in which a person has difficulty in producing speech in a normal, smooth fashion. Individuals with fluency disorders may have speech that sounds fragmented or halting, with frequent interruptions and difficulty producing words without effort or struggle. Neurogenic stuttering typically appears following an injury." (Molt, Lawrence, PhD, 2017.)

"The central control abnormalities in stuttering are not because of disturbance in one particular brain region, but a system dysfunction that interferes with rapid and dynamic speech processing for production." (Ludlow, Christy L., 2003)

The Stuttering Foundation (www.stutteringhelp.org) provides brochures on stuttering, including how therapists diagnose and treat neurogenic stuttering, and the importance of working with a qualified speech pathologist. A speech-language pathologist may provide intervention at any stage across the continuum of recovery.

Vestibular Rehabilitation

"Trauma to the brain can result in abnormal vestibular system functioning, as the brain can receive abnormal signals about the position and movement of the head in space. When vestibular information is inaccurate, the brain most often relies on visual input to stabilize the head on the body. This means that the visual system quickly becomes the most reliable system to assess one's position in space and remain balanced. Relying upon vision alone as the primary source of balance often leads to fatigue and difficulty performing routine daily activities." (Miranda, Nicole, 2022)

The receptors in the neck can be damaged, which creates dizziness and disturbances in control of posture and balance. Vestibular rehabilitation is a means of addressing these balance problems.

Treatment for Visual Problems

- Optometric vision therapy
- Neuro-optometric rehabilitation therapy
- Corrective lenses therapy
- Phototherapy programs (syntonic optometry, light therapy)

In 2014, Dr. Mandelman, Bedford Eyecare, developed a special interest in treating TBI patients when she received a call from Dr. Linda Ferguson, a TBI physician in Truro, looking for a specialist who knew how to treat post traumatic vision syndrome (PTVS). She gave one of her first patients yoked prism glasses and he said it changed his life. He went from living in a dark basement in misery to being able to drive, socialize, live more normally. She was "hooked" and started her journey, taking a myriad of courses to learn how to diagnose and treat PTVS.

The following is an excerpt from an interview I conducted with Dr. Mandelman in 2020.

"Possible visual problems post brain injury: Blurred vision, sensitivity to light, glare sensitivity, reading difficulties, comprehension difficulty, attention and concentration difficulty, double vision, aching eyes, headaches with visual tasks, inability to keep contact or focus, loss of visual field, difficulties with eye movement such as 1. Eye tracking ability, 2. Shifting gaze quickly, 3. Focusing.

"There are two components to the vision system: the focal system used to read or determine what something is, and the ambient system which provides the peripheral awareness to use the focal system. When people have damage to the ambient, symptoms arise like delayed reaction time, difficulty with visually stimulating environments, a tilted centre of gravity causing balance issues, and an inability to walk in a straight line.

"Post traumatic vision syndrome (PTVS) involves a constellation

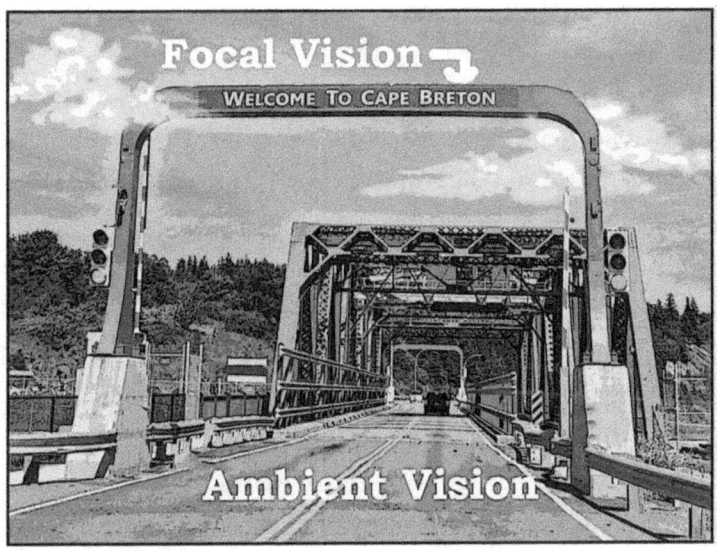

of problems: light sensitivity, double vision, blurred vision, inability to concentrate, multi-task, coordinate eyes, focus, and more. It leads to headaches, difficulty coping in busy, noisy environments, trouble with balance, memory issues, coordination, and speech.

"The focal system allows us to identify objects in the environment with a sharp central vision to pay attention and process details consciously. The ambient system involves peripheral awareness, scaffolding to orient ourselves in space. Researchers propose that injury stretches the fibres of the ambient system, causing a faulty flow of information to and from this part of the brain. Four facts about this system:

"1. It is a great anticipator: always ready for 'what's next.' If I threw an unexpected ball towards a baseball player, he/she/they will catch it. Throw it at a person with a damaged ambient system; it will bounce before they realize what happened.

2. It prevents peripheral visual stimuli from interfering with vision. For instance, a person with an intact ambient system can pay attention to their TV set while children run around. A damaged ambient system cannot cope in busy environments. Peripheral

stimuli are occurring in front, rather than to the side, which can be overwhelming.

3. It helps the body know where it is in space. Senses help us determine where our body is located. We 'feel' the chair; our inner ears give us information about location. If the ambient system provides faulty information to this fine-tuned system, the body may choose a new spot for its centre of gravity, leading to visual midline shift syndrome (VMSS). This displacement of the midline of the body results in a tilted world. To adapt, we develop an abnormal posture and gait.

4. The ambient system is unconscious: If it becomes damaged, the 'thinking part' of the brain attempts to take over its function. The brain has less 'brain power available for activities that require thought.' This results in difficulties with multi-tasking, memory, concentration, speech.

"Neuro-optometric rehabilitation involves a comprehensive evaluation of a patient's oculo-visual system including a careful case history, determination of prescription and binocular vision assessment to determine if the patient suffers from post-traumatic vision syndrome. The patient undergoes extensive gait and posture analysis to determine if a VMSS exists. To treat PTVS, practitioners use prism glasses to rehabilitate the damaged ambient system.

"1. Distance glasses with yoked prisms help offset the 'tilted' world patients perceive, help clients walk with confidence, balance, stability.

2. Near glasses with a reading prescription and base-in prism. These allow patients to read and do computer work more comfortably.

* Yoked prisms: Prism—wedge-shaped piece of plastic, thicker end is called the base, thinner end, the apex. When the base end of the prism for each eye is positioned in the same direction for

each eye, to the right or to the left for both eyes, this is termed "yoked prisms." Base-in prism: When the bases of the prisms for both eyes are closest to the nose, this is "base-in prism."

Syntonics Therapy

In optometry, use of phototherapy to treat visual dysfunction is called syntonics. Patients have an imbalance between the sympathetic and parasympathetic nervous systems. A heightened sympathetic system increases anxiety, oversensitivity to noise, movement, light. Functional visual fields may collapse when the injured try to concentrate causing difficulty in how they process information in their visual field. It causes them to ignore information in their periphery. Syntonics involves focusing on a particular colour to encourage growth of synapsis in the brain, and the use of coloured glasses and light suggested by trained optometrists to improve damaged systems.

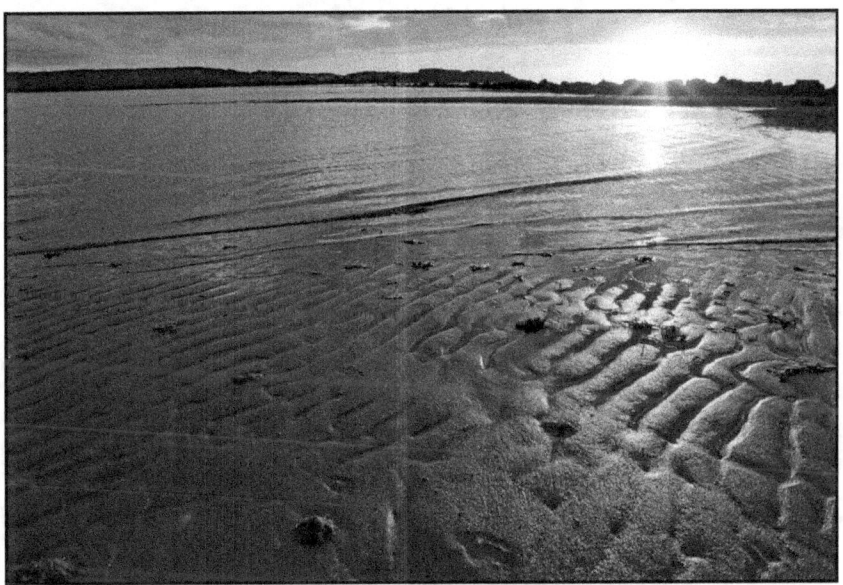

Naturopathic Concussion Treatment

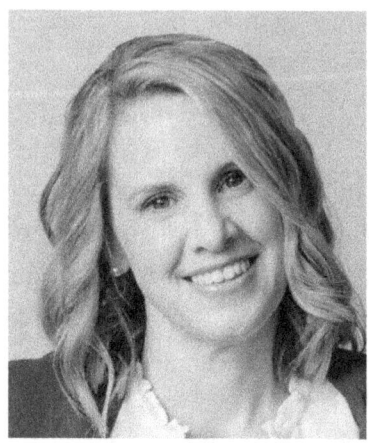

Glenna Calder, Naturopathic Doctor (ND)

"Naturopathic Medicine is an important part of the healing process and many patients with post-concussion syndrome have had tremendous success."

— Dr. Glenna Calder

"Concussions are best treated in an integrative team environment. Naturopathic treatment for concussions focuses on decreasing inflammation of the brain and feeding it with the proper nutrients to heal effectively from the traumatic brain injury. When a concussion occurs, there are several changes that occur rapidly within the brain and nervous system that contribute to increased inflammation, oxidative stress, excessive neuronal stimulation, hormone imbalances, neurotransmitter imbalances, mitochondrial dysfunction, and nutrient deficiencies.

"After experiencing a concussion, it is best to rest physically and mentally: No TV, computers, phones, or video games; no reading or homework, no work or exercise; get lots of sleep; sit or lie in a dark room (if needed). Shortly after, slowly introduce physical activity. Exercise improves blood flow, reduces inflammation and oxidative stress, helps to reduce post-concussion symptoms. It is also important to follow an anti-inflammatory diet. Inflammation of the brain is the first thing a naturopath addresses following a concussion. This typically excludes junk foods, high-sugar foods, dairy products, and processed foods, while incorporating lots of fruits, vegetables, nuts, fish.

"Supplements for individual needs can include N-acetylcysteine (NAC), curcumin (shown to cross the blood-brain barrier), and liposomal glutathione. Water is an essential nutrient and will help remove damaged tissue and speed healing just as dehydration can slow healing. Drink at least two litres a day.

"Once the inflammation calms, the focus becomes supporting the brain to heal, which we do by optimizing nutrition. Brain tissue and all nerve tissue consist mostly of fat. Having adequate amounts of healthy fats in the diet is essential to recovery. Include avocados, flaxseed oil, walnuts, pecans, almonds, pumpkin, sesame, and sunflower seeds. Cook with extra virgin olive oil. Add medium chain triglyceride oil, made from coconut and palm kernel oils to a smoothie with protein powder. Include healthy fats in the diet.

"Nutritional and herbal supplements include glycerophosphocholine (GPC), omega-3 fish oils, acetyl-L-carnitine, and protein powder if having a hard time consuming adequate amounts. Fish oil is a key player in concussion management, as are antioxidant supplements, which combat the oxidative stress that occurs post-concussion. Some examples are Coenzyme Q10 and alpha lipoic acid. Protocols followed are similar for all patients who experience concussions; however, practitioners must treat the person as an individual. Overall health affects healing time. Some may have worsening, pre-existing conditions, contributing to why they are in the ten to twenty percent of people with concussions who do not recover within the normal range." (F. Gillis; Dr. Glenna Calder)

In A Heartbeat

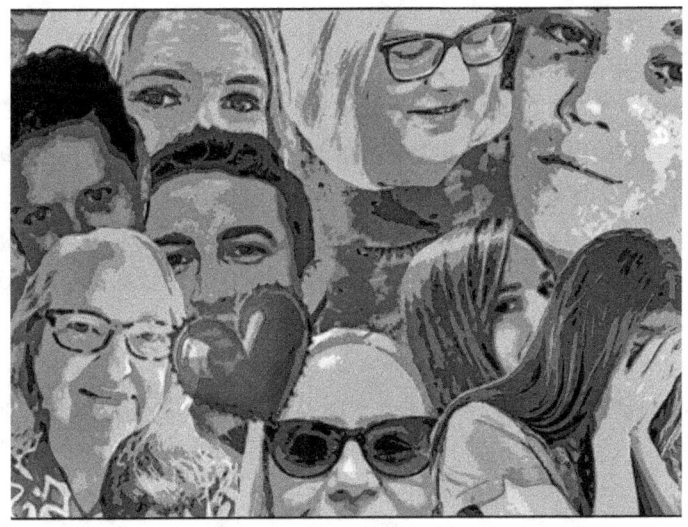

I believe the bad things happen in life to teach us how to look at good things in a whole new light.

— Unknown

Medicine

Medicine must be mentioned as it is an important aspect of treatment, but it is too individualized to detail here. Suffice it to say, a medical doctor will determine medical needs and prescribe accordingly. It is imperative however, that as patients we speak up and not be afraid to say something if feeling unwell, or to discuss our best options as it takes time to get the balance right.

*T*he section, "In A Heartbeat" expands the circle and memoir, shows people how fast injury can happen, incorporating seven stories to inspire as they did me. It is important to tell those we love that we love them. Say, "I love you," not for what they do, but for who they are. Speak it. Say it. Yell it! Whisper it. Do not assume. Make sure loved ones hear, in a heartbeat . . . Before I finish this sentence, a tragic event can happen. Too many haunted my youth, and compel me to write this section.

On a sultry July day, I watched my father work on my baby brother. I vowed to give his life purpose, fixated on how we treat others, remembering his brilliant, giving smile. Seconds forever change lives. We need to tell people how we feel, have no regrets, realize life is fragile.

Years back, my husband displayed symptoms of ALS—falling, bruising, cutting himself without realizing. For upwards of a year, it was his diagnosis. With more testing, the reason for his condition was damage to the spine, and a syringomyelia, or syrinx, a small hole or sac inside the spine, which doctors refuse to touch unless critical. He underwent back surgery for spinal stenosis—the narrowing of one or more spaces within his spine—the first of two. While he was convalescing in hospital, his roommate was a young thirty-something father of two. My husband got to know his wife and mother during his hospital stay. Their story woke me up to the dangers of ice.

This father of two, (now adults), went for a run on a freezing, rainy evening. He headed to his car for a jacket, slipped on the ice, whacked his head on the pavement. A pedestrian heard him moaning on the ground, called an ambulance. Paralyzed from the neck down, he could only move his eyes. He lay unresponsive in the Victoria General in Halifax, head shunts, feeding tubes, IVs, for over a year, as his loyal, devastated, loved ones visited every day. Several infections over long months, his condition precarious, but he was a fighter. From a standing fall, unable to communicate.

But he kept fighting for life and a few years later, was transferred to a rehabilitation centre in Sydney, NS, and regained some function. I hope with all my heart he fully recovered and was reunited with his loved ones. I wanted to share his story as it relates to what we perceive as a simple glance at a cellphone, hurried text, quick turn, fall . . . Life as we know it, can change in a heartbeat.

Outside the clinic in Antigonish, I meet a former student, family friend, Melinda (MacLean) Crawford. Good friends with both my daughters, she played basketball with them in high school. Surprised to see her, I discover that at thirty-two, she had been through the wringer. Off work a year, she noted her eyes were wonky. I told her about my eye therapy. Lots of discussion around prism glasses. I suggested she ask her doctor for a referral. Married, with two small children, she needed to return to her nursing career at St. Martha's Hospital in Antigonish, Nova Scotia. So many unknowns about the brain! Her story morphed, and follows, showing that the symptoms of stroke are another common window into brain injury.

In interviewing people for feature articles, I have come to realize that many enter your heart because their eyes touch you, their smile invites, their demeanour and words say, "you can trust me." They listen and hear the unspoken, see the unseen, understand, accept, and allow authenticity because they have processed life's worst pain.

"There is sacredness in tears. They are not the mark of weakness, but of power. They speak more eloquently than ten thousand tongues. They are the messengers of overwhelming grief, of deep contrition, and of unspeakable love."

— Washington Irving

The Domino Effect

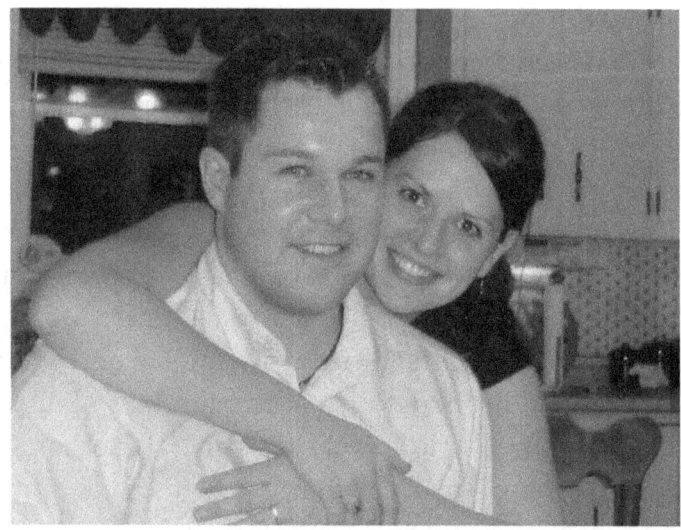

Melinda and husband

"I was screaming for help, but no one was listening. I wasn't being heard!"

— Melinda Crawford

January 17, 2016, is a day burned into Melinda MacLean-Crawford's memory, a drama following on the back of two tragedies, one occurring in September 2015, the other in December. A domino effect, tiles too quickly falling—one onto and into the other, without time to deal with, cope, grieve, understand, rest, recover, or accept.

Melinda comes from a large, tight-knit family of Macleans, mom, and dad (now deceased) living on the farm in Mabou Harbour, Cape Breton, Nova Scotia, parents of five boys and two girls. Caring, passionate, individuals, Big John and Marion have been tried-and-true anchors, community-minded people, salt-of-the-earth souls. Melinda lives with her husband, Jared; son, Colin; and daughter, Sadie in Antigonish, NS. A registered nurse (RN), she works at St. Martha's Regional Hospital, at the time of writing, in ICU. Her two-year hiatus from work is our focus as she too dealt with an invisible injury.

June 6, 2011, through C-section, eight-pound, twelve-ounce son Colin is born. Shortly after delivery, Melinda develops blood clotting in her lungs, known as a pulmonary embolism. The doctor places her on blood thinners, Fragmin injections, and later, warfarin. She stays on the latter for a year. Doctors tell her that having further children would increase the risk of blood clotting issues.

Age thirty-one, she, and her husband decide they want to add to the family. As soon as she discovers she is pregnant, she goes on the same treatment for blood clotting. A controlled pregnancy, she has complete trust in her OB/GYN, Dr. Wescott, a skilled surgeon, now retired. Beautiful Sadie is born, August 1, 2013, seven-pound, twelve ounces of energy. A boy and a girl, everything is perfect.

In 2015, Melinda and Jared decide to go for baby number three, and when pregnant, she resumes the blood-thinning protocol. At twenty-one weeks, September 20, 2015, Melinda goes for her routine ultrasound. A domino tile tumbles, most unexpectedly. No heartbeat. The technician searches, there is none. Melinda's medical brain goes into high alert to protect and distance her from what is happening . . . a baby beyond twenty weeks, dying in utero, is considered stillborn. Melinda and Jared shatter into pieces. She has to go through labour. After two C-sections and the shock of losing her baby; it is excruciating to know her labour is in vain, the result, a parent's worst nightmare.

"That is hard. Thank God, Jared is with me. The doctor induces me at 6 a.m. and I do not deliver until close to midnight. It is rough. A long, long day and understandably impossible to accept. All those razor questions, feelings, flooding in like a bomb: How? Why? We get bogged down in grief, but have tremendous support from family, friends, aunts, uncles, coworkers, extended family. I deliver a baby boy, no birth, and we name him after his two great-grandfathers, Angus Alexander Crawford."

Jared's father crafts Angus Alexander a special wood box, and Mom and Dad take their youngest son home. In Roman Catholicism, it is not customary to bury a stillborn child in its own plot in a graveyard with a headstone. So, what were their options? Their priest, Father Colin, came to the house. They held a ceremony outside, and buried Angus in their yard, with a headstone and angel statue looking over him. Their plans and thoughts—to have someone move his little body to their grave when either of them die. They do that because of the Church's stand, and because they are reluctant to let him go.

"We couldn't deal with it; we were only comfortable with keeping him with us."

Melinda only stays home for three weeks; then goes back to work in October 2015, everything going as fine as it can after such tragedy. To get through, she zeroes in on eating well, fitness, being healthy, to the extreme—she buys a bike, trains for a triathlon, loses thirty-five pounds between October and January. Then, another tile tips.

In December 2015, Melinda's best friend and childhood companion, Becky Beaton, received a diagnosis of late-stage cervical cancer. Always there for each other, they cheer each other on, pick each other up. Back and forth, they travel Antigonish to Halifax and vice versa, offering a hug, support, encouragement on their challenging, unfair journeys. But once a domino tilts, it is only a matter of time before it falls. The tiles come tumbling down.

On Sunday, January 17, 2016, Jared's father's birthday, Melinda wakes up at 6 a.m. to get ready for her twelve-hour, shift starting at seven. She jumps into the shower, the two children, age four and two, sleeping as usual, as is husband, Jared. Preoccupied with a raging snowstorm, Melinda worries about getting to work as a clinical leader, in charge of the registered nurses for the entire hospital of St. Martha's, responsible for adequate staffing each day. Once out of the shower she reaches for a towel, but weirdly, cannot pick it up. Her right hand refuses to work. With her nursing background, she at once thinks stroke, looks in the mirror, sees a right facial droop.

"I am in shock. It lasts several minutes, then goes away. I stare at my reflection and wonder what I should do next. As I putter around the house, I keep thinking, trying to figure it out. It happened so fast, and then it was gone. I figure it is better to go to work, stop in emerge, and get checked—that is the plan."

So, Wonder Woman leaves everyone sleeping, including her husband, barrels through a snowstorm after having a stroke, consumed with getting to work. As one of her RNs gives her report, about to go off shift, Melinda notices the words are not sinking in. She interrupts, and they head to emergency. Once there, she casually tells the people she works with every day her story of not feeling like herself. They stare, deer in headlights.

The doctor on call completes a neuro-physical exam, concludes it could have been a TIA (transient ischemic attack, a temporary blockage of blood flow to the brain). She recommends Aspirin, go home and rest, follow up with her family doctor. Melinda figures she can go back on shift, realizes soon after she forgot to take her aspirin, walks the loop of the hospital back to ER. Within that time, her right hand goes limp, right arm tingles.

They put her in a room, reassess, give her Aspirin. A CT of her head comes back normal. Doctors do not see her as a candidate for the drug doctors normally administer intravenously when symptoms of a stroke remain. They believe it will not be beneficial, but admit her to the stroke unit for observation. When admitted, Melinda finally calls her husband, who knows nothing of the morning's events. She makes light of it, tells him she went to work, and may or may not have had a stroke. Aware of her mother's history he is speechless, and all she worries about is that he packs the right clothes in the right bag.

"God love him! He kept asking me questions. I was trying to answer so he could take it in, but when he landed and laid eyes on me, and I looked and sounded fine, he could not digest I had had a stroke because my symptoms were invisible."

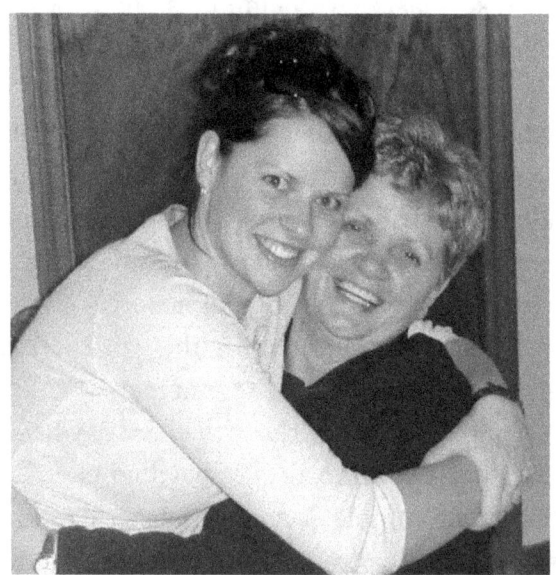

Melinda with her mom

"Then, I call my poor mom . . . God love her! A hard pill to swallow. Reluctantly, I muster, 'Looks like I had a TIA this morning.' I am totally downsizing. The shock and pained disbelief in her voice, I regret calling her, knew because of the blood clots she would feel responsible. Scheduled for an MRI the next day, I told her I would let her know the results. That was the plan. She was in total disbelief, and I was annoyed! After the MRI, Dr. Pereira, who I work with, informs me I did have a stroke. All I can think to ask, 'Do you think I will be off work for a while? So, when can I get going again?'"

Melinda is a racehorse, wanting to get out of the hospital, wondering how she will ever survive without work. She has no other symptoms except pain and tingling. A popular young lady she has tons of visitors. "Watching people come to see me, and the instant relief on their face when they see I am okay—that is my entertainment. Staff and the stroke team are exceptionally good to me. Everyone worries. I am only thirty-four."

They keep her in for a week. She has residual symptoms—her right arm and leg have a lot of burning, nerve pain, and tingling sensations. She realizes the first time she showers in the hospital, she cannot feel hot water and burns her forearm. Neither can she put her arm up to wash her hair or do any prolonged activities as they bring on fatigue, pain, anxiety, and emotional duress.

When Melinda goes home, Jared is *"what the hell"* scared. She is not worried, simply happy she can still walk and talk. After getting home, trying to look after the children and house proves too much for her. She realizes fatigue cripples. "You don't know until you are in it," she says.

She pushes through, struggling until utterly, worn down, she reaches out to an occupational therapist, nurse practitioner, Lena MacDonald, who works through the Heart & Stroke Foundation. Melinda is overwhelmed with her days and Lena helps pace. Melinda realizes she has a window of four hours in the morning when she feels she can get things done and be mentally present for her kids. Her family arranges support so she can rest and sleep. Jared takes on more duties around the house and with the kids. She has to be meticulous about what and where she spends her spoons. "Most of the time, I spent it with the kids, too tired to be mentally present."

Referred to a neurologist in Halifax, she was given the same sad story many women receive. He told her to go see her GP, gave a week's supply of sleeping pills.

"I did not take them. Spinning, my mind refused to stop. Why wasn't he helping me? That was the pinnacle for me—when he said he could not help. Who else would help? I was desperate. I couldn't sleep, couldn't stay on topic, my thoughts raced, spun out of control. What was I going to do? Where could I get help?" A common theme among patients with an mTBI of belittlement—neurologists steering away from the more complicated functional aspects because no structural damage can be seen on scans.

Melinda could not go back to work. She struggled with balancing unimaginable fatigue and pain in her arm and leg, while struggling with brain fog, anxiety, depression, and insomnia. To help, she went on medication. The symptoms lasted for months. The period of being home, she does not remember.

"Jared was my rock, helped me through my struggles and grief. We attempt to deal with deep, personal pain, loss, and my injured brain. From the outside looking in, all seemed right, but behind our smiles, pain lived. It was such a tough time; I don't know if it was left over from the stroke, if too hard on me, or . . . I was stubborn, in denial, defeated. The second year, I crashed and burned. "

And then she visited occupational therapist Jeniffer Hilling.

"The first time I saw her—poor Jeniffer. I wish I could ask if she remembers the conversation; I was struggling so bad. That was the beginning of help. I was screaming; no one was listening. Immediately, she heard me, knew what to do!"

Jeniffer called Melinda's family doctor, who saw her the next day. They postponed rehab while she dealt with and tried to recover from anxiety and depression, left far too long. Melinda did not connect it to her brain injury, finding it difficult to differentiate between the two.

"In between having a stroke and seeing Jeniffer, I remember

thinking, it sounds bonkers. I went to the brain injury group in Antigonish for support."

"I still see their faces when I said, 'I wish I had a major stroke so people could see me!' It is the invisibility of it. People do not get it and I work in health care. It really wears you down. Things happen so quickly. I was trudging through sand and getting nowhere."

— Melinda Crawford

Jeniffer zeroed in on Melinda's visual problems from the stroke affecting her fatigue, referred her to Dr. Sheppard to try yoked prisms. Because she was a stroke victim, the optometrist was unsure what would happen, if she could help because of dead tissue, but was willing to try. Melinda could not wait to get her glasses. She received them in March. By that time Colin had started school and Sadie was in preschool making things easier to manage. She had more time for recovery.

"The glasses were the tipping factor that sped up healing. It could have gone faster had I had known about them earlier. My biggest fear, going back to work—I was scared to fail, look like I could not do my work in front of peers."

Between the yoked prisms and rehab, she was back to work the end of November 2017. Melinda managed, dedicated herself, and earned a promotion. Being on both sides provided insight for Melinda. She worked two days, and two night shifts a week, which accommodated for her fatigue and the need for rest.

On May 14, 2018, Rebecca Maureen (Becky) Beaton, Melinda's dear, best friend, lost her battle with cancer. Melinda was crushed, grief a battle of its own. More challenge and heart-wrenching questions. Her friend was only thirty-six years old and full of vitality. Everyone who knew her loved her, shook their heads unable to understand life's blows. Melinda held on tight to her career.

"I love nursing, hated being a patient. I am happy, healthy enough to be a nurse, even during a pandemic. I work with impressive colleagues: nurses, doctors, dieticians, RTs, PTs, OTs, ward clerks, CCAs. I could not be prouder of both my family and my work family."

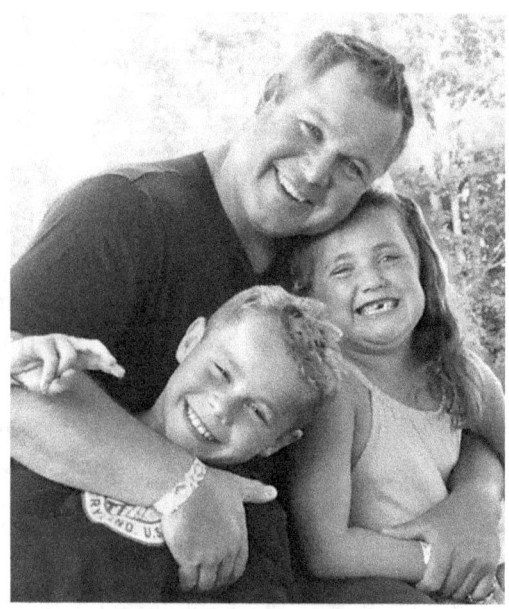

Jared, Colin, Sadie

Echoes of a Younger Woman

*"Don't close the book when
bad things happen in your life.
Just turn the page and begin a new chapter."*
— Unknown

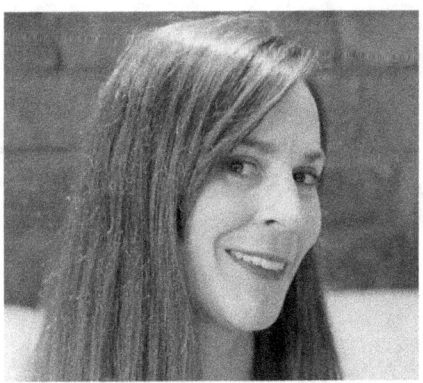

Cara Palmer

*"I was given this comparison which I found best
described a concussion: Your brain is like a filing
cabinet that has tipped over and all the files have
scattered all over the place; it is going to take quite a
while to put them back in order. And some may not go
back to their original place."*
— Cara Palmer

Speaking to Cara after my injury was insightful. Younger folk also get brain injuries, and I knew I had to include her. An inspiration, she kindly shares her story.

"Lots of appointments and specialists! It was all quite draining. In the beginning they were an all-day affair, getting ready to get there, then recovery would take a couple of days. I really had to pace myself. I had an excellent psychologist that I could speak to on the phone. That was difficult to do at first. She really helped me conserve my energy, focus on what I could do as not to get depressed. I slept a lot, listened to my body, tried not to overdo it. She gave me useful tips on how to keep track of things once I started to get more mobile. I wanted to focus on the positive, what I could do, no matter how small, instead of my symptoms which is what I found many concussion clinics do. This is when I noticed a shift in my healing too!

"I saw an osteopath who focused on cranial sacral work and a massage therapist trained under him. I always felt clearer and better after those appointments. I also saw two naturopaths. They provided therapy through vitamins that gave me more energy. A physiotherapist in Halifax used a Chinese medicine approach which seemed quite odd and unconventional, but I really felt better after a few visits with him. I could not do these trips to Halifax until months into the recovery, travel proving too much and then I would have to stay for a few days to recover. My eyes were the last thing to recover, and they gave me issues for a long time. I had to do physiotherapy exercises for my eyes and had a great eye doctor in Antigonish. I got an excellent report on my last visit. My eyes had improved, and I no longer needed visits to the specialist.

"My family doctor recommended that I eat well and avoid junk food. This was the advice I found most beneficial—maintaining proper nutrition. I practised a healthy living program to take down inflammation through a vegan skin care and nutrition company. Later I became a consultant because of my love and passion for their products. It had two meal replacement shakes a day, which I had for breakfast and lunch. Cooking was near impossible in the beginning. I took omega vitamins for brain and eye health.

"Arbonne played a huge part in my recovery—it gave me purpose, joy, and confidence. All my friends and family saw how much it did for my healing. It was wonderful self-care too, something I

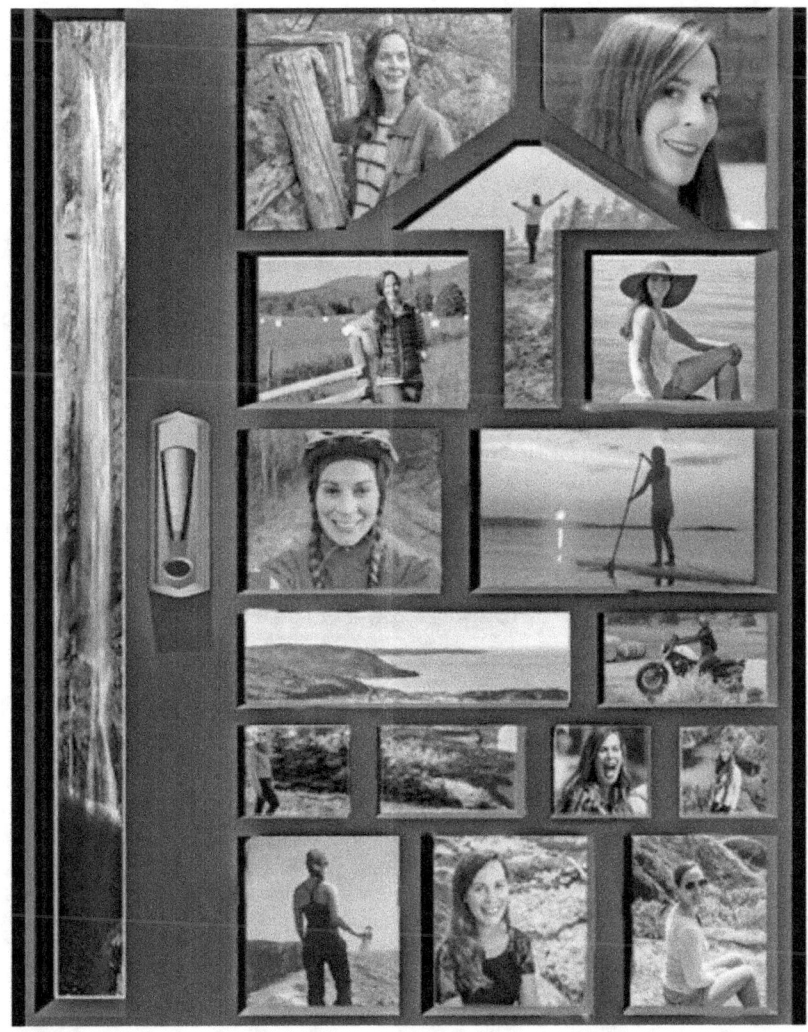

looked forward to when all I could do was shower and that was not every day in early days because it was so tiring. I'd have to lay down and rest after the shower before I could get back up and dry my hair. I did sleep for almost twenty-two hours a day, for the first while.

"I was so thankful to my family and friends for helping with my son during this time as I could barely take care of myself. Noise really bothered me. I had custom-made earplugs that were heaven sent. It made conversation, once too loud, appear normal. I wore sunglasses for a year everywhere, including inside. I could not attend events, walk into restaurants or stores, noise, and conversation too much, I would feel overwhelmed, start to cry. This is what it must be like for anyone with sensory overload issues. It was over a year before I could drive my car. I had a lot of great support and friends even though I could not visit with any of them for a long time after the injury, as conversation was draining. The body is amazing at healing itself. It will take time.

"I wanted the recovery to happen faster than it did, but the pressure and stress I put on myself made it worse. I still have times when I need to slow down, take things off my plate. Stress is the thing that gets me every time and I feel I must step back, rest, and take care of me, even now years later. It does get better; it just takes a while, and it is okay. When I stopped comparing what I used to be able to do and accepted the new me I was able to enjoy life more. Memory is still a bit of a challenge, but I try and relax with it knowing I am doing my best and things will get better, and they have."

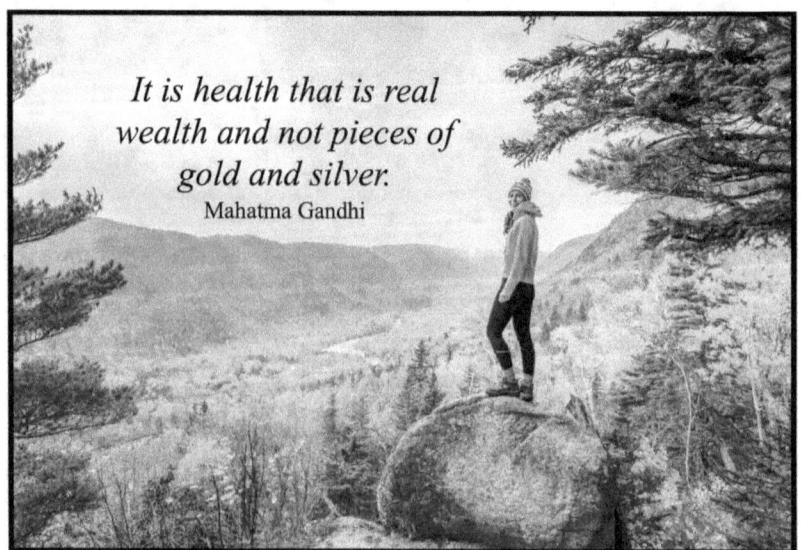

It is health that is real wealth and not pieces of gold and silver.
Mahatma Gandhi

Dreams of the NHL

"In life, you have a choice. You can either look back or look forward. I choose to look forward."

— Ian Malesiewski

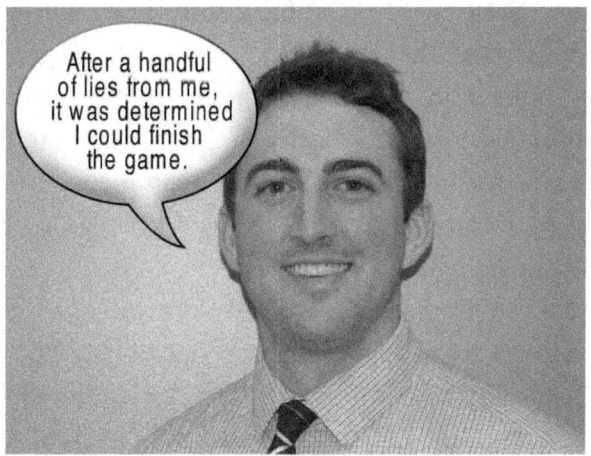

Taylor Lambke

Taylor Lambke was thirty years old when I interviewed him, so we will excuse him if he says anything to implicate me in any conspiracies about the purchase of a black Rogue. I first met Taylor as a keen, car salesperson. Our open personalities allowed us to share a common injury, which altered the course of our trajectories.

Taylor grew up in a family of five in Antigonish, NS, born in the Sydney area to very sports-minded parents. His younger sister, Rebecca, played soccer with Cape Breton University, and younger brother Garrett played hockey. At two, Taylor was on skates, thanks to his dad. And we may forgive him for raising his son to be a huge Buffalo Sabres fan; "A blessing and a curse," says the young man.

Talking to the former hockey star, he was, and is, a driven individual who knows the importance of setting one goal at a time and working hard toward it. His understanding of the importance of an excellent education combined with a love for hockey served him well; he had options post-concussion.

"My goal from an early age was to make the NHL, first being drafted to major junior, which I accomplished. Becoming a captain of a major junior team was also a goal achieved. In my draft year I suffered a shattered collarbone and a broken foot. It was a setback in my career that I could come back from and continue playing in major junior. But when I did not get drafted, my goal switched to education and playing CIS (Canadian Interuniversity Sport) hockey. I took a year off after my major junior career to find where the best fit was for me. Several former teammates and players I had played against reached out to me and helped recruit me to Concordia University in Montreal.

"After a successful first semester at Concordia, my hockey and academic careers were at their peaks, but during an Ottawa vs. Carleton University game my life and hockey career changed forever. A booming, blind side hit knocked me out. I hit my face on the ice and was unconscious for a few seconds. Our two trainers at Concordia assessed me; after a handful of lies from me, medics decided I could finish the game. On the bus ride home, I began to feel dizzy and sick. When we arrived in Montreal the trainers performed more tests and set up an appointment to meet with the head doctor for the athletic department scheduled for the next day. That specialist determined I had sustained a serious concussion, which could have lasting effects. For two weeks I had massive migraines, a tough time getting out of bed. I didn't attend classes for the rest of the semester."

Taylor is unusually calm as he shares what must have been a heart-wrenching time. Well-disciplined hockey players excel in their sport. He continues, "The doctor and our trainers were excellent in monitoring and supporting me through the whole situation.

We tried to create a recovery plan so I might play in the first round of the playoffs. It went well for three weeks, then I had setbacks, started showing symptoms. This time, more severe. Throwing up, major dizzy spells, spending days in bed, I did not go to the rink or classes for about a month. Our team doctor determined my season was over, and potentially my career." He pauses.

"The severe symptoms lasted for about two months. Then, for a period of about six, I suffered from milder effects. I had less severe headaches but could not exercise or do physical activity without falling ill. Prior to the concussion I was in the best shape of my life—winning several fitness tests during training camp and mid-season testing. To this day, I have never felt as good as I did prior to the concussion, physically and mentally.

"I experience symptoms to this day, although not as frequent as I once did, and have not played a game of hockey since that day. I do not have any regrets about my injuries or concussions; it is part of the business and comes with the territory when you are chasing your dreams. Throughout my career I broke bones, had many bruises, but the concussion was the most devastating, because it affected the rest of my life. As a former player, and as a coach, I would tell young people that there is a major risk when playing a contact sport. However, we have come a long way as far as player safety. We have become more knowledgeable about concussions and how to treat them.

"Today I have developed a successful career in the car industry. I coached junior hockey with the Strait Pirates Jr. B team. It allowed me to continue my love of the game and stay around to help young players grow and develop as young men.

"For a long time when my hockey career ended, I was angry and depressed, frustrated because of how it ended, and I had a tough time accepting that. A lot of who I am today is because of my experience on the ice and being around teams, but persevering through the challenging times after my concussion has really given me the character that I have today. It has helped me as a coach and as a person with helping people or players through challenging times. I hope that the worst is behind me and that I can continue to live a long healthy life. However, I would not be surprised if this stays with me forever."

As with all youngsters who play hockey, there are moments that stand out, moments that spark the desire to reach higher, and demand more of self. Taylor had several: winning a high school championship in grade 9; scoring the winning goal in peewee AAA in double overtime; being drafted to major junior; scoring on his first shift of his first major junior game; playing against several NHL players; and last but never least, being roommates with NHL player Matthieu Perrault! Not a bad legacy, to be sure.

As a player and coach, Taylor promoted playing smart, being aware of self and other players in the game. He knows injuries are a part of the fast-paced game, but awareness and education can reduce them. He knows how tough it is to fight, wanting to play in a big game after injury. The tendency to downplay concussion ringing in his and every sports player's mind. He now opts for truth, as secondary injuries to the head can lead to second impact syndrome . . . dangerous if a concussion occurs on top of another that has not had time to heal, making it imperative athletes tell the truth.

Since initially interviewing Taylor, a lot has changed in his life. He switched dealerships and moved to New Glasgow. "I have a beautiful wife, Meghan, and two amazing babies: Kesler and Sophie," he says. He still works in sales and trains and teaches his sales staff, I am sure with his smile and the wisdom of harsh lessons learned.

No Naysayers

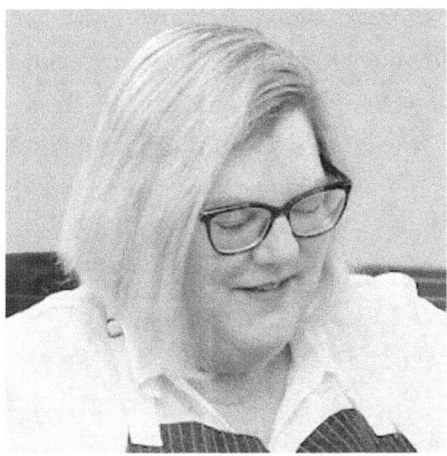

Joanne Schmidt

"I think God created concussions to drive Type A
personalities insane or punish them while on Earth."

— Joanne Schmidt

I taught two teenagers whose mother, Joanne Schmidt, had suffered a brain injury in a vehicular accident. They would talk about how tough life was for her after, but I could not understand her reality. When injured myself, years later, she reached out to me and offered advice, a concussion guru of sorts. Besides headaches and post-concussion syndrome, Joanne suffers from chronic neck pain from whiplash, soft tissue damage, and fibromyalgia, which compounds recovery and leads to bad days, hours, minutes with chronic pain and fatigue stopping her in her tracks. Seems too familiar as we try to avoid hitting the wall—going over or under our threshold. Her story and advice to me follows, as well as her wisdom of prior injury, and post-concussion syndrome.

As Joanne stopped for roadwork, the vehicle behind rear-ended her car, pushing her forward, into the one in front. Her seat broke upon impact, pushed and shook her around the vehicle.

"I was sore for days, could not keep up, could not read afterwards, could not do math, could not carry on decent conversations, could not follow directions. I would sleep all the time. Lights and sound affected me. I was a mess," Joanne says.

"Recovery takes time. You may need weeks, months, years. Allow it. The doctors are skilled at not revealing any agendas whatsoever. But you will want to have some idea. It may take a while. Concussions have their own timeline. Give it rest. Take vitamin D. Get earplugs. Keep sunglasses with you. Speech problems, word dissociations, and aphasia can pop up. Reading can be affected. Do not be alarmed. Try to eat as healthy as possible, and not stress. Give it time. With pushing yourself, it is difficult. You need to take it case by case. You will find lots of little 'hacks.' The biggest thing is not to worry about what others expect you to do. I am only now able to listen to the occasional song. Music was something I could not tolerate for years. So, keep plucking along. Concussions teach patience whether we want it or not. It is hard not to be frustrated.

"I have a cooling eye mask that I put on backwards, so the mask is on the hairline at the top of my neck, and the elastic on my chin. It cools the irritated optic nerves at the base of the neck. They tend to cause a lot of the headaches. In the meantime, make certain to rest, no TV, movies, Netflix, and limited computer. I know . . . boring . . . but your brain needs to heal. Also eat healthy, lots of food with colour, and fish oil, (pills, salmon, sardines, whatever). They also say exercise, but I know for me I had nausea, balance issues, and dizziness. The dizziness is finally starting to ease off. I have only just started getting out for a short walk on a GOOD day!

"Some professionals I have relied on are osteopaths, and a good massage therapist that does therapeutic deep tissue massage. I have been going to an osteopath for years. They finally diagnosed my headaches. It is not chronic migraines, but occipital neuralgia, which is pain radiating from the occipital nerves in the upper neck, on either side of the back of the head. Something to keep an eye out for in case your headaches follow a similar pattern, since your head took a hit to the pavement.

"Since I talked publicly about my brain injury, it has opened more conversation with family and friends. They are more comfortable talking about it. I hope this book helps other families talk about this silent injury."

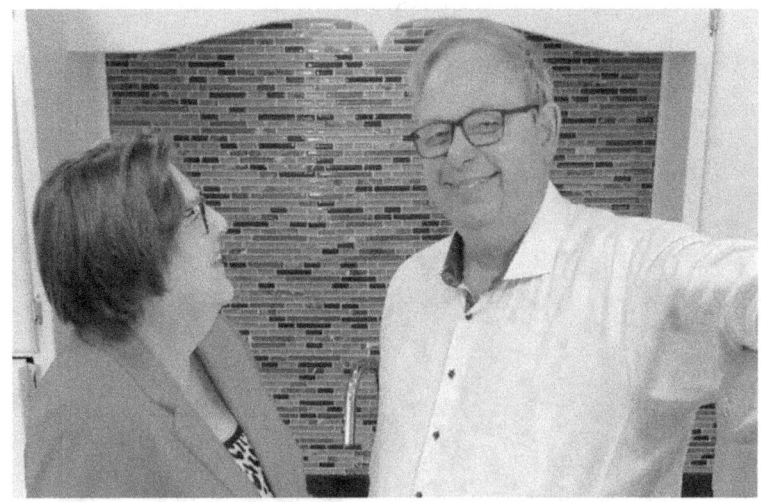

Joanne and Ron Schmidt

Truth be told, I also taught Joanne when I first became a teacher and marvelled even back then at her intellect and drive. One of the strong, she finds whatever mechanism she can to fight life's storms and recover—whatever that means to her. This is the same intelligent, insightful lady (with a brain injury) who became CEO of Galloping Cows Fine Foods—a business she and her husband Ron have run successfully for twenty-five plus years with the help of their two children. Despite her disability, she makes it work the best she can with pacing, help from family, and employees.

Since her injury, Joanne concentrates on less labour-intensive duties as CEO. Her husband does a bit of everything; her mother Annie labelling, and her daughter Courtney oversees marketing, although that may have changed some. The headline in a CBC article, Apr 21, 2017, by Hal Higgins was, "Brain injury hasn't stopped Port Hood woman from crafting successful business." Joanne Schmidt proved naysayers wrong by continuing to run Galloping Cows Fine Foods after her brain injury. She reminds us, "It was not easy!" She had to adapt her environment to work and look after herself. When it comes to livelihood, there is often no choice but to work, and simply do the best you can.

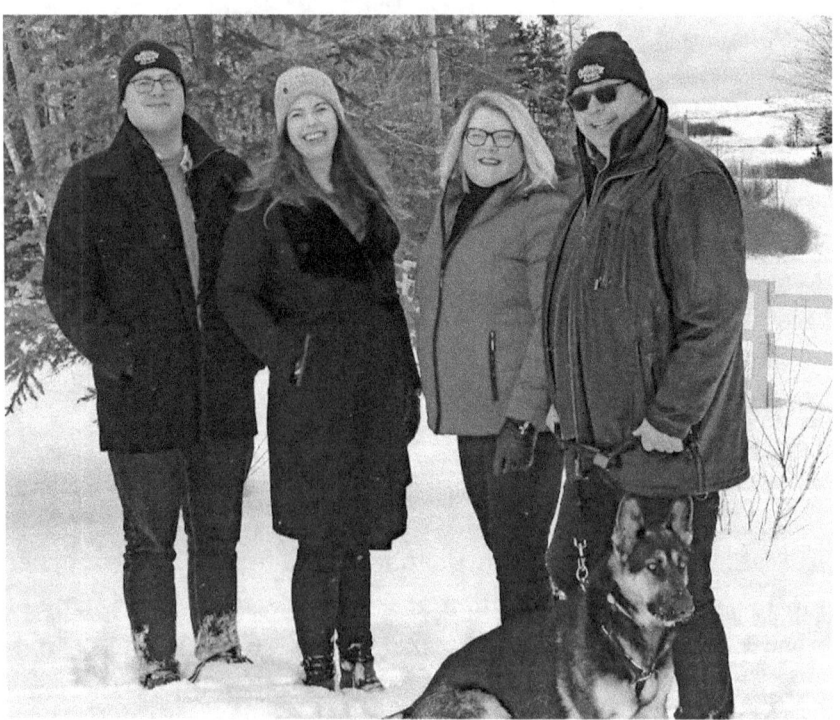

Frank, Courtney, Joanne, and Ron Schmidt

Joanne and her family won several awards over those years, including Entrepreneur of the Year 2017, from the Entrepreneurs with Disabilities Network, sponsored by Royal Bank. The entire family deserves credit for working together and adjusting. My hat's off to every one of them for thriving during challenging times. I admire and respect the tremendous, outstanding woman, wife, mother, daughter, and entrepreneur Joanne became. She did not let a brain injury destroy her dreams. Port Hood, Nova Scotia, is thankful for her, her family, and her business. You can find them at gallopingcow.com. They do all kinds of trade shows and fairs, cater to big events, sell the most delicious jellies and jams, rolls, and ship their products. Joanne is proof that Type A personalities can keep their finger on the pulse of their dreams with education, understanding, pacing, awareness, and discovering diverse ways of managing limitations.

Since interviewing Joanne, life's challenges roared in like a hurricane for her and her family, critical illness adding yet another enormous battle. Some people seem to get hit harder than others and it makes us question and carry the weight of "Why?" It is difficult to complete one battle only to tackle another, but this tight-knit family is managing and continuing to run the business on a smaller scale as the children pursue prestigious goals of their own. They deserve a break if anyone ever did. We send Joanne love, hugs, best wishes, and admiration, and wish her family the best. May the harsh, bumpy road offer a bend, open to the most breathtaking, peaceful scene filled with twittering forest creatures, hummingbirds, and dragonflies to represent hope, peace, and love.

Missing Pages

"No peace lies in the future which is not hidden in this present. Take Peace. The gloom of the world is but a shadow, behind it, yet, within our reach, is joy. Take Joy. There is radiance in the darkness, could we but see—and to see we have only to look.
I beseech you to look.

— Fra Giovanni Giocondo, 16th Century monk,
letter to a friend, excerpt poem, *Take joy*

"I keep a copy in my wallet in case I need it."

—Peggy Ann Bosdet

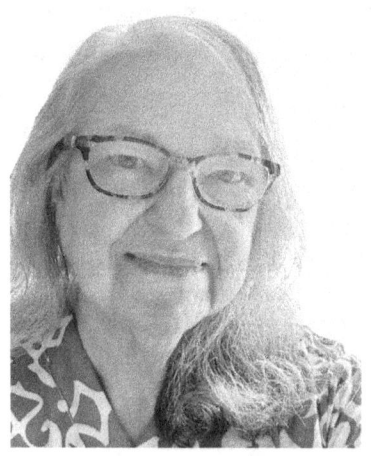

Peggy Ann Bosdet

If ever a human's time on this planet could fill volumes of intriguing reading, it is that of Peggy Ann, and her long-ago, busy-overscheduled, adventurous, independent former self. A horrific accident threatened to strip her of who she was, is, left her with sixteen years of missing pages filling the chapters of what should have been. A traumatic brain injury, or TBI, has immediate effects on a person's brain, ongoing, adverse effects on the person's life. The following narrative shows how important it is to get a head injury treated as soon as possible. In Peggy Ann's case, it was not.

Because it went untreated—many of the after-effects compounded. She discovered a world where specialists recognize TBI symptoms, while others dismiss the obvious, leading to tremendous confusion and duress. It should be shocking, but it is not: failure to recognize a head injury or dismissing the possibility still is too common, yet without a confirmed medical diagnosis, brain-injured patients flounder; the dishonest make everyone else suspect.

October 2024

Peggy Ann's seventy-five-year-old, soft, icy hand touches mine as delicately as her demeanour. She recounts her story, sincere and expressive. Occasional glimpses of humour slip through, trying to mask deep emotion. A kind face, with white hair pulled in a ponytail, rectangular glasses frame her smiling, blue eyes, hinting at a brilliant mind. We are sitting by the fireplace at the Smith Rock Lodge and Chalet Resort, on Fitzpatrick Mountain in Pictou County. We are attending the Tenth Paradise Writers' Retreat put on by OC Publishing. I am in awe of this storyteller, solo world traveller. I hear telltale markers of TBI, am angry for her. She copes with it in a conciliatory manner, pointing out she had severe injuries taking precedence, but wishes all the doctors she came in contact with had validated her brain injury concerns. Glistening eyes show pain caused by the delay.

February 5, 2008

Peggy Ann and Charles were on their way home from Halifax, gentle snowflakes falling when they started out, heavy slush on the road between New Glasgow and Antigonish. "Suddenly I feel us slip, slide, hear Charles behind the wheel say, 'Oh-oh!' I tense up, head-lights coming in the dark distance. The car spins three times. We are out of control on the Trans-Canada. We fly, sail mid-air. Time stops: How long? We aren't moving. Why? Dead silence. Terrible pain. Can't breathe. The right side of my face, eye feels odd. Pressure. Fleetingly, I open my eyes. My husband's face is in front of me. I'm confused. Mouth-to-mouth resuscitation. Why? I try to focus. My neck hurts. He stops, looks up. I'm horrified. Blood on his beard, forehead, cheek! 'He's hurt! Oh, no! Charles is hurt!' I try to ask. He sees my facial concern, answers, 'I'm fine.' I doze off."

Peggy Ann stops, trauma ever-present. I ask if she needs a break.

"No. It's okay. The blood was mine from a cut above my right eye and a deep puncture wound on my right cheek—my face had hit the visor: A BIC pen stored under an elastic band went into my cheek. When I come around, a female holds my hand: 'Peggy—breathe. Deep breath, Peggy.' Too painful. 'Take another breath,' she says. 'Breathe. Again. Breathe.' Charles told me two years later what had happened. We spun across the highway, careened back-wards down a snowy embankment, stopping when the car hit a concrete culvert. The headlights coming at us belonged to her, an off-duty female AEMT (advanced emergency medical technician). She stopped, climbed down through the snow to see if we were okay. We weren't. She called an ambulance, encouraging me to breathe, trying to keep me calm. A miracle she was—right place, right time. What are the odds? Terrified, I told her I was dying. A few months earlier, my beloved mom, who lived with us, had died from pneumonia. The memory of her struggling to breathe increased my mental trauma. In severe pain, I pleaded with her to let me out of the car to get air to breathe."

Peggy Ann does not remember any of it: firefighters, ambulance, paramedics, neck brace, coat being cut off, side door wrenched, backboard, wailing sirens, oxygen mask. Her brain shelters her. Snippets of arriving at the ER, she shares.

"I'm flat on my back. Where is my husband? Is he hurt? Frantic, I open my eyes. 'I'm here, honey.' He stands next to me, holds my hand. 'I'm fine, Peg; you got hurt but they're taking care of you. We'll go home soon.' His voice shakes. I hear snatches of conversations, footsteps, voices, questions. 'Peggy . . . Peggy?' I try to answer, keep dozing off. Let me sleep. 'Peg, be pleasant,' I tell myself. Not polite to say, 'go away,' though I wish everyone would. A lifetime of parental and societal conditioning kicks in, automatic: never show anger, remember your manners."

Peggy Ann stops, takes a deep breath . . . recalls. "I wake, a hand on my shoulder, my husband's. He tells me he loves me. I try to smile, but can't. He asks if it hurts bad. I nod. Someone asks me to open my right eye. It feels odd. A doctor nearby talks to a nurse. I feel the bandage on my cheek pull, lift. 'She needs this stitched right away; call Dr.?' (can't remember name), 'she does smaller stitches, better for this lady's face, less scarring.' I am 'this lady.' My chest hurts both sides, front and back. The oxygen mask does not help, can't breathe. I try a deeper breath: Ribs explode! PAIN! Agony! 'Don't do that again!' My chest, excruciating pressure, ribs, boobs? I need to throw up. Nurse rushes over, hands me a small plastic bowl. Cleans me up. Just liquid."

Curious the mind's focus when traumatized. Peggy Ann spiels, releases the horror.

"I doze and wake, want to leave . . . 'Honey, honey . . . your collarbone's broken. They're keeping you on oxygen overnight, 'til you can breathe easier.' 'No, I want to go home!' Panic. 'Please don't leave.' 'I'm here, Peg, it's okay.' 'Honey; Peg, wake up. Peg, look at me.' Charles looks tired, worried, more than earlier. 'Are you okay? Can we go home now?' 'No, the doctor is here; he wants to talk to us.' I look up. 'Peggy, you're going to be fine; you'll stay with us a while: you have a broken back.' I try to take that in. My husband looks rattled. I don't understand: it was a broken collarbone, now it's my back? A nurse in ER, says I should sleep, doctor wants me here until I am stable. I'm confused: stable? I start to cry. 'Your husband is leaving for home.' Home! He's going home! 'It's near 5 a.m.,' she says. 'You've been here since 8 p.m., nine hours. His friend is here to pick him up—he's exhausted; you've both been through a lot.' She gives me a shot for pain, dims the light."

All this dear lady has been through floors me; testament to the strength of the human spirit. Once stabilized, she is transferred from St. Martha's in Antigonish to the QEII in Halifax. It is the beginning of ten painful, subsequent ambulance trips back and forth for various procedures—needing morphine shots each time en route.

"It isn't easy. A TBI changes you in odd ways—not your intelligence, but the ability to think the same—you lose track of time, have trouble with schedules, cannot remember numbers or instructions for even a minute after reading them. The deficits manifest to both the patient and those living with them. It was tough for my husband to understand I was not being difficult, obtuse, or unaware of my deficits. I knew they were there all too well. After I returned home from the hospital, I had to deal with debilitating, clinical depression. Still do."

Peggy Ann spent three months in hospital in a back brace, two flat on her back, six months in a rented hospital bed at home on the first floor. I shake my head. Peggy Ann thinks she should lighten things. "Years after the accident I asked our GP, 'How was it the two of us in the same car, Charles only had a bruised back, yet my body was broken?' Our doctor grinned and replied, 'When the rear of the car hit the concrete, it stopped cold. You, the passenger, slammed against the steel door and visor. He hit air, and you, and you are much softer than a steel door.' I remind Charles I saved his life! He owes me." She laughs. It is good to see her experiencing joy. "I loved being independent, open to the unexpected, meeting people in new cultures, enjoying their arts and food."

She offers fleeting pieces of background, enticing me to know more, as only a well-written book can. I smile, trying to imagine

Peggy Ann as a feisty young dynamo. Born in Chicago, a self-assured, artistic city girl, full of questions, her mind absorbed facts. She attended university, but disillusioned dropped out her first year. Two weeks past her nineteenth birthday, she travelled for one year, encircling the world entirely on her own, the best education she could ever have had.

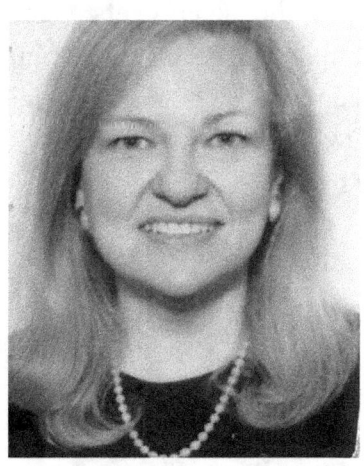

After that epic trip ended, Peggy Ann married after a whirlwind romance, stayed in an unhappy relationship for twenty-three years, then divorced; that book left closed for now.

After her big trip, she started an export/import business, allowing her the freedom and the income to travel abroad, off and on, for three more years. In 1976 she became a celebrity pastry chef and chocolatier, a fascinating, surprise career.

"I did the inaugural cake for the governor of Illinois, a cake for President Gerald Ford, a birthday cake for Bob Hope, and custom chocolates of his famous profile (face) to give his guests. I was nominated to audition for the 1982 World Culinary Olympics (U.S. Pastry and Chocolates division), and wrote a weekly column on food design for a chain of newspapers. This 'sweet life' came to a screeching halt later in 1982."

At age thirty-two, ten years after headaches and other health issues, doctors diagnose Peggy Ann with a macroadenoma—large brain tumour between her pituitary and hypothalamus. She has surgery at the Brain and Spine Hospital of the University of Chicago; it is non-malignant. After a long hospitalization and lengthy recovery, she has no further problems. During recovery time, Peggy Ann writes. She finishes a manuscript and sends it to an American publishing house and gets a contract to write three books, still in print, but NOT the one she originally sent. Recently an interested party contacted her, and that original manuscript will be published by 2026. Outstanding! Never say never. Glimpses of the missing coming back.

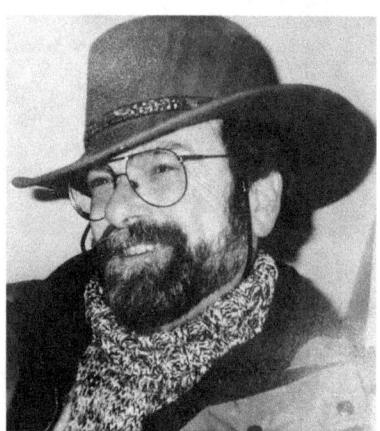

Charles

Continuing her story, Peggy Ann meets Charles in 1995, a Canadian citizen working in the United States as a journalist and business consultant. He longs to return to his Canadian roots in Nova Scotia, on a small island off Cape Breton called Isle Madame. They make two trips; find Nova Scotians courteous and welcoming. In 2002, they buy a house. A city girl: Chicago, New York, Paris, Mumbai, (formerly Bombay), Philadelphia, and Southern California. The switch to living in a rural area is a culture shock. "Isle Madame is so friendly, a complete change. We had never felt such kindness." Her husband is thrilled, and that is enough for her.

Peggy Ann looks out the expansive window of the lodge, the autumn colours glorious over the long vista; she too is in the autumn of her life. Perhaps she wonders at the vibrant colours after so much barren grey, her spring and summer missed. She peers back at me. "It's a strange coincidence meeting you here: our first trip to Nova Scotia, we stayed at this very lodge. Winding through the forest on unmarked roads, we wandered lost for three hours, extremely low on fuel. The owner waited up to 11 p.m.—gracious about the late hour. Amazing place, Nova Scotia."

She is on a roll. "When heading back from that first trip to Nova Scotia, by Boston to Los Angeles, we were late arriving in LA. Over the intercom, the pilot announced seven passengers needed to connect to a flight to New Zealand, asked everyone to let them off first. When the seatbelt sign turned off, hundreds jammed the aisle, standing like sardines. Charles looked at me, and said, 'That would never happen at the Halifax International Airport.' He was right."

"In 2008, doctors in Nova Scotia did everything they could to save me. Was my continual vomiting—several times a day during the months in hospital—a red flag? They did countless tests on my stomach, but nothing showed, yet I vomited for months, and at home several times a day. Was it from head injury or heavy pain meds? God bless the doctors who never give up. I threw up three times in one doctor's office. He flagged it, said, 'I know you had a TBI. How could you not with the severity of your injuries?' I felt immediate relief, my issues validated. He said I needed cognitive therapy. I couldn't do the things I used to; he reassured me they were *there*. 'You take the scenic route instead of a straight line.' I started to cry. I was finally going to get real help."

Peggy Ann had a loss of equilibrium, ongoing severe proprioception, balance issues. Discharged from the hospital, she saw a parade of specialists. An ENT doctor, neurologist, cognitive therapist, neuropsychologist, physical therapist, and balance specialist concluded she had a TBI. But insurance doctors displayed scepticism throwing her into a dark world of mind games. She experienced tremendous grief from third-party doctors hired by insurance companies, knew her brain had changed, struggled.

An insightful occupational therapist suggested a psychologist Peggy Ann should contact to accept life's new challenges. "I did not want to go, was in denial a long time, fully expecting to return to a competent, independent, former version of self. My symptoms were real. Why were they sending me to a psychologist?"

The psychologist suggests Peggy Ann has PTSD, and it needs to be dealt with. Peggy Ann replied, "No, I don't. Do not put that on me! I was not in a terrorist attack, war, or shot at. I don't have PTSD!" Her understanding, only war, murder, or terrorism causes it. The therapist firmly told her, anything exceptionally traumatizing can lead to PTSD and pointed out Peggy Ann had a life-threatening experience. Half her face had fallen; she couldn't breathe, almost died. Her head injury triggered traumas. The brain compartmentalizes to protect. Her psychologist said Peggy Ann was adept at shoving trauma into boxes, never to be opened. But the accident collapsed her life so fully, she could no longer keep those boxes hidden and closed. When damaged as she was, too many pages flew open, thoughts, memories flooding from Neverland.

"Many significant experiences led to a productive, full life. I wanted to remember only that. In my mid-forties, I met a man I adore, who adores me. I never focus on difficulties, times I was embarrassed or harmed, kept them inside, didn't believe I could be traumatized—but the accident, that's what happens with PTSD. It sneaks up on you. Took me forever to accept hyper-vigilance— extreme startle reflex, irrational fear, smelling smoke, vehement reaction to unexpected noise, aversion to crowds. People tromp or whistle in the house, so their presence does not startle me."

She shakes, puts her hand to her chest; a physical reaction. Peggy Ann went from a vivacious, independent, world traveller and entrepreneur, to being completely dependent on others. It tore her adventurous spirit, stripped her of who she was. Prior to her accident, she built a retail store, The Candy Shop, in Port Hastings, at the rotary of the Canso Causeway; largest candy store in Canada; its sister company, a chocolate factory, both under the same corporate umbrella. Peggy Ann started in Arichat; needing the space, opened in Port Hawkesbury, turning out handmade premium chocolates. The two ventures, combined under one corporate name, employed thirty people in an area that sorely needed well-paying, year-round jobs. On November 16, 2007, she hosted the store's grand opening. On February 5th, 2008, her world shifted.

A remarkable person, Peggy Ann speaks French (poorly, she says, but reads it very well) and has studied basic Hindi. Her interests are eclectic: Oriental art, antiques, musical instruments, and cooking. She used to give lectures about art and cultural history at universities and art museums on the evolution and usage of garment buttons, tracing them back into the 1600s.

"My life before does not minimize my experience, but I miss what I lost." She stops, a silent tear slipping down her cheek, holds in a lot. Her next few words hold more pain than they have a right to witness. "I never saw my store, factory, or offices again; overnight I went from a perfectly healthy fifty-nine-year-old businesswoman to someone with infirmities of old age with no transitional, or gradual entry. I'm at peace now, but I regret what happened. I had to close my store, lay off employees, almost lost everything. The decade was a complete wipeout. Where was I? Lost, it seems. I'd always believed your sixties were the last hurrah. Hard not to feel sorry for myself. I know better. Many people suffer invisible illnesses and don't show it—far more than we realize. Everyone has something, no matter how blithe and unconcerned they may act, or look. I fight depression on many levels. Having PTSD puts a monumental strain on life in insidious, hidden ways, affecting the sufferer, family, and friends."

Plagued with fatigue and pain, Peggy Ann lost interest in what had defined her, isolated herself socially, felt incompetent. She loved to play jazz piano, lost that skill—a major, personal loss she finds daunting. It was her muse, comfort, confidante. Fiction books remain challenging, but she can read non-fiction. She could not write professionally or string words together, but with time, she regained that ability. She cannot drive, and as an independent person, loathes asking for help.

In the beginning, Peggy Ann had a nursing aide/caregiver five hours a day, five days a week, for three years; then switched to three hours each weekday for five years. Now she has an aide for one hour each weekday. Before her accident, she taught formal food design, intricate pastries and cakes, and the Japanese art of Okimono (the art of fanciful complex vegetable and fruit carving). She also taught clay sculpture classes, but lost those abilities the first few years. Her healing brought a desperate search for her true self, questioning the whereabouts of the real Peggy Ann. A speed reader, she lost that ability as well, a frustrating journey to getting it back.

A long-time friend in Vancouver called long after the accident to ask what she was up to. She said, "Nothing," and meant it. She rarely left the house except to go to a doctor, or a hospital for tests, and even stopped going to the library. "I love libraries, was once a publicly elected board member of a large suburban library system."

And she did more. Of course, she did . . . From 2000 until her accident in 2008, Peggy Ann was a member of a group of four volunteers who helped thousands of "Lost Canadians," obtain their rightful citizenship through the courts. Don, in Vancouver, and Peggy Ann's Manitoba-born husband, were two of those affected. "A few years ago, after the accident, Don flat out told me I needed something to do; he could hear it in my voice. A legal crusader, he started asking, 'Peg, can you edit this? Research this?' He helped me regain a part of myself. Controlling my hours to avoid exhaustion, and visual setbacks, I began. He was right, I needed to know I was capable. I re-strengthened those skills, becoming their researcher (pro bono) for historic legal issues contested in Canada, for the group he heads. With Don's urging, I wanted to do some good, find the me who was independent, travelled the world alone, loved to drive coast to coast, just to see—everything!"

The missing pages, ripped from her life for sixteen years, present a doleful comparison to a woman who was once so autonomous. Her current life clashes monumentally with the woman who lived young into her late fifties. Her husband is supportive, even when he doesn't understand those difficulties he can see, and the others she hopes he never will. He's her rock—she never wished him to be. He tells her he is there for her, always. Perhaps her greatest blessing is his marvellous sense of humour, which surrounds her: his silliness, surprises, and Chaplinesque talents make her laugh, her best medicine and most joyful therapy.

Another tear falls from Peggy Ann's eye. She takes a moment to wipe it. Here she is in her mid-seventies, staying alone in a country lodge, attending a writers' retreat. It is her first outing and over-night trip away from her husband or nurse's aide in sixteen years. Friends help. What an inspiring, courageous lady, smart as a whip.

"What helped tremendously—a cognitive therapist demon-strated to us what was happening in my brain, how my mental pathways differed from before. She drew a large circle; before my brain would solve by going from point A at the top of the circle, directly to point B at the bottom. After, the signals have to take a more circuitous route with curves and twists before getting to point B. Thus, everything I did, or thought, was slower. Understanding my brain's new operating method helped us understand when con-versing. Scatterbrained, I wandered off topic. My husband quietly steers me back with our pet phrase, 'You're 'rabbit-trailing.' I had trouble with my vocabulary, using wrong words in sentences; that cleared up. My sense of timing remains haywire."

Gifted with an IQ of 169, it dropped twelve points after the accident, discovered through examinations by a neuropsychologist. With brain injuries, what doctors must consider upon presentation besides the injury itself, is the vast diversity in human brains—whether a person is predominantly right or left-brained; their intelligence level; age, how exercised, formed, and developed their brain is; in what capacities, what it retains and experiences. Impossible to compare apples to candy, emphasizing the need for individualized diagnosis and treatment. We have only tapped the profound, mystical complexities of the human brain.

Peggy Ann recalls the headlines of January 7, 2011, when the Penguins announce Crosby suffered a concussion. "At that moment, it all made sense. If it weren't for Sidney Crosby and his story, I would never have clued into what my head injury entails. I saw myself in his symptoms. He was famous, so people stopped and listened.

"Understanding head injury accidents and insurance claims is complicated—the misbelief, no evidence on film, some doctors negate the existence of concussion, mTBI or TBI; the pangs of rejection, ridicule, and suffering caused. My opposing lawyer's doctor said, 'You didn't hit your head hard enough to have had a concussion.'"

Peggy Ann's voice drops, stops. Eyes glisten. Not hard enough? She had worse than a concussion, a TBI, traumatic brain injury! Her right eye black and swollen shut, a cut above her eyebrow, scratched cornea, cracked tooth. She had continuous vomiting, double vision, a severed nerve causing half her face to drop. Spinal fractures of the mid-back: sixth, seventh, and eighth thoracic vertebrae, and fractured sixth cervical (neck) vertebra. Contusions in the lungs, a pneumothorax in one, a small collapse in the other, broken ribs on both sides, broken collarbone, sprain of one shoulder, tear in the other, internal injuries, right-side hairline skull fracture. She needed to learn to walk again, had years of physiotherapy a few times a week to rebuild her muscles and help her cope with pain. And once all was settled, years later, cognitive and traumatic eye therapy.

"The way the legal system was run; I got even more depressed. When I went to one insurance-selected neurologist he said, 'That looks like overkill.' I didn't know what he was talking about, soon realized he meant my cane. He even suggested I'd stopped at the drugstore on the first floor, to purchase it. My cane was well-used. He snapped pictures of the centre section, questioning the legitimacy of my injuries, skewed facts and evidence, doing everything in his bizarre manner to discredit me. I was distraught, knew something was up, stopped at my lawyer's office on the way home, explained what had happened. He took pictures of the handle which looked like holy hell, the cracked bottom rubber cap sorely in need of replacing. Later, they faced off about the cane issue, quite combatively. Mine won."

Peggy Ann stops, trembles, stabs of ridicule not healed. Her voice maintains its unassuming tender flow. Her face opens wide like a book with blank pages, well-worn dog ears marking years of suffering and tragedy. She wonders where those precious years went. I get it. Love her for her courage. Although private, she allows the ink to flow in the hope it will help others with similar symptoms or battles to not feel so lost.

In 2016, after missing more timely chances because of court battles, she follows the road of physiotherapist, ophthalmologist, optometrist, goes to the Bedford Eye clinic for eye trauma. Dr. Erin Sheppard said she should have seen her far earlier. Over her time with Dr. Sheppard, she receives four pairs of glasses with yoked prisms to steady her balance.

She reminisces about good times: "I loved travelling; that was my life. When I lost it, I felt like I was nobody, lost my income, independence, all I could do before."

Peggy Ann is a sweet and forever, quizzical visionary. I marvel, sit in amazement, wonder what the delicate lines etched on her worldly face could tell me, what she would have done with those years stolen from her. More than I could ever write.

"Do you come here often?" The playful question comes from an older gentleman strolling nonchalantly into the room where we sit. A striking man, well-groomed with salt and pepper hair, moustache, and beard, stands tall, with a cowboy hat positioned just so. A twinkle in his eye, he observes the gal beside me. So cute is the loving glance between them. I immediately know he is her husband, here to pick up his date. Another salt-of-the-earth gentleman. For years, Peggy Ann could not climb stairs or return to their shared bedroom. They eventually afforded a chairlift to at least one floor, tired of asking her husband to grab the blue top from upstairs and him bringing down four.

Is that a wink I see from him, easily displaying a confident swagger, quick sense of humour? I would never have known this amazing intellectual, or her story, had we not arrived at the same retreat and started talking. Seems that is true of a great many stories. A fascinating lady and couple, what an unexpected treasure! They deserve credit for their love and respect, especially him for staying. A comforting chapter in the making. I hope Peggy Ann gets back those missing pages. I'd like to read about her three weeks alone in a Bombay hospital; the time she got lost in Athens, where no one spoke English or French, and she got help from the wrong person; her time abroad when a Catholic priest strolled into her room expecting to give her last rites, yet she was not dying.

Another writer at the phenomenal retreat beautifully sums up this gracious lady: "Peggy Ann embodies a sense of wonder with tales of days lived well. Stories of far-off journeys coupled with the tantalizing audacity to be well ahead of her times, she is a testament that women can be kind, compassionate, and disruptors—allowing women to show up fully as they are." (Sheri Godfrey, November 8, 2024).

I concur; Peggy Ann is beginning to fill those missing pages.

Flipping Life's Adversities

"Once you choose hope, anything's possible."
— Christopher Reeve.

This was one of the first stories to inspire me to kick myself in the backside. Although Rachelle's disability is visible, what she overcame was not. Making her a woman of inspiration. Her story spurs us forward to not give up. I was impressed with her dynamite attitude and unwillingness to give up on her dreams. As we recover, we learn and grow from that which provides life lessons.

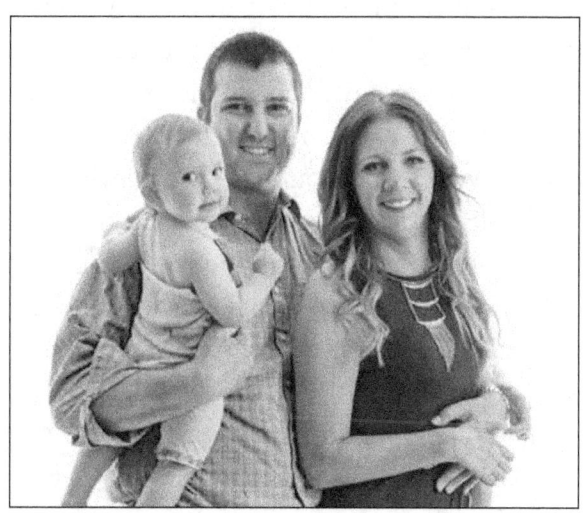

Chris, Rachelle, and Kaylee Chapman

TLC documented Rachelle Friedman Chapman's journey on January 23, 2017. As I watched spellbound, I cried, smiled, and cheered all within one hour. Hers is a heartbreaking story of love and loyalty, overcoming adversity, and following your dreams. In a heartbeat, Rachelle's life changed.

In 2010, four weeks before her wedding, at her bachelorette party the unthinkable happened. During an after-party swim, one of Rachelle's best friends playfully pushed her and she fell into the pool. Her head struck the wrong way. She broke her neck and has been paralyzed from the chest down ever since. Through the ordeal she understandably lost a friend, although Rachelle affirms if someone unintentionally hurts you, it is important to forgive, even if it means moving on.

As horrendous as her accident was, she never gave up! Life is too short—one of her mottos. The television show focused on one of her dreams. She always wanted to have children; that was a primary goal. The doctors informed her that her condition, medication, and circumstances made giving birth dangerous, so she had yet another dream stripped away. But that did not stop her.

With the help of her husband, Chris, and family members during rehabilitation, Rachelle pushed through the challenges and obstacles to be as well as she could be, and slowly adjusted to life as a quadriplegic. She and Chris married a year after the accident and began revisiting the concept of having a family. Her college friend Laurel Humes offered to be a surrogate, and in May 2015, Rachelle and Chris fearfully and joyously brought home their baby girl, Kaylee.

Raising their daughter is a team effort. Rachelle's mother, Carol Friedman, lives with the couple, mostly to help her daughter get out of bed and into her wheelchair in the mornings after Chris leaves for his job as a school science teacher.

"Even though my fingers do not work, I have found a way to manipulate my hands to do a lot of things. I can hold Kaylee. I feed and play with her while Chris is washing bottles or whatever. We have a system that works for us," Rachelle says.

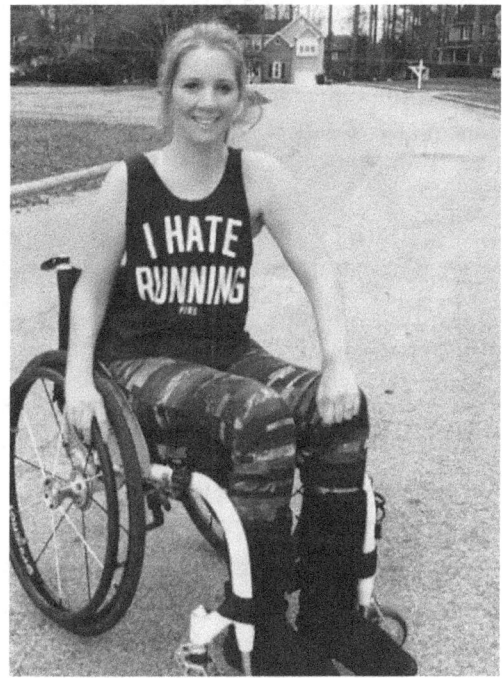

Rachelle

Her ambition is to become as independent as she can, even adding driving to her goals. She has become a motivational speaker, blogger, and author. After the accident, she became known as the paralyzed bride; she recently published her memoir, *The Promise: A Tragic Accident, a Paralyzed Bride, and the Power of Love, Loyalty, and Friendship*. I've read excerpts but I look forward to slipping between the pages of inspiration when able to absorb an entire book. One message Rachelle promotes is how much a quadriplegic is capable of, and that perhaps society should not see them as broken, simply changed. Hers is a quest to educate and make people aware of spinal injuries. Our goals intersect. At the time of writing, she, Chris, and Kaylee happily live in Knightdale, North Carolina, where they hope to build on their family. Maybe, someday, Kaylee will have a baby brother or sister. Power to them and their advocacy! Makes me smile and shed tears at their courage and tenacity. Rachelle also has a sense of humour so needed during tough times, and a splendid attitude, splendid because it goes beyond positive; her outlook carries no ill will, only a gratefulness for what she has and what she can do. A lesson we all could learn.

I feel humbled and blessed to have permission to include such an incredible story. This young woman is living proof that determination combined with love can conquer daunting odds. Rachelle and her family refuel my gas tank. When tired I look at her smiling face, or that of her daughter or husband and life is good again, very much what we make it, although we need help—people helping people. It warms the heart to see glimpses of the massive good in the world, especially as news and television focus on the dark side. We need sparks of inspiration, such as Rachelle's story, shared because she wants to help others who suddenly suffer life-changing injuries.

Deep down, we are the same once we strip away the crud; we are emotional beings who feel, breathe, yearn, aspire, love. To shift my anger and resentment of what I could not prevent, I view the glowing faces of Chris, Rachelle, and Kaylee Chapman. They make me smile. In them I see sunshine.

I visit Rachelle's Instagram or Facebook page. An insightful blogger she shares valuable life lessons. She helped me put things in perspective, thus the need to include her story. Several documentaries and videos of Rachelle exist online on YouTube, and various television networks. My favourite documentary on Rachelle on YouTube, originally on NBC, is "EMOTIONAL Changes for INSPIRING Bride and Groom," an episode of *George to the Rescue*, January 26, 2020. So heartwarming, it made me cry. George and a team of community members pitch in to create a beautiful and—most importantly—more quadriplegic-accessible home for Rachelle.

Pure Resilience

"Be patient— sometimes you have to go through the worst to get to the best. Give time some time."

— Karen Salmansohn (Daily Inspirational Quote)

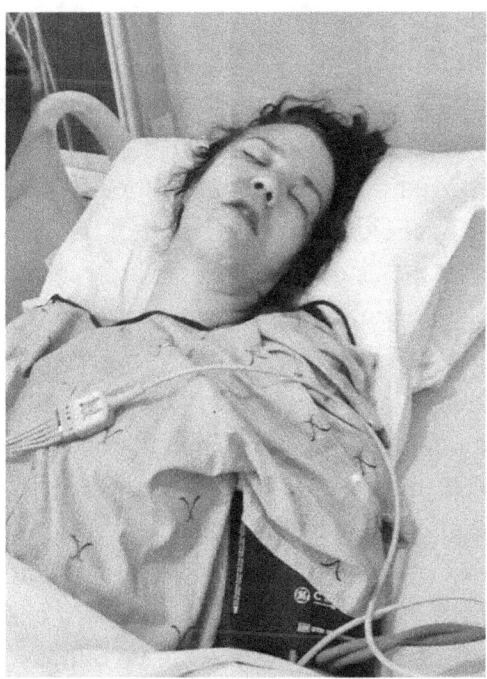

Rhiannon Chisholm, Day of Accident

You are thirty-two years old, and everything is going your way. You secure employment three hours from your family home in a physically demanding trade you enjoy. You take care of your body through exercise, eat a clean, healthy diet, seldom drink alcohol. You make one of the biggest investments a person can make—you buy your first house in June 2022, which makes you proud of your discipline, hard work, and accomplishments. You are a strong, independent woman who stands proud of your successes. But . . .

September 12, 2022, is a rueful day as Rhiannon Chisholm tells it. "We are heading to work, early morning, from Sackville where I live, through Magazine Hill and Burnside into Dartmouth, Nova Scotia. My boyfriend is driving. He makes an odd sound, slumps back over the headrest. In panic mode, split seconds, I shake him, try to wake him and move his leg, get his foot off the gas pedal. I grab the wheel, steer from the passenger seat. For six bands of telephone poles, I fight to regain control. We are going too fast; he unaware! We thunder into a telephone pole, snap it in two, tires screeching, metal crunching, glass breaking as we crash into rocks. The mangled truck screams, stops with a revolting jolt near an Irving building. We hit the ditch going at least 150 kilometres per hour. The passenger side takes the brunt of the impact. I remember hitting my head. Dad figures I smoked the rear-view mirror and was knocked out cold."

The ambulance rushes the seriously injured couple to the QE II Halifax Infirmary, where neurosurgeon Dr. Lutz Weise hurries Rhiannon into emergency surgery, spends twelve hours trying to put her back together. It is touch and go. Once he opens her up, he has to put everything back in its place, her spine severed at her L3 vertebra. He repairs her discs at L3 and L4, fuses them with two titanium rods connecting the L2 to L4 vertebrae. Once out of surgery, he places her in an induced coma. She has a crack in her skull, right-side forehead, causing a brain hemorrhage and brain swelling. Her face swells and her spine leaks fluid. She broke blood vessels in her nose, banged and bruised her right knee and ankle, broke her radius, and has a tear in her shoulder, scheduled for surgery the next day if she is stable. Her then boyfriend sustains less serious injuries. While she is heavily sedated, the hospital notifies her mom and dad in the dreaded moment all parents fear. Rhiannon's mom reacts.

"When the phone call came, we were frantic! A three-hour drive, we did not know if we would make it in time. We threw our suitcases together. All we could think—What is going to happen to our baby girl?"

Rhiannon's parents, Lynn and Cyril, face the unknown on that dreadful trip from Port Hood to Halifax pushing worst-case scenarios away. Hearts shattered and petrified. What was in store for dear Annie? (Rhiannon's nickname), the extent of their baby girl's injuries? Would she know them, remember what happened, be able to speak, walk, survive?

Five excruciating hours they wait in the common room as Rhiannon's doctors fight to stabilize their baby in ICU. In a surreal haze they listen as doctors tell them they are monitoring a brain bleed as she recovers from emergency spinal cord surgery. How do they process it all? Their baby girl has not a clue she was mangled.

The surgeon asks Lynn and Cyril to come back the next morning to see if she will know them. He takes her out of her coma. They are terrified. "Please God let our baby recognize us," Lynn prays. First thing, she leans into her daughter and says, "Hi Annie." Her heart skips a beat while she waits, clinging onto her daughter's hand for the longest minute in history. Fear of brain damage shrieks in everyone's mind. What if her daughter does not know her? What if there are major neurological deficits on top of paralysis? In early morning knots, they watch, wait, witness groggy eyelids flutter, open, pray she knows them. They hold their breath, scared to breathe. Sluggish, Rhiannon turns toward them. They brace . . .

"Mom? You're here!"

Lynn cannot contain herself as she takes in sorrowful, puppy-dog eyes, reaches out with utmost tenderness and hugs her girl.

"Of course, I am."

Next, she turns to her father. "Hi, Dad. Knew you would be here with Mom!" Cyril reaches over to give her a gentle kiss, blinking tears away before she can see.

"Do you remember what happened?" Lynn asks.

"Bang! Screaming metal, can't . . . feel my legs!"

"Swelling from surgery, hon. Give it time."

"Airbags exploded. Jolted."

"Protected you."

"Tried to steer away from oncoming traffic. Burning rubber. Were folks hurt?"

"No. You did well!"

"Sooo tired."

"You are going to be okay. We'll fight this."

The medical staff are amazed with her exceptional memory of the accident. The doctor sedates her again, to give the brain and spine time to heal. Lynn knows her daughter's determination is born from her own fire, and she does not want to crush her hope.

"'Paralyzed from the waist down,' Dr. Weise reiterates to us, 'extremely low chance of her ever walking. Her bowel and bladder might come back but chances not.' Our hearts broken, all we can do is stand by her bed and pray, let the hundreds of concerned people know she is resting. I instruct those assisting Rhiannon in ICU to keep quiet about the severity of her injuries and the possibility she will never walk."

For the Chisholms it is a brutal first week, Rhiannon in ICU in a controlled coma, the brain given a chance for the swelling to go down. "We go from gratitude, she is alive, to angst, dreading what her future might hold. Her severed spine and swelling in her brain, major concerns. It takes a couple of weeks for her to come around, her body fighting to heal itself. As sedation lessens, nurses and doctors test her daily for neurological deficits. Rhiannon does not fully understand the risk and danger she is in."

Rhiannon takes over. "Every morning, nurses ask about the day and date, who I am, when I was born. It annoys to no end. I almost tell them off. They bombard me with questions, bug me, every day the same. I get cocky, refuse to answer. Nothing is wrong with my brain; I will prove it. Their questions remind me of what could be, and waves of depression and fog take over. I want to stop my meds; figure I do not need them; they made me loopy."

The bionic woman, is she trying to prove it to the medical staff, or to herself? Doctors explain the protocol for the medications to prevent infection, reduce swelling, manage pain levels. They cut back where they can, start getting her out of the hospital bed, show her how to use a transfer board to move to a wheelchair. Brain fog and headaches slow her down. Fear races through her mind, plays Ping-Pong back and forth, back, and forth. Will she recover?

> "My momma is my rock, snapping me out of shit . . . she takes me for a 'walk,' and encourages me. 'You can do this, Annie, I believe in you.' The surgeon told me paralysis was expected after major spinal surgery; the hope, I will regain feeling as the swelling decreases, and I heal."

Rhiannon sinks to her lowest point when nothing will move in her lower extremities, no matter how much she wills it. She pushes herself up in the bed, dying to get out of it for good. Her mind may be ready, but her body is not. As days morph one into another, her dad's heartbreak carves into a serious countenance and faraway expression. He is too scared to look close in case his face crumbles. He has to be strong for his baby girl. And so, he keeps busy, helps get her house ready for when the doctors release her, builds a ramp, renovates the bathroom so it is wheelchair assessible, returns to his job in Port Hood. Her work union generously pays for the house ramp. Her father's deep love carries her when she cannot carry herself.

Digesting the devastating developments, her mom and dad say little about the wheelchair, each waging their own mental war, refusing to accept her future might entail moving with wheels instead of legs. Her momma refuses to consider the possibility and cheers her on. Rhiannon believes it fuels a resilient mindset and recovery. Their steadfast encouragement, prayers, and presence are her backbone while hers heals; they hold her together as she fights the war of her life. She searches inside, digs deep, as one battle brings on another, and another as her broken body mends.

Rhiannon does not remember much of those first weeks in hospital. Graduating takes on a new meaning as she transitions from bed to wheelchair. "I sit on the chair and feel like I am on a marshmallow, my brain not receiving the message I am paralyzed. I know it, but I don't, which is weird, right?"

Her parents protect her, so she will not go too far down a hole she cannot climb out of. The brain bleed continues to be of concern. Doctors place her in a private room, less noise and stimulus; they do not want to overwhelm her brain or give it too much information. It needs quiet to heal.

On October 7, 2022, they transfer her to the Nova Scotia Rehabilitation Centre into a private hospital room. When discharged from the QEII Infirmary, they transport her to rehab in the wheelchair that had been her life for weeks. Unbeknown to her, the file that goes with her is for the rehabilitation team to train her in life skills to live in a wheelchair.

With COVID-19 the rehab is strict about visitors; her older sister Genna, husband Adam, children: McKinley, Deacon, and Grady, not allowed in, which she finds super tough. Then unexpected, but not, Rhiannon and her boyfriend break up. She has a war to fight and needs her energy. "I'm okay, figure I'm going to be on my own, have a lot to be thankful for, and need to conserve my energy for healing."

She tires easily; lights and sounds hurt, she is more emotional, forced to face a new reality—life forward in a chair, although her mother would poo-poo that away, make her look out toward the glorious, mystic sunset, walk toward it on Port Hood beach, each tomorrow a new day. For months Rhiannon fights with everything she has. Her physiotherapist tells her progress will be wheelchair to walker, cane, and eventually, no cane at all.

"The senior physiotherapist at the rehab, Carolyn Cowan, was Rhiannon's miracle and angel until discharge," says Lynn. "Our baby made so much progress with her. Carolyn commented that in her twenty years, she had never seen anyone gain the success Rhiannon did, never saw such determination and focus. Most would have considered giving up but not our baby."

To her advantage, before the accident, Rhiannon worked out, had a healthy body and mind, was determined to get back to where she was. Therapists affirm for her that family and loved ones can help bring you back. Through her powerful will, many prayers, and steadfast family pillar, Rhiannon's life begins turning in rehab. With physio every morning, she improves mobility. Her mom spends hours keeping things positive, praising her, wheeling her down the streets of Halifax, taking her window-shopping, while her dad works on her house. Her parents endure and remain resilient, despite substantial burdens.

Adrenalin powers Lynn: she keeps herself busy in the hopes of not having to face her daughter's truth. If negative thoughts slip in, she bulldozes them out. Thanksgiving weekend, 2022, Cyril and Lynn are on their way from Port Hood to Halifax, Rhiannon texts. "Mom, when are you coming?" She is antsy, battling the what-if game.

"We'll be there soon, hon. Don't worry," Lynn texts back, sad for her baby girl, scared it is becoming too much with little sign of advancement in several weeks. It is the anniversary of Lynn's brother's death, a young man killed in a vehicular accident. While Cyril drives, she silently prays to her brother from the passenger seat, eyes squeezing tight. *I need you, Jason. Please, please, please send me a sign our little Annie will be okay. Please. If you're in*

Heaven, do this for us. I'm sure you don't want to see her in a wheelchair the rest of her life.

Very unlike her, Cyril asks why she is so quiet. "I'm praying for Jason to send me a sign he heard me, and that she'll be okay."

Cyril, nods, looks ahead. Is that a tear Lynn sees rolling down his cheek? At the hospital, Lynn goes in and asks, "Hey, hon, how ya doing?"

"Mom, you'll never believe. My big toe moved. It moved, Mom! I'll show you."

When your spine starts to regenerate, bursts of life come back, like freezing, then thawing. Rhiannon concentrates hard; her big toe twitches. "Oh my God, I can't believe it," Lynn exclaims. "The toe moved right in front of my eyes."

Cyril bursts into the room, Lynn sits on the chair, flabbergasted. Rhiannon shows her dad, although getting the toe to move a third time, more difficult. Lynn stays seated, overcome with a deep, radiating peace for the first time since the horrific accident.

"I silently thank my brother Jason, and press, 'Can you get her back on her feet?'"

That first month, second, third; Rhiannon contends with mountains, including the piercing embarrassment of being a young woman unable to take care of grooming, bodily functions, showering, bathing, dressing. It weighs on her. Before, she had been her own boss, and very, very independent.

Lynn follows her daughter every step of the way, walks for her baby girl until she can walk for herself. It takes months, the future unsure, but with a never-ever-give-up attitude, Rhiannon pushes herself; that is her nature. As her body heals, inspirational quotations resonate and give her something to hang onto in a bleak environment.

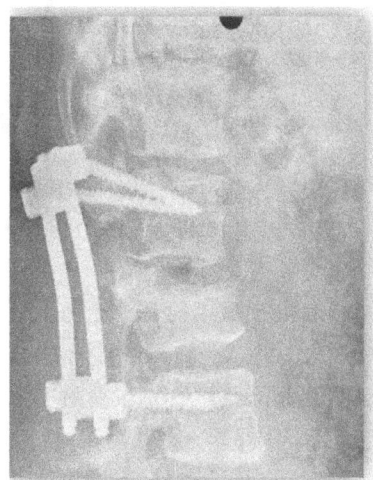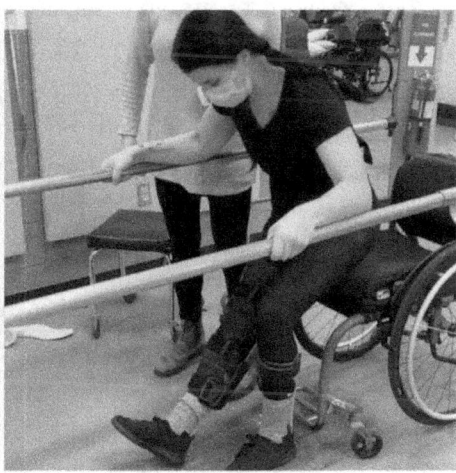

Rhiannon's First Step

Rhiannon refuses to appear weak, keeps secrets in relation to how she truly feels, as her fears balloon into tears and angst, an undeniable mental and physical fight to get to the finish. She shows her mettle and resilience, time and time again. With the parallel bars, on November 29, 2022, "I take my first step. I did it! I am a wild beast in my hospital bed, reaching one side to the bed rail, pulling myself up, even as my body heals from spinal fusion. Nothing is going to keep me down."

Doctors discharge her from in-patient rehab on December 9, 2022, but she remains in her wheelchair as her body gains muscle and mobility from long therapy sessions where she gives her all. When they go back to her house, a wheelchair, walker, braces, mobility contraptions fill her living room. The evening of December 9, when settled in, Lynn broaches the elephant skirting the room. "Rhiannon, your dad, and I have something to tell you. I pray you won't be upset with me."

Rhiannon's big brown, frightened eyes look at her mother. "I won't be upset."

"Dr. Weise told us you had an extremely low chance of ever walking. It broke our hearts; we couldn't say anything. I told the staff not to tell you. They were under my strict orders. I wanted to give it a chance, help you fight . . ."

"That's why they were weird around me, even at rehab. Thank you, Mom. I'm glad I didn't know. It would have slowed me up, just the thought of it."

Doctors recommend against a busy Christmas for Rhiannon's well-being. The family keep it quiet, the three of them celebrating a most blessed holiday, video calling Genna and Adam and the little ones.

Lynn travels back and forth to Halifax, every week by herself for six long months, as she tries to keep up with her employment responsibilities and duties as a municipal counsellor for the County of Inverness. She takes a leave from her job as a teacher's aide, for the Strait Region, shortly thereafter retires. When she comes home at the end of tiresome months, in private she crashes. Rhiannon is out of the woods, or so they think.

Five months after her first life-saving surgery, X-rays reveal that she had been "walking" around with a broken back; little holding her spine together. She must once again have major surgery on her spinal cord. February 1, 2023, she goes under the knife again and Dr. Weise removes the broken rods in two same-day, marathon surgeries. The first with her on her belly, as he removes the broken rods, replaces the damage with pins and new rods. Next, they roll her to a second operating room and position her on her left side for a right-side procedure. Dr. Weise takes out her floating rib, allowing him a better view as he goes through a muscle to get to the vertebrae. Once there, he puts in a cage—piece of metal hardware to replace the damaged disc. He then bone crafts L2 and L4 together, with the L3 cage in the middle. She is back in a hospital bed recovering a mere three days, when they send her home in throbbing pain, to heal and catch up to where she was before.

A trooper, she comes through the second and third operations, laughing at the fact she managed to break titanium rods. After healing, she returns to outpatient rehab and receives a back brace. She wears it for two and a half months. Lynn is constantly by her side, taking Rhiannon to rehab every morning until, December 2023, one full year later.

"My back feels like a welded unit. It does not move, and makes my movements stiff, creates pain if I sit or stand too long. The L5 controls my right knee and limp, which continues to improve. An awkward gait, small cost for being able to walk. The one provocative, haunting question I have is not answered. What happened to the driver to cause the accident and my near death? Scans taken showed he had no neurological issues. So why did he pass out while driving the truck in the middle of chaotic traffic? Knowing what happened would bring me closure, help someone before or in case it happens again. Not knowing haunts and terrifies me."

Lynn expresses her appreciation for the health care Rhiannon received. "Dr. Weise did both spinals . . . he was excellent, and the follow-up meetings were beautiful because he was so happy to give us good news. He said he was going to Germany on sabbatical that June and he jokingly said he was taking Rhiannon with him as part of his study, amazed by her progress and recovery in such a brief time."

Life is sometimes prophetic. Months before Rhiannon's accident, on July 1, 2022, Lynn and Cyril went to visit Rhiannon, who was working at the shipyard in Levi, Quebec. While in the province, they visit the famous Sainte-Anne-de-Beaupré Shrine in Quebec, known for miracles performed. Lynn (a locally well-known musician) buys two bottles of blessed holy oil and fervently sings in Saint Anne's cathedral. She posts about her visit and video of her singing on Facebook. A week after Rhiannon's accident, late September, I find the post. Chills run down my spine, tingle the back of my neck, raise the hairs as the words uncannily fit.

Lynn's strong, lilting voice sings out in the majestic cathedral, reverent notes holding the syllables, "A-ve Ma-ri-i-a, Oh, my love, my love, this can really be, that someday you'll walk, down the aisle with me."

If that is not prophetic, I do not know what is. Tears stream down my face as I watch the video in its new context, cry and pray for Rhiannon and her family, a glimpse from where their strength comes. Fate and faith intercede. The girl I taught now teaching me to never give up.

Lynn shares, "Not a day missed rubbing that very same holy oil on Rhiannon's legs, and I prayed to Father Archie MacLellan, a saintly deceased priest known for healing people in Inverness County."

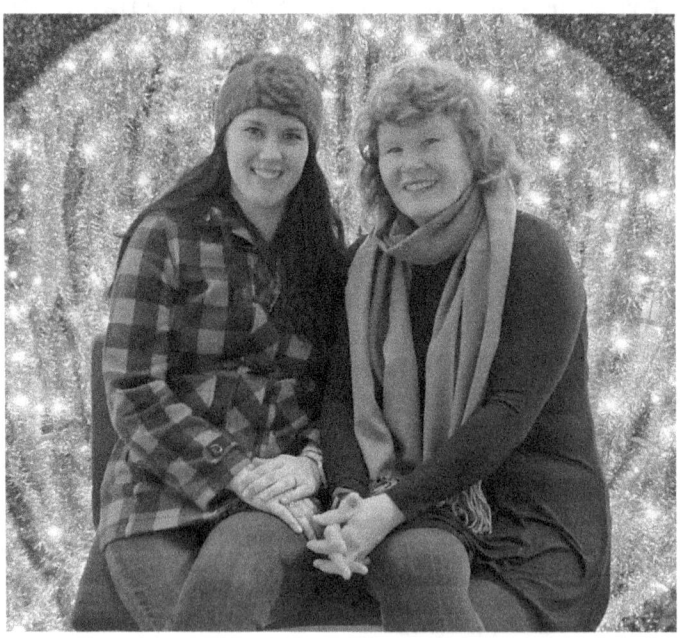

Rhiannon and her mom, Lynn Chisholm

Rhiannon acknowledges the after-effects of her brain injury and back surgery. "At first, I felt overwhelmed. Lights and noise bothered me. Turning my head felt like I was shaking my brain. Nerve damage in my nose affected smell and taste for the first year. PTSD slipped in. It is rough, reliving the horror and sensations of the crash. I still deal with that. Lots of adjustment. Certain sounds, sights trigger, put me right back. I get mad, find it hard to control my emotions. If I hear popping balloons, my eyes roll back and I slip into another world . . . loud noises cause it . . . it's weird, knocks me out of reality. PTSD strikes when anything reminds me of the airbags going off."

Paralysis and near-death will not deter this vivacious trooper, with a robust constitution. She believes what does not break you, strengthens you. Having hit the lowest low, she realizes how important little things are. She appreciates the gift of life; her zealous work paying off. Brain fog is not too bad, unless tired, or she pushes it.

Following tragedy, we root for the underdog, hope for their happiness. Symbolic of endings and beginnings, the stars line up as this courageous fighter wrestles the odds, shocks her doctors. In October 2023, a year after her accident, she finds a text message from a guy she used to see around work. Coty James MacRoberts messages and asks her on a dinner date. Shocked, she agrees. At dinner she finds out he followed her journey on Facebook and wanted to meet her.

"It is interesting how he came into my life a year later when the knee brace came off and that challenging part of my life was done. Pretty magical when you think about it." When she tells me this, I detect a glow and see a big smile.

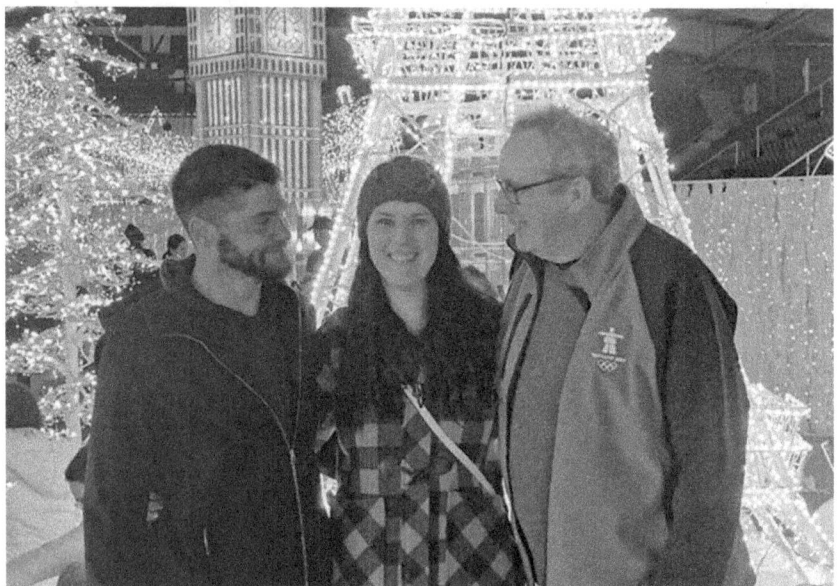

Rhiannon standing with Coty James and her dad, Cyril.

His is a tragic story as well, the thread that brings them together, the fact someone else understands the pain we as humans endure. On July 1, 2020, a horrendous car accident claimed the life of Coty's girlfriend and mother of their three children: Samantha, nine; Madison, seven; and Matthew, five. That right there, puts life into perspective, fast. It is rough—mentally and emotionally—trying to console, soothe three wee ones while dealing with the stark reality you will never see your partner, your children's mother, again. Coty's mother Rose, and father Darren, take over, help their son and grandchildren. Their rock and angels, they love them through grief and sadness, as Cyril, Lynn, and Genna love Rhiannon through hers. Tight-knit families are the greatest support.

Rhiannon gains a dose of wisdom. "The doctor said a brain bleed can last up to a year, so I had to take it easy. Not in my vocabulary, although I do have to pace."

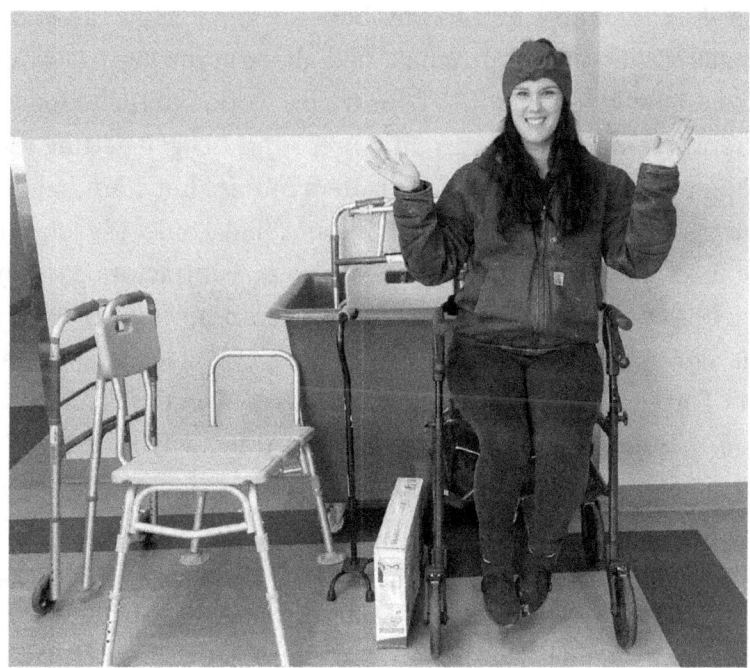

Last Day of Rehab

"December 19, 2023, my last day of physiotherapy, I went outside and yelled to no one and everyone, 'I did it!'" According to Lynn, Jamie Muir, a physical therapist, was their rock and angel in outpatient rehabilitation.

On December 21, 2023, Rhiannon finishes her second physiotherapy in Sackville for her torn shoulder. Two different physio appointments completed, fourteen months later. "I did it!" she exclaims again, overjoyed she succeeded. Against all odds. As she walks out the door, no chair, crutches, canes, she yells, "Only Rhiannon left!"

"I believe in good and bad karma," she says. "Everything I went through I was supposed to. I believe in angels. On February 1, 2024, I donated my medical aids to the Red Cross. Boy, it felt good!

Times I figured there was no way, but look at me! How can I not be changed? While in rehab, concerned about going back to work, I realized I could not handle labour trades work, but the union contractor offered me the job as union rep, and I began getting ready at the end of June 2023. Work is demanding, but I am handling it. I am a union rep for Painters Union Allied Trade. My job is full time. I collaborate with members, workers, contractors, go on job sites, help with issues or concerns that crop up. I work with the same workers so that is nice." She pauses. "I had leadership training in Toronto, March 7, 2024, which was cool, and was in Quebec, May 5-9, 2024. It is demanding, involves travel and learning. That tires me out, but I am doing okay, considering. I can't run a marathon, but I can prepare for one. It's different from before; my body gets stiff and sore, and my mind tires, so I pace, and rest, work my eight hours a day, even if not in the traditional sense of consecutive hours, as weekends also slip into the mix. I fight off the bad days a substantial amount of time, then get back at it."

A year and a half after her accident, Rhiannon Chisholm looks back with peace in her heart. Once weighed down, now it dances, a melody of joy in every guarded, calculated step. Her gait may appear uncertain, her pace slow and robotic, but she exudes courage, continuous healing, and a triumphant spirit. A champion, she beat the odds, and if she has her way, nothing will stop her.

> "I got my warrior scars to remind me of battle wounds. My steadfast attitude, family, Mom—they're 100 per cent my rock. My ability to be disciplined turned on even more when I needed it most. I have gratitude I didn't have before, feel people's pain. I've been there, came out of a hole, the accident, the most chilling experience ever. Having those lowest points in life makes you a better person, changes your perspective. I think I found the definition of pure resilience!"

"Do you feel like your old self?" I ask.

"No, I believe I am a better version!"

That dinner date must have gone well; Coty and Rhiannon beam, together ever since, (time of writing, November 2024). Rhiannon claims Coty's children are the absolute sweetest. Is it possible for the worst in life to flip into the best with a twist of fate, faith, a resilient attitude, and willingness to never give up?

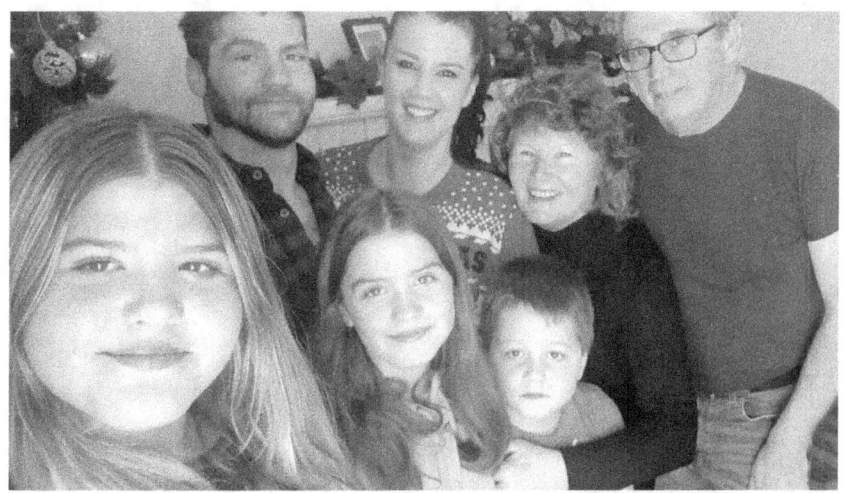

Rhiannon with new family: Coty, Lynn, Cyril, Samantha, Madison, Matthew

Finding Myself

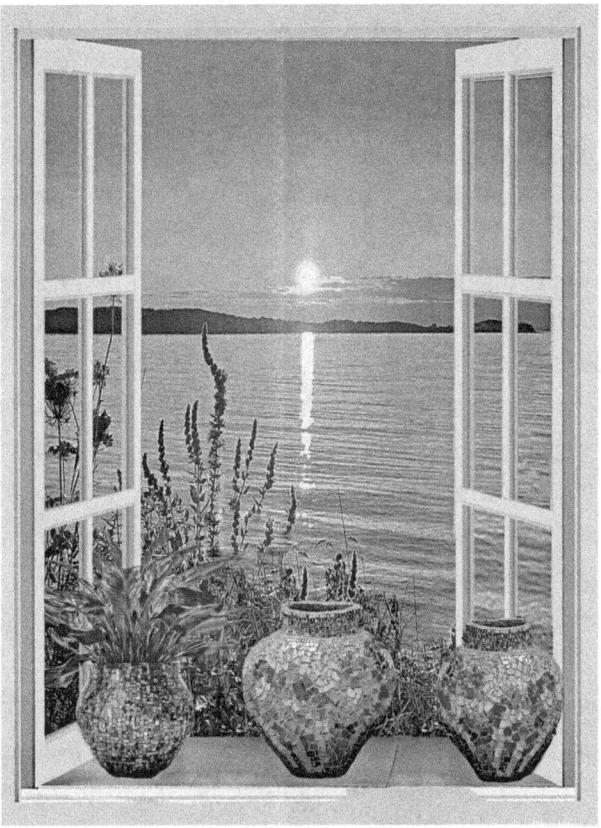

"You may encounter many defeats, but you must not be defeated. In fact, it may be necessary to encounter the defeats so you can know who you are, what you can rise from, how you can still come out of it."

— Maya Angelou.

*D*awn is brighter than dusk, fewer particles in the air, less pollution. A long, hard journey is now in my rear-view mirror; I venture onto fresh paths and adapt to rejoining life. So many things I want to do and say. Pacing lets me rediscover this wondrous world. Sure, I forget, but it no longer leads to frustration. I've learned to manage change, avoid going below 30 per cent energy level, a good principle for anyone to follow. When fatigued or overloaded, we fall prey to our worst selves. Awareness helps us refuel. If I write, visit, or care for my grandbabies, I need rest, although hugs and kisses and smiles warm my heart, have me wanting to live forever. I build wellness into my schedule, rise above the muck. It's necessary every day to step back and refill the gas tank, especially if I deplete my energy on a new project. If overstimulated in a crowd I wear sunglasses and earplugs.

As of 2024, I still wear yoked prisms in my eyeglasses, which have a slight blue tint, but have *normal* glasses as well. They ground me. I have also developed glaucoma making me wonder if there is a connection to mTBI. As we age, we must take care of our body, rather than take it for granted. My television records various shows so I can watch in stages. A musician, my husband loves blasting tunes. He has been waiting for my head to heal and for me to adapt. No longer am I on a boat, tossing and turning in tumultuous waves. Those swells have subsided. I have gained, inch by inch, confidence in my recovery and my brain. My plan each day is to walk, stroll, and enjoy the scenery, listen to the lapping waves as they tell their secrets. The spectacular view now seen from a unique perspective, I have regained independence, freedom, and appreciation. My lens centres on surrounding plenitude.

Despite my damaged confidence, and resurfacing trauma, I do not let them define me. I am done worrying about judgment, work towards self-love. I appreciate what my body does for me. Time to focus on my health and well-being, change my sedentary lifestyle.

My brain and body need activity, healthy food, lots of water. The recipe seems easy, yet we have trouble following it. I learned my lessons. Expert advice and staying within my limits makes life good. We owe it to ourselves to give it our best shot!

Anniversary dates of my accident no longer upset me. My threshold is not as high as I would like, but that is okay. I challenge myself. Through the stories of others, I gain strength on bad days. If they can do it, so can I. My nose keen, I sniff out my bullshit, bury it. Dangerous how we talk ourselves out of challenges, make excuses, keep ourselves cocooned where comfortable, no chance of change or growth. I recognize when I am feeding myself BS! Hopefully, it does not sneak in to stink everything up.

I enjoy my patio, sitting under the shaded enclosure, my ocean companion, but not in the same way as before. I accept I have persistent post-concussion syndrome (PPCS), but it does not control me. Most of my therapies have ended. I cannot express enough how grateful I am. I have come a long way, baby! Might be slow as a turtle, but I won the race.

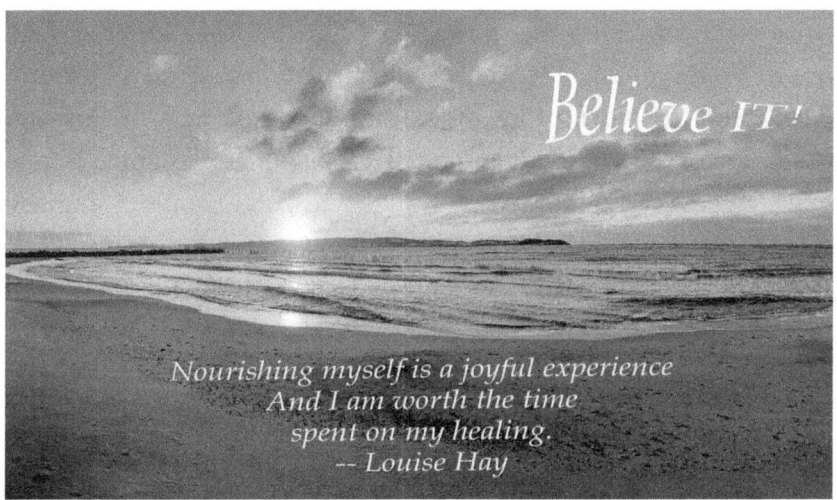

Believe IT!

Nourishing myself is a joyful experience
And I am worth the time
spent on my healing.
-- Louise Hay

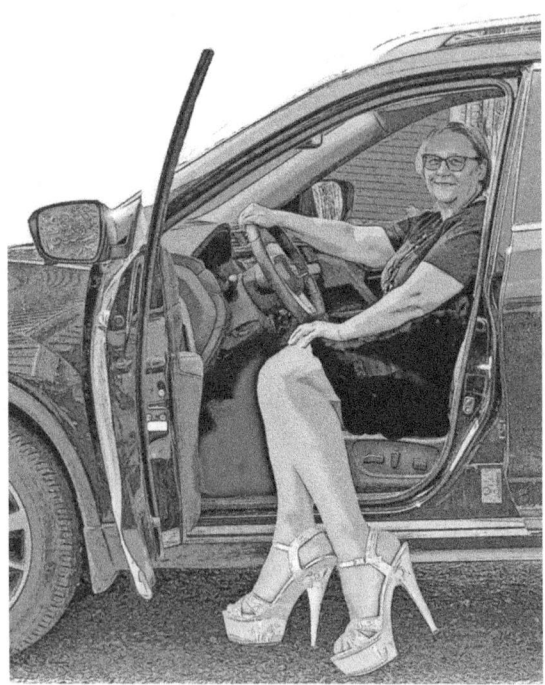

Francene Driving

And I am driving! So excited, freedom once again. I go on short runs; each time increase the distance. If I become fatigued, I do not drive. Acceptance is not only of my injury, but of PPCS and PTSD, and the person I have become. I am not weak, but strong, different yet the same. My life involves challenge. My spirit bursts alive, kicking, grateful for tiny things and good people. I manage the difficult moments.

I have learned from Indigenous people, hold them in high regard, admire their sacred teachings, respect for the environment, love of nature. The privilege was mine of teaching many Indigenous youth at Dalbrae Academy in several of my English and Advanced English-12 courses and studying with First Nations students during my master's program, Multicultural Diversity, Administration & Leadership, at St. Francis Xavier University from 2012-2014. I wish everyone could treat people from different

ethnic backgrounds equitably; differences enrich, a theme reinforced in my master's program. We have much to learn from
each other.

I will thrive, blessed with family, friends, my home community of Port Hood, and the county of Inverness as we make great
cheerleaders for one another. May those who journey with me
receive blessings and grace. One of my early medical practitioners
informed me I had a mountain to climb, thus my analogy. And now,
I have climbed it. The views are spectacular, rays of light spreading
over a dark, ominous road. See it! Believe it! I know how to navigate, hold the compass, recognize what direction I want to travel,
and with daily modifications, my toes edge into the ocean. When
overwhelmed, I revisit my own words, practise my breathing, slow
hyperactivity. Oh, how I fought at first! We must learn to accept
knowledge and wisdom where we can find it.

Time rolls around so fast I cannot keep track of the days.
Writing and rewriting requires tremendous concentration; I am
slower than I used to be. The beast has left me with deficits, but it
takes longer for the claw to squeeze. Manuscripts written prior to
my fall need to be published. As energy allows, I will find homes
for them. With a controlled environment, I manage the computer.
These improvements bring happiness, my soul and my identity
coming out. I want to pursue educational opportunities, publish
high school curriculum materials written during my career. My
passion for teaching remains. I can continue to teach through
words and resources.

Still, out of shape, I must be honest with myself. Positive
thinking, Fran! Shift perspective. See losing weight as a game or
challenge to overcome. Make it fun and competitive, reward small
successes. We need to taste success—especially when healing.
Motivation is a great catalyst. Baby steps. One step forward . . .
then another, and another. My slow journey to recovery is an
eye-opener. We rarely learn about the unfamiliar until forced. If it

resonates with others, then I found purpose amidst debris, which I now control instead of it controlling me. Empowerment. Thank you, to all my therapists. Progress. Yippee! We worked hard and made it through. May we always find laughter in the rain and look for the sunshine.

A harsh, judgmental world is making people clam up, keeping struggles and invisible injuries to themselves. Too many suffer alone. When we strip away filters of difference, we discover we are the same, needing emotional and mental encouragement. My hope is everyone experiences support. A slight gesture like offering to drive, run errands, cook, or visit can make an enormous difference in someone's day. May we listen to the messages we send, let our goodness show as in spring's first breath, summer's sunny smile, autumn's magnificent splendour, and winter's snow angels.

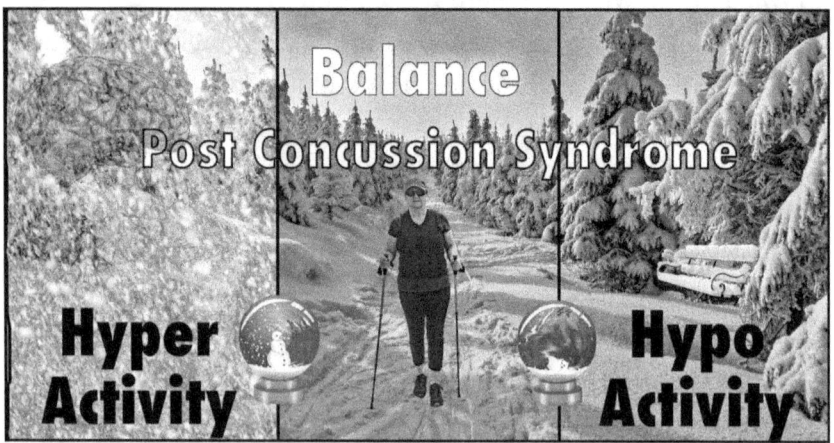

It helps to be aware of our body, how we react, our emotions, beliefs. None of us is perfect; we need to stop trying to prove we are. As humans, we are tough on ourselves. Letting go, giving ourselves a break, showing ourselves grace and kindness develops a mindset of perseverance. It means not giving up when trees fall, the climb too steep, a seagull craps on our shoulder. Being happy is a state of mind. To offer the best possible chance, we can accept, forgive, appreciate, believe in something bigger, have faith, and a desire to better ourselves without fault finding. Those who enter our lives are precious gifts. Life's choices rest in where we put our efforts, who we devote our time to, where and how we distribute it. Thank you for allowing me to share mine with you.

With tremendous effort and help, I received tools, tricks, tips, resources, hacks, and placed them here, in one place for later use. I needed to make it easier, reminders and advice most valuable. The brain is an immense superhighway of electrical impulses still being discovered. As these pages become a book, it will sit at my table to remind me of challenging days—that we can pass through the eye of a needle with faith, good people, and a positive mindset. The individuals I have talked about here remind me of that! I hope family members and friends of the injured or sick pick up a copy as prevention, and encouragement for those who need education, comfort, or inspiration.

The title for this book evolved once I decided I would share my experiences. My initial thought was *Who would have believed?* This intimidating beast caught me off guard, its symptoms left me in shock. Next, I contemplated *Robbed.* Then I softened it, picked *Stolen.* Both show movement, focus on what the fall took from me. Curious, I changed it to *Acceptance* to show growth, a far cry from previously considered. It promoted permanency, a transformative mind shift, was not true; I was not "there" yet.

And now, the "i" has returned to "I" and I understand when and how she disappeared. I fought hard to get her back, different but the same, for we are more than our occupation, our roles; they simply reflect who the world see us as. My self-esteem still requires work, but it has not taken away my confidence. Now my aim is to educate the unaware; families, high school teachers, youth who sit close to my heart, coaches, the young and old. I hope that universities use the musings within to educate their health science students, not as a medical reference, but from a patient perspective, a glimpse of how to treat the whole person. I believe it can be a valuable resource for health care practitioners, including physiotherapists, speech pathologists, occupational therapists, nurses, doctors. My hope is for these pages to offer an opportunity for classroom discussions about brain injuries, patients, treatments, profundity of the human engine that allows us to function. Do not cast those with inexplicable symptoms aside.

Writing is my therapy of choice. It enables me to express my thoughts and emotions—unravel my fears, loss, anger, doubts, questions, disbelief, shame, guilt, and sadness. Through lessons and a tumultuous journey within these pages, I can reflect on where I was, where I am, where I want to go. I can drive now so no distance is off limits, if done in stages. At least on paper, I get there. In creativity, the spirit soars free. We must find our passion; integrate it into our lives, discover good people who share our interests. Words cannot describe my husband's undying support; it was hard on him as it is with all caregivers. They deserve many, many thanks.

Through awareness, we move on. I notice the signs of lingering symptoms creeping over my threshold, the need for silence to rejuvenate. When I turned sixty-five I decided I would do some things just for me like go to a salon once a month to get manicures or pedicures. Secrets Spa & Hair Design, owner Denise England and her gracious staff have in two years become friends who know of my inhibitions around physical appearance. With Denise's encouragement I have skin rejuvenation I should have had decades ago but was too scared to even broach the topic with anyone. Their slogan of making everyone look beautiful holds true as receiving help in areas that hold you back is freeing and builds confidence. It is worth saving those pennies. The way I am going, I will look better at age seventy than I did in previous decades. I am laughing. I have learned that women matter. We matter. And we need to take the time for self-care.

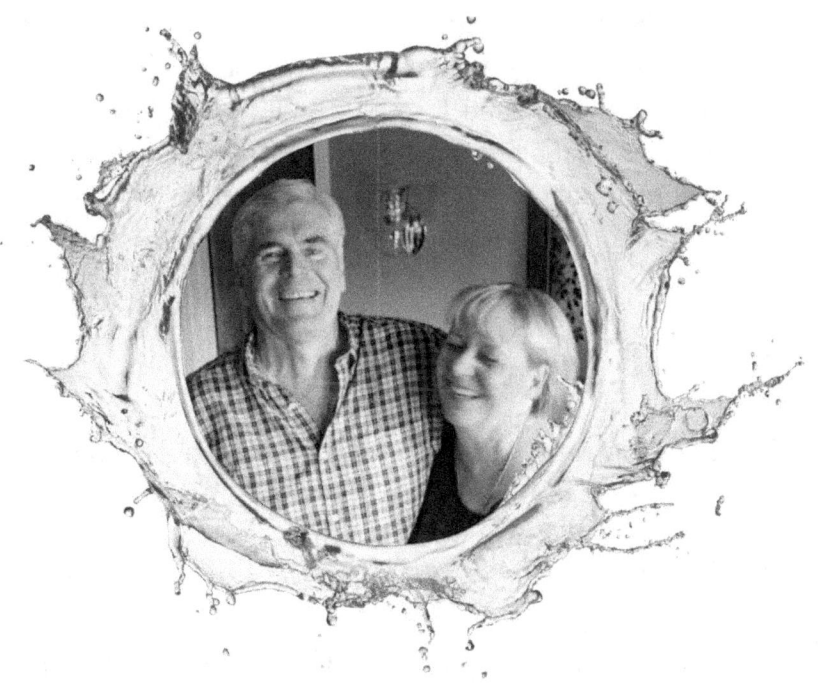

Sandy & Francene

It wasn't until the fall of 2024, after a few years of practice that I was able to drive to Port Hawkesbury, no issues. Yay! Now, I am overjoyed behind the wheel. In October, I did a week-long Paradise Writers' Retreat where I spent time with people I met from the year before and six new people, and the writing within burns. I forced myself to walk instead of taking drives and I made sure I did not miss any of the sessions, up at seven-thirty in the morning. I took the half-hour I needed for myself, showered, had breakfast, and contributed during the sessions more than I should have, but after isolation I was hungry for human interaction. Inside me lives a passion for anything and everything that means something to me.

When I see people suffering, it ignites a fire within to help that lonely girl on the beach as she watched her father trying to bring her baby brother back to life. If I provide healing tears or boost that desire to help others, then I will have carried out my purpose in life. For the first time in ten years, I crossed an item off my bucket list—to go to a live concert! You read correctly. My husband, sister-in-law, and I went to Halifax, Nova Scotia, to see Celtic Thunder, a fabulous, professional group of male, Irish singers. A big undertaking involving three days, and I even managed to shop for Christmas. I rested up for a day, then my husband and I babysat our wee granddaughter.

The Sunny Side

In late 2024, I learned an important lesson that I did not realize for six years was even of consideration. Doctors often prescribe medication that they hope will work, but the onus is on us as patients to speak up if we are not seeing the results we hoped for. With a head injury it is tricky as the side effects may not be physical but emotional or mental. It was very difficult for me to handle the frustration of not being able to do what I could before, or when under my 30 per cent energy level. Because of chronic fatigue I did not have the wherewithal and was unable to handle overload. Uneducated in head injuries I did not know what was a symptom of my injury or a side effect of medication.

For years I fought to find ways to handle difficulties, sometimes with success, sometimes with miserable failure, triggered to overreact and funnel down a dark, black hole. I did not realize I was not on the best medicine for me. It took six years of putting up with not being myself and finally saying *enough already* to discover, I did not have to put up with the emotional gong show. A brutal lesson learned the hard way.

It was then that my nurse practitioner put me on new medication, and within weeks I started feeling the old me coming back. What a grace! I could not believe I could feel this way again. I felt like myself. I cried and bawled and cried some more, only this time, the first in a long time, my tears were happy ones. Tears well in my eyes even as I write this. We don't have to suffer. I can see the sun shining brighter than ever through the dark. We need to look for it and advocate, especially at the bleakest times, and not give up. We are ongoing beings, growing, learning, renewing ourselves. By being true to who we are we gain the most satisfaction, and now I have that chance again. I knew I was off, but I did not know how to "fix" it . . . such a weak verb. Please remember storms and left-overs will plague but with the knowledge, education, awareness, support, and tools, we can see the sunny side.

My goal is to live each day without self-criticism. That is accep-tance. It is okay to not be okay. I want to stress the valuable lessons learned through therapists and the importance of being open to what they say. We may think we have the answers, but the perspec-tive of someone with expertise in a particular field can make the difference between a good or bad day. Living with a concussion, head injury, or invisible illness is no picnic and there will be times when we want to throw in the towel; this book is not meant to dis-courage, but to help manage symptoms along the way, so we do not feel like we are going crazy.

My mTBI shortfalls still have me controlling my environment, pacing, knowing I will need to rest after doing too much, asking people to speak slower and lower, sitting with my back to the wall, turning off lights, moving slowly, steady on my feet, and always trying to keep the balance between too much and too little, but that is okay.

God gifted me with the opportunity to teach, and although classroom teaching was stripped away, I can teach in other ways and share resources and lessons learned. I thank Anne and OC Publishing for the opportunity to publish my memoir plus. May it provide solace, information, awareness, and a place to start. I reit-erate that it is in sharing stories, experiences, and anecdotes that we help each other without ever knowing or realizing we touched someone in a profound way. Isn't that remarkable! Through our facial expression, twinkle in the eye, smile, we affect others. Surrounded by nourishing people, we grow as individuals. My journey does not end but begins.

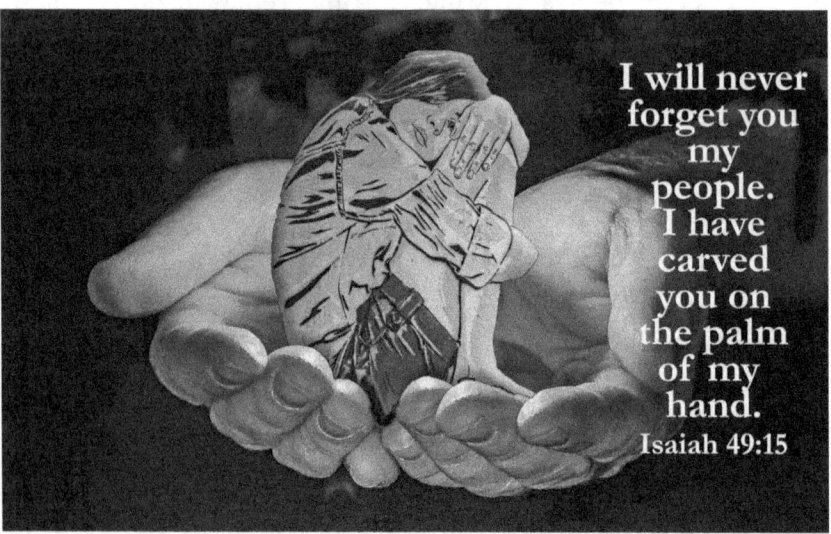

I will never forget you my people. I have carved you on the palm of my hand.
Isaiah 49:15

Relaxing by my patio door, I listen to outdoor merry melody. A dusky sky, scarlet red over the horizon ideal for reflection. We need music, song, and people in our lives. Among the sounds of joviality, I realize the importance of celebrating moments, discovering interests, hobbies, pastimes to make us smile. "Quit" is not a word in my vocabulary, although it crosses the mind when daily, chronic pain flares, or my claw squeezes. We look for answers even when there are none. We keep going, keep plugging, keep swimming across the ocean or climbing that steep mountain, because that is the spirit that burns inside. I have found myself, a collection of fragments, remnants, echoes, footprints, scattered pieces. I pick up the pieces, examine, rearrange, replace, better than before, glue them back together in a self-mosaic.

May you the reader feel something within. My absolute best to each and every one who finds and takes home, *Where Did i Go*. We will always be a work in progress, each day a new opportunity to love and be loved. I suspect that is the secret to living a happy life, one where we can find satisfaction. I always remember the wonder, tenderness, and life-giving love of a child. If only we could focus on love and its many dimensions, we might just have the secret to living a happy life. May we look for the sunshine, continue to hug those we love and those we appreciate.

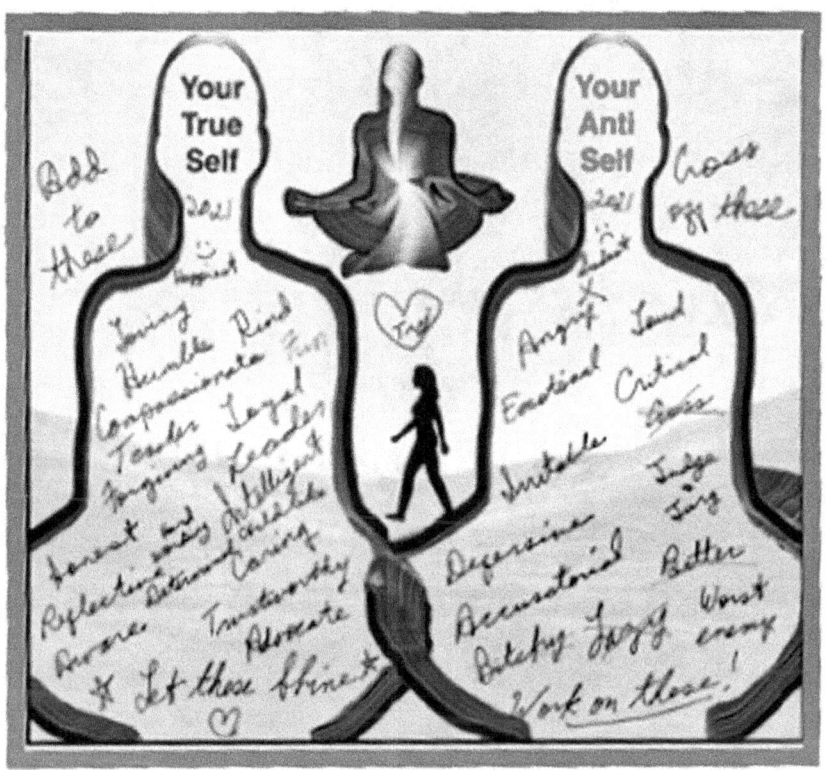

A web series that began on January 9, 2024, has most everything I would want or need from the experts. The 2024 CCC Webinar series starts with a most knowledgeable, Dr. Charles Tator, neurosurgeon and director of the Canadian Concussion Centre. Every second Tuesday, there is another renowned speaker. Dr. Tator says using the terminology mTBI is an insult to anyone with symptoms that last beyond the normal expected time of thirty days, especially when symptoms last years. I concur.

*Our lives
are continual
metamorphosis
where we discover
who we are,
and all
we can be.*

*Wings
are simply
those
we meet
along the way
who help us
fly!*

Francene Gillis

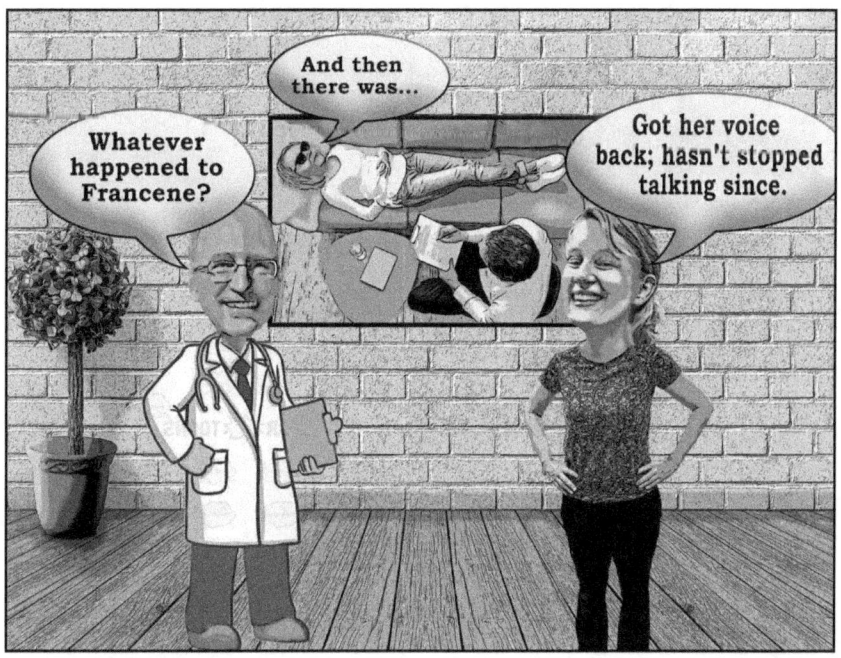

References & Resources

"A Guide to Help Parents and Families Re-Connect the Pieces through Education and Recovery Strategies." 2014. Back in Action: Physiotherapy Whistle, Concussion/Mild Traumatic Brain Injury: A Whole-Body Condition. June 1, 2014. http://www.backinactionphysiotherapy.com.

ABI Association of Nova Scotia, https://www.nshealth.ca/clinics-programs-and-services/acquired-brain-injury-abi-home.

Ackerman, Courtney. 2018. "What Is Neuroplasticity? A Psychologist Explains." PositivePsychology.com. July 25, 2018. https://positivepsychology.com/neuroplasticity/.

Acabchuk, R.L., Brisson, J.M., Park, C.L., Babbott-Bryan, N., Parmelee, O.A., & Johnson, B.T. (2020). "Therapeutic Effects of Meditation, Yoga, and Mindfulness-Based Interventions for Chronic Symptoms of Mild Traumatic Brain Injury: A Systematic Review and Meta-Analysis." *Applied Psychology: Health and Well-Being, 13(1)*, 34-62. (Headway, Brain Association, 21 Mar 2022)

American Physical Therapy Association, "Dry Needling by a Physical Therapist: What You Should Know." 2019. Move Forward, Physical Therapy Brings Motion to Life, June 28, 2019. http://www.moveforwarddpt.com.

Arden, John B. Arden, *Rewire Your Brain: Think Your Way to a Better Life*

Back in Action Physiotherapy, "Reconnecting the Pieces: A Guide to Understanding Symptoms and recovery Strategies for Patients and Families," June 1, 2014, https://backinactionphysiotherapy.com

Bolte Taylor, Jill, *My Stroke of Insight: A Brain Scientist's Personal Journey*, 2016, New York, Penguin Books

Bosdet, Peggy Ann, interview by Francene Gillis, *Where Did i Go?* October/ November 2024

Boyd, Lara, "After Watching This, Your Brain Will Not Be the Same," TEDx Vancouver, 2015, https://www.youtube.com/watch?v=LNHBMFCzznE.

Brain Canada Foundation, Traumatic Brain Injuries, September 5, 2024, https://braincanada.ca/i-am-not-my-tbi/

Brain Injury Alliance, Colorado; Brain Injury Facts & Figures. https://biacolorado.org/brain-injury-facts-figures/

Brain Injury Association of America, The My Brain Injury Journey Campaign, Brain Injury Awareness in News and Media, 2024. https://www.biausa.org/public-affairs/public-awareness/brain-injury-awareness

Brain Injury Association of Nova Scotia, "Concussion." Accessed Apr 19, 2024. https://concussionns.com

Brain Injury Association of Nova Scotia. Accessed May 22, 2024. http://braininjuryns.com/about-us/

Brain Injury Association of Nova Scotia. n.d. Accessed March 24, 2022. http://braininjuryns.com

Brain Injury Association of Waterloo—Wellington. Accessed Sept 19, 2017. http://www.biaww.com

Brain Injury Canada, Canada's Resource Website, Government of Canada, 2024, braininjurycanada.ca

Brain Injury Canada, "Mental Health," Government of Canada, 2022, https://braininjurycanada.ca/en/mental-health

BrainLine, "Three Minute Breathing," December 8, 2009. Reviewed July 25, 2018. *Adapted by Melissa Felteau from Williams, M., Teasdale, J., Segal, Z., Kabat-Zinn, J. (2007), "The Mindful Way Through Depression," New York: Guilford Press.* https://www.brainline.org/article/mindfulness-meditation-and-prayer-after-brain-injury.

BrainLine, WETA-TV, the flagship PBS station in Washington, D.C. (https://www.brainline.org/about-us, accessed August 2024.)

Brainworks Neurotherapy, "What is neuroplasticity? Brain plasticity explained." https://brainworksneurotherapy.com/what-is-neuroplasticity/

Canadian Association for Suicide Prevention, CASP, Media Guidelines, Entertainment, Public Service Announcements and Social Media; Public Service Announcements, https://suicideprevention.ca/media/media-guidelines/

Canada Public Health Agency, "The Government of Canada announces the winner of the Detecting Concussions Using Objective Indicators Challenge," News release, June 13, 2024, Ottawa, Ontario, Public Health Agency of Canada; https://www.canada.ca

Canadian Mental Health Association, Alberta Division. Aboriginal Youth: A Manual of Promising Suicide Prevention Strategies; Centre for Suicide Prevention; https://scholar.google.ca/scholar?q=Aboriginal+Youth:+Manual+of+Suicide

Carroll, Ryder therapist, "Resilience—bouncing back when facing adversity," Genius Recovery Blog, https://geniusrecovery.org/resilience-bouncing-back-when-facing-adversity/?gad

CBC news story, "Concussions Raise Long-Term Suicide Risk Three to Fourfold, Says New Canadian Study," February 8, 2016. https://www.cbc.ca/news/health/concussion-suicide-1.3439209

CDC, United States government, "Traumatic Brain Injury & Concussion," Centers for Disease Control and Prevention. US Department of Health and Human Resources, February 13, 2016, http://www.cdc.gov.

CDC, United States government, "Traumatic Brain Injury & Concussion," TBI Data, May 16, 2024, https://www.cdc.gov/traumatic-brain-injury/data-research/index.html

Cervical Whiplash | Trauma. N.d. www.youtube.com. Accessed June 17, 2023. https://youtu.be/jgMdL7vEga8.

Chambers, Cathrine E. MEd, CCC, RCT-C; March 06, 2018; Counselling Therapist.

Chapman, Rachelle, 2021. Interview by Francene Gillis. *Where Did i Go?*

Chisholm, Lynn. 2024: The Ordeal, Interview by Francene Gillis. *Where Did i Go?*

Chisholm, Rhiannon, 2024. TBI and Spinal Cord Injuries in a Young Woman. Interview by Francene Gillis.

Complete Concussion Management, Cleveland Clinic, "Whiplash, Neck Strain," 2024, https://completeconcussions.com/; https://my.cleve-landclinic.org/health/diseases/11982-whiplash

Concussion Legacy Foundation, n.d. Accessed October 4, 2022. https://concussionfoundation.org.

Concussion Management: Return to School Guidelines for Children & Youth, a Concussion Is a Brain Injury and Must Be Taken Seriously! McMaster University. https://canchild.ca/system/tenon/assets/attachments/000/000/291/original/MTBI-return_to_school_brochure.pdf.

Cognitive fx, Fong, Dr. Alina, PhD, "Post-Concussion Syndrome: Persistent Symptoms, Diagnosis & Treatment," July 16, 2024. Medical Rev Dr. Mark Allen, https://www.cognitivefxusa.com/blog/post-concussion-syndrome-and-post-concussion-symptoms

Cudmore, Dr. David, and Tara Sutherland CATI). n.d. "A Concussion Clinic: The Antigonish Model." CATA Canadian Athletic Therapists Association.

CTV News, "Rowan's Law Passes in Ontario, Aim to Prevent Youth Concussions." June 7, 2016, www.ctvnews.ca.

Doctors of NS, DNS Your Doctors, "Dr. Cudmore tackles Concussions Head On," May 13, 2015, http://www.yourdoctors.ca/.

Elliott, Clark, *The Ghost in My Brain: How a Concussion Stole My Life and How the New Science of Brain Plasticity Helped Me Get It Back*, 2016, New York: Penguin.

Foojan, Zeine, Nicole Jafari, Mohammad Nami, Kenneth Blum, Science Direct; "Awareness integration theory, A Psychological and genetic path to self-directed Neuroplasticity," *Health Sciences Review*, Volume 11, 2024,100169, ISSN 2772-6320, https://www.sciencedirect.com/science/article/pii/S2772632024000229

Foundation, Betty Clooney, Chart on How TBI Affects Behaviour, 2017 online resources, https://www.facebook.com/BettyClooneyCenter/.

Fran, J., and T. Hart, "Depression after Traumatic Brain Injury," in collaboration with the Model Systems Knowledge Translation Center, 2010, MSKTC Factsheets, https://msktc.org/lib/docs/Factsheets/TBI_Depression_and_TBI.pdf

Government of Canada, Concussion: Symptoms and Treatment, July 23, 2018, https://www.canada.ca/en/public-health/services/diseases/concussion-sign-symptoms.html

Grech, Ron, "Head injury expert invited to speak in wake of rise in concussions," *The Timmons Daily Press*, Dec. 2, 2018

Guidelines for Concussion/Traumatic Mild Brain Injury & Prolonged Symptoms, Second Edition, 2013, Ontario Neurotrauma Foundation, https://concussionsontario.org/

Hampton, Debbie, "What Your Brain Needs to Know about Neuroplasticity," April 14, 2019, The Best Brain Possible, https://thebestbrainpossible.com/neuroplasticity-brain-mental-health/#google_vignette

Harris, Dr. Russ, *The Happiness Trap,* introduction, https://www.actmindfully.com.au/wp-content/uploads/2021/^{10}/2nd-edition-of-The-Happiness-Trap-chapter-1.pdf

Healthline: Medical Information and Health Advice You Can Trust, 2019, http://www.healthline.com

Hempstead, Doug, "Inquest Called into Death of Ottawa Rugby Player," February 15, 2015, www.ottawasun.com

Honourable Jane Philpott, P.C., MP Minister of Health, 2016; "Government takes action to develop national guidelines for concussion management," Government of Canada. https://www.canada.ca/en/public-health/news/2016/10/government-takes-action-develop-national-guidelines-concussion-management.html

Hurley, Katie, LCSW; Everyday Health, Resilience Resource Centre, "Resilience: A Guide to Facing Life's Challenges, Adversities, and Crises," July 29, 2024, Medically reviewed, Seth Gillihan, PhD; https://www.everydayhealth.com/wellness/resilience/#resilience-theory

Johnson, Shannon, "Whiplash Injury Overview," Healthline, medically reviewed by Angela M. Bell, MD, FACP, updated on June 22, 2023, https://www.healthline.com/health/whiplash

Kamala Institute, Centre for the Integrated Treatment of Trauma and Anxiety, 2018, Cathrine Chambers, Counsellor

KANTAR TNS, "Baseline Survey on Understanding and Awareness of Sport-Related Concussions," Public Health Agency of Canada, POR # 021-17, Contract # HT372-173253/001/CY, Government of Canada, July 09, 2017. Accessed, February, 2024

Kennedy, Mary B, "Synaptic Signaling in Learning and Memory," *Cold Spring Harbor Perspectives in Biology,* vol. 8,2 a016824. 30, Dec. 2013, doi:10.1101/cshperspect. a016824

King, Nigel S., *Overcoming Mild Traumatic Brain Injury and Post-Concussion Symptoms—A self-help guide using evidence-based techniques,* Brown Book Group (UK), 2015

Lambke, Taylor. n.d. Concussion in a Young Male. Interview by Francene Gillis. *Where Did i Go?*

Lazarus, Dr. Russel; What Is Syntonic Phototherapy? Optometrist Network, December 20, 2020, https://www.optometrists.org/vision-therapy/neuro-optometry

Lloyd, Brenda, "I'm Clawing My Way Back from a Brain Injury, so Please Be Patient," personal essay, *The Globe and Mail*, August 9, 2019

Lovett, Esther. n.d. "Esther Lovett: My Story and My Legacy," Concussion Legacy Foundation, Boston. Accessed October 5, 2022, https://concussionfoundation.org/en-ca/personal-stories/inspiring-stories/esther-lovett-pcs-blog/my-story-my-legacy/

Love Your Brain, "Research-based LYB Tips to access your resilience," https://www.loveyourbrain.com/tips

Ludlow, Christy L., and Torrey Loucks, "Stuttering: A Dynamic Motor Control Disorder," *Journal of Fluency Disorders,* 28 (4): 273–95, https://doi.org/10.1016/j.jfludis.2003.07.001

Lyubomirsky, Sonja, (professor of psychology), "Happiness takes work," *Greater Good Magazine*, The Science of a Meaningful Life series, July 2010, https://greatergood.berkeley.edu/video/item/happiness_takes_work

MacDougall, Jolene, interview, Francene Gillis, "Feeling Spring's First Breath," *Inverness Oran*, March 29, 2023

MacLean/Crawford, Melinda, interview, Francene Gillis, MTBI after a Stroke 2021.

Massage Therapists' Association of Nova Scotia (MTANS), www.mtans.ca.

Mandelman, Dr. Toby, interview on CTV Atlantic, January 28, 2016, https://www.ctvnews.ca/lifestyle/article/seeing-clearly-how-post-trauma-vision-syndrome-affects-concussion-patients/

Mandelman, Dr. Toby, June 2020, interview by Francene Gillis

Mason, Michael Paul, *Head Cases: Stories of Brain Injury and Its Aftermath*, April 28, 2009, Farrar, Straus and Giroux, LLC.

McDermott, Prof. Kevin, and Clark Elliot, "Public Perspective: Author '*The Ghost in My Brain*' explains how his brain damage was cured by a new set of eyeglasses and some puzzles," 2015, YouTube, https://www.youtube.com/watch?v=7dxrustpXdQ

McDonough, Victoria Tilney, senior editor, BrainLine, "Mindfulness, Meditation, and Prayer After Brain Injury," https://www.brainline.org/article/mindfulness-meditation-and-prayer-after-brain-injury

Middleton, Jackie, "Prevention & Recovery, the Impact of Concussions," *Canadian Living*, April 7, 2014, https://www.canadianliving.com/health/prevention-and-recovery/article/the-impact-of-concussions

Miranda, Nicole, PT, DPT, "What Happens to the Brain and Vestibular System After a Traumatic Brain Injury?," Article, 019, Vestibular Disorders 07, 2022; VEDA Life Rebalanced, Traumatic Brain Injury (TBI), https://vestibular.org/wp-content/uploads/2022/07/Traumatic-Brain-Injury-TBI_19.pdf

Molt, PhD, Lawrence, and J. Scott Yaruss, PhD. n.d., "Neurogenic Stuttering Guides," The Stuttering Federation, Memphis, Tennessee. Accessed May 22, 2021. https://www.stutteringhelp.org/sites/default/files/Migrate/0111neur.pdf

Morgan, "JP," John Pierpont, July 13, 2023

Muradov, Jamil, PhD Candidate, Killam Scholar, Department of Medical Neuroscience, Faculty of Medicine, "Living with traumatic brain injury: Proposed legislation supports nationwide strategy for care," Dal News, Dalhousie University, July 5, 2024.

Murray, Sandra, BEd, MCP, RCT, interview, Francene Gillis, October 28, 2024

Nacanulli, Mia, "How the Food You Eat Affects Your Brain," TED Talks, 2020, https://www.ted.com/talks/mia_nacamulli_how_the_food_you_eat_affects_your_brain

National Academies of Sciences, Engineering, and Medicine, *Traumatic Brain Injury: A Roadmap for Accelerating Progress*, Washington (DC), National Academies Press (US), Feb 1, 2022, https://www.ncbi.nlm.nih.gov/books/NBK580077/

National Institutes of Health (NIH), Turning Discovery into Health, U.S. Department of Health & Human Services, 2024, https://www.nih.gov/about-nih/what-we-do/nih-turning-discovery-into-health

Neff, Kristin, "Self-Compassion: Theory, Method, Research, and Intervention," *Annual Review of Psychology*, 2023, 74. 10.1146/annurev-psych-032420-031047.

Neuman, D., S.R. Miles, A. Sander, and B. Greenwald, "Irritability, Anger, and Aggression after TBI," Model Systems Knowledge Translation Center (MSKTC) Fact Sheets, February 2021, https://msktc.org/sites/default/files/MSKTC-IrrAftTBI-Factsheet-508.pdf

Niftyadmin, "Mild TBI Symptoms," Traumatic Brain Injury, 2019. http://www.traumaticbraininjury.com/symptoms-of-tbi/mild-tbi-symptoms/

Mild TBI Symptoms, Traumatic Brain Injury. Accessed April 21, 2024, http://www.traumaticbraininjury.com/symptoms-of-tbi/mild-tbi-symptoms/.

Nunes, Julia, "Life in the Shadows of the Concussion Debate," *The Star*, June 5, 2016, www.thestar.com.

ONE Team, ONE Family aiming ONE GOAL, YouTube video, Nov. 2023, https://fb.watch/ukmx7BQwr-/

Ontario Brain Injury Association | Education, Awareness, & Support | OBiA." n.d. Ontario Brain Injury Association. Accessed March 16, 2023. http://www.obia.ca

Ontario Neurotrauma Foundation, 2013, *Guidelines for mTBI and Persistent Symptoms: Second Editio,* P.46.

Palmer, Cara, Post-Concussion Syndrome in Younger Women Interview by Francene Gillis, 2021.

Parachute – "Preventing Injuries. Saving Lives." n.d. Parachute.ca. Accessed September 30, 2016, https://www.parachutecanada.org.

Parachute Canada, Video, 1E9, Concussion: It's Not All in Your Head, Jan 26, 2023.

Parachute Concussion Ed app, parachute.ca/concussion; download Concussion Ed for free in the App Store and Google Play Store.

Parachute Canada, "Potential lost, potential for change: The Cost of Injury in Canada," 2021; Data from 2018. parachute.ca/costofinjury.

Parachute Canada, Popping the Bubble Wrap, on Apple and Spotify podcasts, YouTube, https://www.youtube.com/watch?v=A4BOL9ZCS3s, and Story Studio Network, www.storystudionetwork.com.

Pink Concussions. n.d. Pink Concussions, Female Brain Injury, https://www.pinkconcussions.com. Accessed March 23, 2020.

Ray, Marie B, "Who is Marie Beynon Ray," *Fort Francene Times*, March 2010, https://fftimes.com/news/who-is-marie-beynon-ray/

Roehr, Bob, "Concussions Affect Women More Adversely Than Men," Scientific *Scientific American*, a Division of Springer, Nature America, Inc., March 9, 2016, Copyright 2016 *Scientific American, Inc.*

Schmidt, Joanne, Post-Concussion Syndrome Advice, interview by Francene Gillis, 2020.

Schwartz, PT, DPT, CSCS, Dr. Jessica B. n.d., PT2Go (website/blog), tremendous resources for patients, clinicians, doctors, educators, medical personnel, http://www.pt2go.co/

Seale, Gary S., PhD, LPA, LCDC, CBIS-T, "Suicidality and Suicide Prevention following Brain Injury," *Psychiatric Times*, July 10, 2024.

Sentis, "Neuroplasticity," YouTube Video, 2012, https://www.youtube.com/watch?v=ELpfYCZa87g.

Shergill Y, Côté P, Shearer H, Wong J. J, Stupar M, Tibbles A, Cassidy D.J, "Inter-rater reliability of the Quebec Task Force classification system for recent-onset Whiplash Associated Disorders," *Journal of the Canadian Chiropractic Association*, 2021:65(2):186-192.

Sherring, Susan, "Inquest Recommends Rowan's Law for Concussion Management," *Ottawa Sun*, June 1, 2015, https://ottawasun.com/2015/06/01/inquest-recommends-rowans-law-for-concussion-management

Sherring, Susan, "Rowan would be 'very impressed': mom," *Ottawa Sun*, June 3, 2015, https://ottawasun.com/2015/06/03/rowan-stringer-coroners-inquest-jury-returns-with-48-recommendations

Shetty, Jay; author, podcaster, 2024, https://www.brainyquote.com/quotes/jay_shetty_1118675

Shetty, Jay: bestselling author; 2024, https://www.jayshetty.me/about-jay

Smith, Jessie, "13 Concussion Therapy Exercises You Can Do at Home," Neural Effects, Feb. 25, 2022, https://neuraleffects.com/blog/concussion-therapy-exercises/#physical-exercise

Smith, Marlee, 2024, Community Navigator, interview by Francene Gillis.

Speech and Hearing Association of Canada, n.d. Shans.ca. Accessed May 22, 2020, http://www.shans.ca/our-professionals/speech-language-pathology/.

SportsMedBC, "New Protocols for Concussions Advised for All Sports in Canada," Sportmedbc.com, July 2, 2019. http://sportmedbc.com.

Stella Center, DC, "What Is the 333 Rule for Anxiety?" 2024, https://stellacenter.com/resources/333-rule-for-anxiety

Sterling, Dana, owner, Sterling Structural Therapy, 2024, website, https://sterlingstructuraltherapy.com/about-us/

Stone, Dr. Jon; MBChb FRCP PhD, "Functional Neurological Symptoms," University of Edinburgh, Scotland, 2009, http://www.neurosymptoms.org

Sunnybrook Health Science Centre, "Mild Traumatic Brain Injury/ Concussion: Your Guide to Recovery," March 2019, https://sunny- brook.ca/content/?page=bsp-concussion

Sutton, Jeremy, PhD, "18 Effective Thought-Stopping Techniques (& 10 PDFs)," PositivePsychology, 2024, https://positivepsychology.com/ thought-stopping-techniques/.

Tator, Dr. Charles; Middleton, Jackie, "The Impact of Concussions," *Canadian Living Magazine*, April 7, 2014.

Tator, Dr. Charles, neurosurgeon and director of the Canadian Concussion Centre, CCC Webinar Series, January 9, 2024 on YouTube.

TED, "Michael Merzenich: Growing Evidence of Brain Plasticity," YouTube, 2009, https://www.youtube.com/watch?v=Z41BTeAU7DI.

The American Veterans Health Administration (VHA); Department of Defense (DOD); Health Information Management, Office of Informatics and Analytics, "Fact Sheet, Coding Guidance for Traumatic Brain Injury (TBI)," effective as of October 1, 2015, http:// www.rstce.pitt.edu/va_tbi/documents/11192015/11192015_03.pdf

The Mighty, Mighty Proud Media Inc., An Online Growing Health Community, https://themighty.com/

The Healthline, http://www.healthline.com/health/ best-traumatic-brain-injury-blogs#1

Mayo Clinic, www.mayoclinic.org, February 28, 2018

Tsao, Jack W., *Traumatic Brain Injury: A Clinician's Guide to Diagnosis, Management, and Rehabilitation*, Cham, Switzerland: Springer, 2020.

Ubelacker, Sheryl, "Concussions Raise Long-Term Suicide Risk Three to Fourfold, Says New Canadian Study," *The National Post*, February 8, 2016, https://nationalpost.com/health/concussions-raise-long-term- suicide-risk-three-to-fourfold-says-new-canadian-study.

UPMC: Life Changing Medicine, a MODEL for Understanding Concussion Assessment, 2016. Chart on Trajectories. http://rethinkconcussions. upmc.com.

University of Queens, Australia, Brain Institute, "Concussion tests and diagnosis," https://qbi.uq.edu.au/concussion/concussion-tests-and- diagnosis#:

Web MD, A Visual Guide to Concussions and Brain Injuries, Medically Reviewed by Jabeen Begum, MD on March 27, 2024.

Webster, Barbara J., "Lost & Found: What Brain Injury Survivors Want You to Know," BrainLine, July 28, 2011, https://www.brainline.org/article/lost-found-what-brain-injury-survivors-want-you-know.

Webster, Barbara J., "A Brain Injury Support Group Could Be One of the Best Things That Ever Happens to You," Brain Line. Accessed April 17, 2017. brain line.org. https://www.brainline.org/story/brain-injury-support-group-could-be-one-best-things-ever-happens-you.

Weightman, Margaret M, Mary Vining Radomski, Pauline A Mashima, Borden Institute (U.S, and Carole R Roth. 2014. Mild Traumatic Brain Injury Rehabilitation Toolkit. Department of the Army.

WETA, Preventing, Treating, and Living with Traumatic Brain Injury (TBI), BrainLine | All about Brain Injury and PTSD, WETA, 2015, http://www.brainline.org.

"What Is Syntonics?" n.d. CSO, College of Syntonic Optometry. Accessed May 2022, http://www.csovision.org.

Whitefawn, Sharon, "Self-Nurturing Meditation," YouTube, 2014, https://www.youtube.com/watch?v=5IW_mFwqORU.

William C. Sheil Jr., MD, FACP, FACR, MedicineNet.com, Neuroplasticity, 2017.

Wiltshire, A.E., There actually is a Science of Happiness; Lasting Changes, 2023

Wylie, G. R., & Flashman, L. A., "Understanding the interplay between mild traumatic brain injury and cognitive fatigue: models and treatments," *Concussion (London, England)*, *2*(4), CNC50. https://doi.org/10.2217/cnc-2017-0003

Wilder, Lisa, "Anxiety and Stuttering Treatment," CSA Canadian Stuttering Association, 2015.

William, C, and Jr. Sheil, "Neuroplasticity: The 10 Fundamentals of Rewiring Your Brain," Reset.me, 2017, http://reset.me/story/neuroplasticity-the-10-fundamentals-of-rewiring-your-brain/.

Williams, Dr. Vernon B., "Three Concussion Myths Busted," *Sports Neurology & Pain Medicine*, March 2, 2017. http://www.vernonwilliamsmd.com.

Wu, Aiguo, Zhe Ying, and Fernando Gomez-Pinilla, "Omega-3 Fatty Acids Supplementation Restores Mechanisms That Maintain Brain Homeostasis in Traumatic Brain Injury," *Journal of Neurotrauma* 24 (10): 1587–95, https://doi.org/10.1089/neu.2007.0313.

Zellmer, Amy, The Blog, Healthy Living, Traumatic Brain Injury, "5 Things Every TBI Survivor Wants You to Understand," Dec 6, 2017, https://www.huffpost.com/entry/5-things-every-tbi-survivor-wants-you-to-understand_b_6800984.

Zellmer, Amy, *Faces of TBI; Embracing the Journey: Moving Forward After Brain Injury*, CreateSpace Independent Publishing Platform, Feb. 9, 2018, https://www.braininjurymn.org/annual_conference/CONF-2019-presentations/AmyZellmer.pdf

Zellmer, Amy, *Life with a Traumatic Brain Injury: Finding the Road Back to Normal*, CreateSpace Independent Publishing Platform, Nov. 2, 2015.

Zinn-Kabat, Jon, Wisdom Trove; Jon Kabat-Zinn Quotes, wisdom trove. com (Awesome Quotations).

www.ingramcontent.com/pod-product-compliance
Lightning Source LLC
Chambersburg PA
CBHW071704120626

46550CB00001B/102